Campylobacter

EDITOR
D. G. Newell

SUB-EDITORS
M. J. Blaser (C.D.C., Atlanta)
J. G. Cruickshank (PHLS, Exeter)
J. Davis (PHLS, Colindale)
R. A. Feldman (C.D.C., Atlanta)
A. D. Pearson (PHLS, Southampton)
M. B. Skirrow (PHLS, Worcester)
D. J. Taylor (University of Glasgow, Glasgow)

ORGANISING COMMITTEE
J. B. Butzler
D. G. Newell
R. W. A. Park
A. D. Pearson
D. A. Robinson
M. B. Skirrow
T. J. Trust

Campylobacter

Epidemiology, Pathogenesis and Biochemistry

Edited by

D. G. NEWELL

Public Health Laboratory Service,
Southampton General Hospital,
Southampton, England

Proceedings of an International Workshop on Campylobacter Infections held at University of Reading 24–26th March 1981 under the auspices of the Public Health Laboratory Service

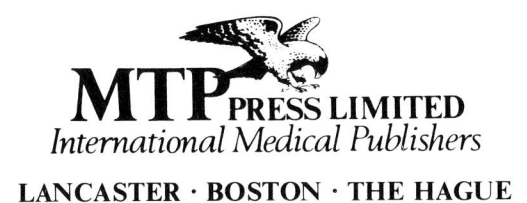

MTP PRESS LIMITED
International Medical Publishers

LANCASTER · BOSTON · THE HAGUE

Published in the UK and Europe by
MTP Press Limited
Falcon House
Lancaster, England

British Library Cataloguing in Publication Data
International Workshop on Campylobacter Infections
(*1981: University of Reading*)
Campylobacter.
1. Enteritis—Congresses 2. Campylobacter—Congresses
I. Title   II. Newell, D. G.
616.3′44   RC862.E47

ISBN 0-85200-455-9

Published in the USA by
MTP Press
A division of Kluwer Boston Inc
190 Old Derby Street
Hingham, MA 02043, USA

Library of Congress Cataloging in Publication Data
Campylobacter, Epidemiology, Pathogenesis, and Biochemistry

Includes Bibliographical References
1. Campylobacter infections—Congresses.
2. Campylobacter—Congresses. 3. Epidemiology—
Congresses. I. Newell, D. G. (Diane G.) [DNLM:
1. Campylobacter—Congresses. 2. Campylobacter
Infections—Congresses. QW 154 161C 1981]
QR201.C25C27   616.3′4400145   82-11

ISBN 0-85200-455-9   AACR2

Copyright © 1982 MTP Press Limited

All rights reserved. No part of this publication
may be reproduced, stored in a retrieval
system, or transmitted in any form or by any
means, electronic, mechanical, photocopying,
recording, or otherwise, without prior permission
from the publishers.

Typeset by Speedlith Photo Litho Limited, Manchester
and printed by Redwood Burn Limited, Trowbridge

Contents

Acknowledgements		vi
Foreword *J. E. M. Whitehead*		vii
List of participants		ix
Introduction		xvii
SECTION	I Geographical epidemiology	1
	II Taxonomy and typing	33
	III Growth requirements and culture media	67
	IV Serology and serotyping	87
	V Clinical aspects	127
	VI Pathogenesis	161
	VII Molecular biology	205
	VIII Epidemiology and environmental aspects	247
	IX Discussion on public health measures	303
	X Campylobacters – where do we go from here?	307

Acknowledgements

I wish to express my gratitude to the following sub-editors who helped to co-ordinate and prepare parts of this publication.

    A. D. Pearson
    J. G. Cruickshank
    R. A. Feldman
    M. B. Skirrow
    J. Davies
    D. J. Taylor
    M. J. Blaser

I would also like to thank the members of the organising committee, Professor J. P. Butzler, Dr R. W. A. Park, Dr A. D. Pearson, Dr D. A. Robinson, Dr M. B. Skirrow and Professor T. J. Trust who ensured the smooth running and success of the meeting and Oxoid Ltd., who provided the financial support essential to the meeting.

D. G. Newell

Foreword

Two influences appear to have contributed to the surge of interest in campylobacter infections that has occurred during the past 5 years. The first is the enthusiasm and success with which microbiologists, previously discouraged by their inability to identify the microbial cause of many cases of acute enteritis, have been able to demonstrate these new enteric pathogens in a wide variety of settings and occasions. The second is the fascination that unravelling the complexities of a new communicable disease holds for many others in the medical, veterinary and biological fields. The combined effect has been that work has progressed rapidly but with varying degrees of corroboration, and in so many directions, that the general picture of these infections had become increasingly blurred. By 1980, the point had been reached at which it seemed to workers in the Public Health Laboratory Service (PHLS) and elsewhere that an effort should be made to bring cohesion to a scene that might otherwise become chaotic, and so it was decided that the PHLS should sponsor the first International Workshop on Campylobacter Infections at the University of Reading in March 1981.

A workshop format was chosen for the meeting to allow work still in progress to be described and to facilitate presentation of technical details. The meeting was attended by 137 participants and confined to those actively working in the subject. Those participating were drawn from several countries besides the United Kingdom and included Australia and Japan. Aspects of campylobacter infections were considered in separate sessions devoted to molecular biology, taxonomy, biotyping, growth requirements, clinical aspects, pathogenesis, serology and epidemiology.

The editor has adopted the wise course of selecting papers and abstracts together with edited discussions and comment. Published proceedings that are simply collections of papers with transcripts of the discussions added to them usually make dull and lengthy reading, for they lack the benefit of the immediacy of the circumstances in which they were delivered. The form in which these proceedings have been published offers the reader a comprehensive and readily assimilable insight into the 'state of the art' in the study of campylobacters and the infections they cause, as perceived at the time of the first International Workshop.

J. E. M. Whitehead
Director of the Public Health Laboratory Service

List of participants

Dr J. D. ABBOTT
Public Health Laboratory
Withington Hospital
Manchester M20 8LR, England

Mr T. N. ALLSUP
Veterinary Investigation Centre
Government Buildings
66 Ty Glas Road
Llanishen, Cardiff CF4 5ZB, Wales

Mr R. R. AL-MASHAT
University of Glasgow
Veterinary School
Bearsden Road
Bearsden, Glasgow G61 1QH, Scotland

Dr C. M. ANAND
Provincial Laboratory of Public Health
Southern Branch
PO Box 2490, Calgary, Alberta, Canada
T2P 2M7

Mr M. ANSFIELD
Veterinary Investigation Centre
Block C, Government Buildings
Whittington Road
Worcester WR5 2LQ, England

Mr M. S. BAIN
Veterinary Investigation Centre
Riseholme
Lincoln, England

Dr A. BASKERVILLE
Centre for Applied Microbiology and Research
Porton Down
Salisbury, Wilts. SP4 0JG, England

Dr R. A. BASSETT
PHLS Headquarters Office
61 Colindale Avenue
London NW9 5EQ, England

Mr J. BENJAMIN
Department of Pathology (Microbiology)
Worcester Royal Infirmary
Castle Street Branch
Worcester WR1 3AS, England

Dr M. J. BLASER
Enteric Diseases Branch, Bacterial Diseases Division
Bureau of Epidemiology
Centers for Disease Control
Atlanta, GA 30333, USA

Professor V. D. BOKKENHEUSER
St. Luke's Roosevelt Hospital Centre
Amsterdam Avenue at 114th Street
New York, NY 10025, USA

Mr. F. J. BOLTON
Public Health Laboratory
Royal Infirmary
Meadow Street
Preston, Lancs. PR1 7PS, England

Mr. J. L. BRANDMEYER
Marion Scientific Division
Marion Laboratories Inc.
PO Box 9627, Kansas City, MO 64134, USA

Mr D. BRUCE
Public Health Laboratory
County Hospital
Hereford HR1 2ER, England

Dr J. H. BRYNER
National Animal Disease Centre
PO Box 70, Ames, IA 50010, USA

Professor J. P. BUTZLER
Microbiology Laboratory
University Hospital of St Peter
322 rue Haute
1000 Brussels, Belgium

LIST OF PARTICIPANTS

Mr T. CHEASTY
Central Public Health Laboratory
175 Colindale Avenue
London NW9 5HT, England

Dr A. A. CODD
Public Health Laboratory
Institute of Pathology
General Hospital
Westgate Road
Newcastle-upon-Tyne NE4 6BE, England

Dr A. O. COKER
Department of Microbiology and
  Parasitology
Lagos University Teaching Hospital
PMB 12003, Lagos, Nigeria

Mrs A. O. COKER
Department of Microbiology and
  Parasitology
Lagos University Teaching Hospital
PMB 12003, Lagos, Nigeria

Dr J. G. CRUICKSHANK
Public Health Laboratory
Church Lane
Heavitree, Exeter EX2 5AD, England

Mr M. A. CURTIS
Public Health Laboratory
County Hospital
Hereford HR1 2ER, England

Dr J. V. DADSWELL
Public Health Laboratory
Royal Berkshire Hospital
Reading, Berks. RG1 5AN, England

Dr V. DANIELIDES
Infectious Diseases Hospital
Department of Bacteriology
Thessaloniki, Greece

Mr G. P. DAVID
The University of Liverpool
Department of Veterinary Preventive
  Medicine
Field Station 'Leahurst', Chester High Road
Neston, Wirral, Merseyside L64 7TE, England

Dr J. R. DAVIES
Public Health Laboratory Service
61 Colindale Avenue
London NW9 5EQ, England

Mr M. De BOECK
Microbiology Laboratory
University Hospital of St Peter
322 rue Haute
B-1000 Brussels, Belgium

Miss S. A. De GRANDIS
Department of Bacteriology
The Hospital for Sick Children
555 University Avenue
Toronto, Ontario, Canada M5G 1X8

Dr J. DEKEYSER
National Institute for Veterinary Research
Groeselenberg 99
B-1180 Brussels, Belgium

Dr P. De MOL
Department of Microbiology
University Hospital of St Peter
322 rue Haute
B-1000 Brussels, Belgium

Dr F. KIJS
Biological Laboratory, Department of
  Microbiology
Free University
Amsterdam, The Netherlands

Dr J. DOLBY
Northwick Park Hospital
Watford Road
Harrow, Middx. HA1 3UJ, England

Dr E. FALSEN
Institute of Medical Microbiology
Department of Clinical Bacteriology
University of Göteborg
Guldhedsgatan 10
S-413 46, Göteborg, Sweden

Dr R. A. FELDMAN
Enteric Diseases Branch, Bacterial Diseases
  Division
Bureau of Epidemiology
Centers for Disease Control
Atlanta, GA 30333, USA

Dr I. R. FERGUSON
Public Health Laboratory
County Hospital
Hereford HR1 2ER, England

Professor B. D. FIREHAMMER
Veterinary Research Laboratory
Department of Veterinary Science
Montana State University
Bozeman, MT 59717, USA

Dr P. C. FLEMING
Department of Bacteriology

LIST OF PARTICIPANTS

The Hospital for Sick Children
555 University Avenue
Toronto, Ontario, Canada M5G 1X8

Mr D. F. GIBBONS
Veterinary Investigation Centre
Crown Street
Liverpool L6 6EH, England

Mr K. P. W. GILL
Central Veterinary Laboratory
New Haw
Weybridge, Surrey KT15 3NB, England

Dr P. GILL
Public Health Laboratory
Glyde Path Road
Dorchester, Dorset DT1 1XD, England

Dr R. GLASS
International Centre for
  Diarrhoeal Disease Research
PO Box 128, Dacca-2, Bangladesh

Professor A. A. GLYNN
Central Public Health Laboratory
175 Colindale Avenue
London NW9 5HT, England

Dr. F. W. GOLDSTEIN
St Joseph's Hospital
6 rue Pierre-Larousse
75674 Paris, France

Dr M. GUBINA
Institute of Microbiology
61105 Ljubljana, Yugoslavia

Ms H. GUNNARSSON
University of Göteborg
Guldhedsgaten 10
S-413 46 Göteborg, Sweden

Dr B. J. HARTOG
Keuringsdienst van Waren Enschede
Vlierstaat 111 Postbus 777
750 AT Enschede, The Netherlands

Professor T. HOFSTADT
Department of Microbiology
The Gade Institute
MFG-byget
N-5016 Haukeland sykehus, Bergen, Norway

Dr R. HOLBROOK
Unilever Research
Colworth Laboratory, Colworth House
Sharnbrook, Beds MK44 1LQ, England

Dr R. HOLLANDER
Staatl. Medizinal-Untersuchungsamt
Alte Poststrasse 11, Postfach 3852
D-4500 Osnabruck, West Germany

Mr M. HUDSON
Central Public Health Laboratory
175 Colindale Avenue
London NW9 5HT, England

Mr W. R. HUDSON
Agricultural Research Council
Meat Research Institute
Langford, Bristol BS18 7DY, England

Mr D. HUNTER
Animal Health Centre
Quarry Dene
Westwood Lane
Leeds LS16 8HQ, England

Dr D. N. HUTCHINSON
Public Health Laboratory
Royal Infirmary
Meadow Street
Preston, Lancs. PR1 6PS, England

Dr T. ITOH
Tokyo Metropolitan Research Laboratory of
  Public Health
24-1, Hyakunin-cho, 3-chome, Shinjuku-ku
Tokyo 160, Japan

Dr A. E. JEPHCOTT
Public Health Laboratory
Myrtle Road
Kingsdown, Bristol BS2 8EL, England

Dr E. JIRILLO
Department of Microbiology
Bari University Medical School
70124 Bari, Italy

Mr J. JOHNSSON
Institute of Medical Microbiology
Department of Clinical Bacteriology
University of Göteborg
Guldhedsgatan 10
S-413 46 Göteborg, Sweden

Dr D. M. JONES
Public Health Laboratory
Withington Hospital
Manchester M20 8LR, England

Dr P. JONES
Central Public Health Laboratory,
Division of Enteric Pathogens

LIST OF PARTICIPANTS

175 Colindale Avenue
London NW9 5HT, England

Dr K. JORGENSEN
Institute of Hygiene and Microbiology
13 Bulowsvej
DK-1870 Copenhagen V, Denmark

Dr B. KAIJSER
Institute of Medical Microbiology
Department of Clinical Bacteriology
University of Göteborg
Guldhedsgatan 10
S-413 46 Göteborg, Sweden

Dr M. KARMALI
Department of Bacteriology
The Hospital for Sick Children
555 University Avenue
Toronto, Ontario, Canada M5G 1X8

Dr M. S. KHAN
Warwickshire Area Health Authority
Pathology Laboratory
Lakin Road
Warwick CV34 5BJ, England

Dr M. KIST
Institute for General Hygiene and
  Bacteriology
Hermann-Herden-Strasse 11
Postfach 820, D-7800 Freiburg, West Germany

Professor H. J. KOORNHOF
The South African Institute for Medical
  Research
Hospital Street
Johannesburg 2001, South Africa

Dr T. U. KOSUNEN
Department of Bacteriology and Immunology
University of Helsinki
Haartmaninkatu 3
00290 Helsinki 29, Finland

Professor D. W. LAMBE Jr
East Tennessee State University
Department of Microbiology
Box 19870A, Johnson City, TN 37614, USA

Dr T. LAMBERT
24 rue Jeanne d'Arc
926000 Asnieres, France

Mr K. P. LANDER
Central Veterinary Laboratory
New Haw
Weybridge, Surrey KT15 3NB, England

Dr A. J. LASTOVICA
Department of Microbiology
Red Cross Childrens Hospital
Rondebosch, Cape Town 7700, South Africa

Dr S. LAUWERS
Microbiology, Free University
Laarbeeklaan 101
B-1090 Brussels

Dr G. H. K. LAWSON
Department of Veterinary Pathology
Royal (Dick) School of Veterinary Studies
Veterinary Field Station
Easter Bush, Roslin, Midlothian, Scotland

Mrs S. LEAPER
National Collection of Type Cultures
Central Public Health Laboratory
Colindale Avenue
London NW9 4HT, England

Dr H. LIOR
National Enteric Reference Centre
Bureau of Bacteriology
Laboratory Centre for Disease Control
Tunney's Pasture, Ottawa, Ontario K1A OL2, Canada

Dr N. LUECHTEFELD
Veterans Administration
Medical Center
1055 Clermont Street
Denver, CO 80220, USA

Dr B. M. LUND
ARC Food Research Institute
Colney Lane
Norwich NRF 7UA, England

Mr H. H. McBRIDE
Public Health Laboratory
Southampton General Hospital
Tremona Road
Southampton, Hants. SO9 4XY, England

Dr D. B. McGECHIE
Department of Microbiology
Fremantle Hospital
PO Box 280, Fremantle 6160, Western Australia

Dr A. MADDOCKS
Department of Bacteriology
St Mary's Hospital Medical School
Wright-Fleming Institute
London W2 1PG, England

LIST OF PARTICIPANTS

Dr A. MAELAND
Microbiological Laboratory,
Ulleval Hospital
Oslo 1, Norway

Dr B. K. MANDAL
Regional Department of Infectious Diseases
University of Manchester School of Medicine
Monsall Hospital, Newton Heath, Manchester
M10 8WR, England

Mr P. A. MANSER
Veterinary Investigation Centre
Coldharbour, Wye
Ashord, Kent, England

Dr S. L. MAWER
Public Health Laboratory
Hull Royal Infirmary
Anlaby Road
Hull HU3 2JZ, England

Dr L.-O. MENTZING
Länslakarorganisationen
761 86 Karlstad, Sweden

Dr B. MERRELL
Naval Medical Research Institute
Bethesda, Maryland, USA

Dr G. MIRAGLIOTTA
Bari University Medical School
70125, Bari, Italy

Professor P. MOUTON
University Hospital
Rijnsburgerweg 10
2333 AA Leiden, The Netherlands

Mr J. NELSON
Veterinary Investigation Centre
Elmbridge Court, Cheltenham Road
Gloucester GL3 1AP, England

Dr D. G. NEWELL
Public Health Laboratory
Southampton General Hospital
Tremona Road
Southampton, Hants. SO9 4XY, England

Dr G. NYSTROM
c/o Lansladarorganisationen
751 86 Karlstad, Sweden

Mr P. A. OLUBUNMI
University of Glasgow Veterinary School
Bearsden Road
Bearsden, Glasgow G61 1QH, Scotland

Dr J. OOSTEROM
Laboratory for Zoonoses and Food
  Microbiology
Antonie van Leeuwenhoeklaan 9
Postbus 1, 3720 BA Bilthoven,
The Netherlands

Dr R. J. OWEN
National Collection of Type Cultures
Central Public Health Laboratory,
Colindale Avenue
London NW9 5HT, England

Dr C. E. PARK
Microbiology Research Division
Bureau of Microbial Hazards
Health Protection Branch, Health and Welfare
Canada
Ottawa, Ontario K1A OL2, Canada

Dr R. W. A. PARK
Department of Microbiology
University of Reading
London Road
Reading, Berks. RG1 5AQ, England

Mr P. PARKINSON
North West Water
Dawson House
Great Sankey, Warrington, Lancs. WA5 3LW
England

Dr L. PATRICK
Public Health Laboratory
Odstock Hospital
Salisbury, Wilts. SP2 8BJ, England

Dr D. J. H. PAYNE
Public Health Laboratory
St Mary's General Hospital
Milton Road, Portsmouth, Hants. PO3 6AQ,
England

Dr A. D. PEARSON
Public Health Laboratory
Southampton General Hospital
Tremona Road
Southampton, Hants. SO9 4XY, England

Dr J. L. PENNER
Department of Medical Microbiology
Faculty of Medicine
University of Toronto, Banting Institute
100 College Street
Toronto, Ontario M5G 1L5, Canada

Dr Y. PIEMONT
Bacteriology Laboratory

LIST OF PARTICIPANTS

Faculty of Medicine
3 rue Koeberle
67000 Strasbourg, France

Dr P. PIOT
Institute of Tropical Medicine
Nationalestraat 155
B-2000 Antwerp, Belgium

Dr J. F. PRESCOTT
Ontario Veterinary College,
Department of Veterinary Microbiology and
 Immunology
Guelph, Ontario, Canada N1G 2W1

Dr A. B. PRICE
Northwick Park Hospital
Watford Road
Harrow, Middx. HA1 3UJ, England

Mr H. H. RAZI
Department of Microbiology
University of Reading
London Road
Reading, Berks. RG1 5AQ, England

Dr S. RILEY
Public Health Laboratory
Plymouth General Hospital
Greenbank Road
Plymouth, Devon PL4 8NN, England

Dr L. ROBERTS
Veterinary Investigation Centre
Mill of Craibstone
Bucksburn, Aberdeen, Scotland

Dr M. ROGOL
Government Central Laboratories
Ministry of Health
PO Box 6115, Jerusalem 91060, Israel

Dr B. ROWE
Division of Enteric Pathogens
Central Public Health Laboratory
Colindale Avenue
London NW9 5HT, England

Mr P. J. SEAMON
Veterinary Investigation Centre
The Elms, College Road
Sutton Bonington, Loughborough, Leics.
LE12 5RB, England

Dr W. P. J. SEVERIN
Area Laboratory for Pathology and
 Microbiology
Burg, edo Bargsmalan 1
7512 AD Enschede, The Netherlands

Mr I. G. SHAW
Veterinary Investigation Centre
Block C, Government Buildings
Whittington Road
Worcester WR5 2LQ, England

Dr. M. SHMILOVITZ
W Hirsch Regional Microbiology Laboratory
Kupat Holim, Haifa and Western Galilee
PO Box 4934, Israel

Dr N. A. SIMMONS
Guy's Hospital
St Thomas' Street
London SE1 9RT, England

Dr M. B. SKIRROW
Department of Pathology (Microbiology)
Worcester Royal Infirmary
Castle Street Branch
Worcester WR1 3AS, England

Dr J. B. SOLOMON
Grampian Health Board
The Laboratory
City Hospital
Aberdeen AB9 8AU, Scotland

Dr V. STICHT-GROH
Institute for Hygiene and Microbiology
Josef-Schneider-Strasse 2
Bau 17, Würzburg, West Germany

Dr P. STOVELL
Animal Pathology (Pacific Area)
Agriculture Canada
3802 West 4th Avenue
Vancouver, BC, Canada V6R 1P5

Mr W. G. SUCKLING
Public Health Laboratory
Southampton General Hospital
Tremona Road
Southampton, Hants. SO9 4XY, England

Dr R. SUTTON
Diarrhoeal Diseases Control
World Health Organization
1211 Geneva 27, Switzerland

Dr A. SVEDHEM
Department of Clinical Bacteriology
University of Göteborg
Guldhedsgatan 10
S-413 46, Göteborg, Sweden

Dr C. E. D. TAYLOR
Public Health Laboratory

LIST OF PARTICIPANTS

Addenbrooke's Hospital
Hills Road
Cambridge CB2 2QW, England

Dr D. E. TAYLOR
Department of Bacteriology
The Hospital for Sick Children
555 University Avenue
Toronto, Ontario, Canada M5G 1X8

Dr D. J. TAYLOR
University of Glasgow Veterinary School
Bearsden Road
Bearsden, Glasgow G61 1QH, Scotland

Dr W. A. TELFER-BRUNTON
Public Health Laboratory
Royal Cornwall Hospital (City)
Infirmary Hill
Truro, Cornwall TR1 2HZ, England

Dr P. THOMPSON
Public Health Laboratory
New Cross Hospital
Wolverhampton WV10 0QP, England

Professor T. J. TRUST
Department of Biochemistry & Microbiology
University of Victoria
PO Box 1700, Victoria, BC, Canada V8W 2Y2

Dr P. C. TURNBULL
Central Public Health Laboratory
Colindale Avenue
London NW9 5HT, England

Dr H. W. van LANDUYT
Department of Microbiology
A Z St Jan van het O C M W
Ruddershove, B-8000 Brugge, Belgium

Dr R. VANHOOF
Department of Medical Microbiology
Institute Pasteur
Stoomslepersstraat 28
B-1040 Brussels, Belgium

Mr B. VEAL
Public Health Laboratory
Southampton General Hospital
Tremona Road
Southampton, Hants. SO9 2XY, England

Dr M. VERON
Faculty of Medicine Necker-Enfants Malades
146 rue de Vaugirard
75730 Paris, France

Dr M. WALDER
Department of Clinical Bacteriology
University of Lund
Malmö General Hospital
S-214 Malmö, Sweden

Dr J. G. WALLACE
Public Health Laboratory
St Anne's Road
Lincoln LN2 5RF, England

Dr W.-L. L. WANG
Veterans Administration
Medical Center
1055 Clermont Street
Denver, CO 80220, USA

Miss S. WATERMAN
Department of Microbiology
University of Reading
London Road
Reading, Berks. RG1 5AQ, England

Dr K. C. WATSON
Lothian Health Board
Central Microbiological Laboratories
Western General Hospital
Crewe Road
Edinburgh EH4 2XU, Scotland

Dr R. WEAVER
Department of Health and Human Services
Centers for Disease Control
Atlanta, GA 30333, USA

Dr S. WELKOS
Eastern Virginia Medical School
Department of Microbiology and
 Immunology
PO Box 1980, Norfolk, VA 23501, USA

Mrs J. G. WELLS
Enteric Diseases Laboratory Section
Epidemiologic Investigations Laboratory
 Branch
Bacterial Diseases Division
Centers for Disease Control
Atlanta, GA 30333, USA

Dr D. G. WHITE
Public Health Laboratory
Royal United Hospital
Combe Park
Bath, Avon BA1 3NG, England

Dr. P. J. WILKINSON
Public Health Laboratory
Plymouth General Hospital

LIST OF PARTICIPANTS

Greenbank Road
Plymouth, Devon PL4 8NN, England

Sir ROBERT WILLIAMS
Public Health Laboratory Service Board
61 Colindale Avenue
London NW9 5EQ, England

Dr A. M. M. WILSON
20 Merchiston Avenue
Edinburgh, Scotland

Dr E. P. WRIGHT
Public Health Laboratory
Luton and Dunstable Hospital
Lewsey Road
Luton, Beds. LU4 0DZ, England

Dr A. M. YAKUBU
Department of Medical Microbiology
A B U Hospital
Zaria, Nigeria

Dr S. E. J. YOUNG
Communicable Disease Surveillance Centre
61 Colindale Avenue
London NW9 5EQ, England

Introduction

In 1957 King[1] identified related vibrios (heat tolerant campylobacter) as being pathogenic to man but only since the establishment of techniques for their isolation from faecal material[2,3] have campylobacters been recognized as a major cause of gastroenteritis in man.

Over the last 5 years or so, a plethora of papers have been published on campylobacter infections and considerable information has become available on the epidemiology and clinical presentation of the disease. However, confusion in the areas of taxonomy and isolation techniques had occurred and appeared to be restricting advances in epidemiology, pathogenicity and molecular biology. It, therefore, seemed an opportune time to co-ordinate resources, initiate an international exchange of information and provide a basis for collaboration.

The International Workshop on Campylobacter Infections was held under the auspices of the Public Health Laboratory Service and with the financial support of Oxoid Ltd. The three-day meeting took place at Reading University during March 1981, and comprised eight workshops and several discussion groups in which 137 clinicians, veterinarians and scientists from 21 countries participated.

These proceedings include all the contributions given during the meeting either in the form of abstracts submitted prior to the meeting or extended abstracts and invited papers. The workshop structure has been retained in these proceedings for ease of editing and, I hope, clarity. Generally the papers are included in the workshop during which they were presented but it is acknowledged that many of the sections were overlapping in content.

The discussions of individual papers and any general discussion were recorded and the editor has summarized relevant discussion points at the end of each paper. Editorial summaries of each workshop have also been undertaken where attempts have been made to establish, in the opinion of the editor, advances in information, their significance and areas of future work. Where possible references to published work have been included.

In an attempt to clarify the problems of nomenclature the *Approved List of Bacterial Names*[4] has been used (Figure 1), except where previously published material is referred to or where comparisons of reference strains, with old nomenclature, would be confused by adoption of the approved names.

It is the intention of the editor that these proceedings should prove an up-to-date source of research and applied information in a rapidly moving field of bacteriology.

INTRODUCTION

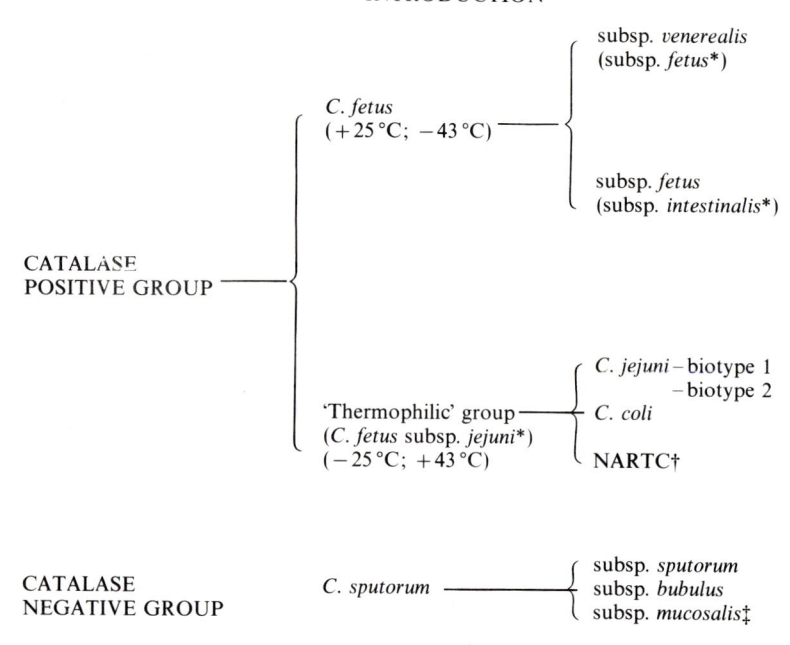

```
                        ┌─ C. fetus          ┌─ subsp. venerealis
                        │  (+25 °C; −43 °C)  │  (subsp. fetus*)
                        │                    │
                        │                    └─ subsp. fetus
CATALASE       ────────┤                       (subsp. intestinalis*)
POSITIVE GROUP          │
                        │                    ┌─ C. jejuni – biotype 1
                        │                    │            – biotype 2
                        └─ 'Thermophilic' group  ─ C. coli
                           (C. fetus subsp. jejuni*)
                           (−25 °C; +43 °C)  └─ NARTC†


                                              ┌─ subsp. sputorum
CATALASE              C. sputorum  ───────── ─┤  subsp. bubulus
NEGATIVE GROUP                                └─ subsp. mucosalis‡
```

Figure 1 Classification of genus *Campylobacter*. Nomenclature is that of the *Approved List of Bacterial Names* (1980) except where indicated

* Smibert (1974), † Nalidixic acid-resistant thermophilic campylobacter – Skirrow and Benjamin (1980b), ‡ Lawson and Rowland (1974)

I hope that such a collection of papers will be useful to medical and veterinary bacteriologists and researchers interested in enteric diseases but wish to emphasize the preliminary nature of much of the work reported.

D. G. NEWELL

References

1. King, E. O. (1957). Human infections with vibrio fetus and a closely related vibrio. *J. Infect. Dis.*, **101**, 119
2. DeKeyser, P., Gossuin Detrain, M., Butzler, J. P. and Sternon, J. (1972). Acute enteritis due to related vibrio. First positive stool culture. *J. Infect. Dis.*, **125**, 390
3. Skirrow, M. B. (1977). Campylobacter enteritis: a 'new' disease. *Br. Med. J.*, **2**, 9
4. Skerman, V. B. D., McGowan, V. and Sneath, P. H. A. (1980). Approved List of Bacterial Names. *Int. J. Systemic Bacteriol.*, **30**, 270

SECTION I
GEOGRAPHICAL EPIDEMIOLOGY

Co-chairmen: R. A. Feldman and A. D. Pearson

1	Epidemiology of endemic and epidemic campylobacter infections in the United States M. J. Blaser, R. A. Feldman and J. G. Wells	3
2	Campylobacter enteritis in Tokyo T. Itoh, K. Saito, Y. Yanagawa, S. Sakai and M. Ohashi	5
3	*Campylobacter jejuni*: A common cause of diarrhoea in Sweden B. Kaijser and A. Svedhem	13
4	Acute enteritis due to campylobacter – an epidemiological study M. Walder and A. Forsgren	14
5	Some epidemiological features of campylobacter infections in Oslo A. Maeland	16
6	Human campylobacter infections 1977–1980 National Data based on routine laboratory reporting S. E. J. Young	17
7	Campylobacter enteritis in Hong Kong and Western Australia D. B. McGechie, T. B. Teoh and V. W. Bamford	19
8	*Campylobacter jejuni* as an aetiological agent of diarrhoeal diseases in Israel M. Shmilovitz and B. Kretzer	22
9	Campylobacter enteritis in Northern Greece V. Danielides, P. Agoustidou-Savvopoulou, S. Manios, G. Sidira and A. Kanzouzidou	25
10	Campylobacter enteritis in developing countries P. de Mol	26

11	Epidemiological features of campylobacter enteritis in Bangladesh *R. I. Glass, I. Huq, P. J. Still, G. Kibriya and M. J. Blaser*	28
12	Campylobacter enteritis in Zaria *A. M. Yakubu and C. S. Bello*	30
13	Editorial discussion	32

1
Epidemiology of endemic and epidemic campylobacter infections in the United States

M. J. BLASER, R. A. FELDMAN and J. G. WELLS

Centers for Disease Control, Atlanta GA, U.S.A.

Only 11 states are now routinely reporting campylobacter isolates to CDC, but even within these states reporting is not mandatory. Data from Oregon suggests that there are as many campylobacter isolates as shigella or salmonella. During a 2 year study of 2670 faecal specimens submitted to the laboratories of three hospitals in Denver, from patients with gastrointestinal illnesses, campylobacter was isolated from 4.6% (Table 1). The rate of stool positivity was highest during the summer and lowest in the winter. There was no significant difference in the positivity rate for males (5.2%) or females (4.0%). The highest age-specific positivity rate was from patients 10–29 years of age and the positivity rate was 22% for males of that age during the summer. In a still-continuing study of campylobacter infection, data from hospitals in eight different areas in the United States were collected over a one-year period (Table 2). The preliminary stool positivity rates ranged from 9.4% (Michigan) to 1.2% (Georgia) (mean 5.7%). Only 6% of the campylobacter isolates were from children less than one year of age although 14% of stool specimens were from this age group. 39% of the campylobacter isolates were from persons 20–29 years old and this group had the highest age-specific stool positivity rate.

Table 1 Rate of isolation of three enteric pathogens from faecal specimens submitted to three Denver hospitals, by age of the patient, March 1978–February 1980

Age (yr)	Number of faecal specimens	Campylobacter	Salmonella	Shigella
<1	875	1.3	4.0	0.2
1–9	656	3.0	2.9	6.9
10–29	554	12.1	3.6	3.1
30–49	252	6.7	2.0	3.2
50–69	204	2.9	2.0	0
≥70	73	1.4	4.1	4.1

Positive faecal specimens (%)

Table 2 Rate of isolation of three enteric pathogens from faecal specimens by hospital, eight-Hospital Collaborative Study, January–October, 1980

Location of hospital	No. specimens examined	% with Campylo-bacter	% with Salmon-ella	% with Shigella
Oregon	402	6.2	2.7	0.7
Colorado	351	5.7	1.4	0.9
Michigan	366	10.1	1.1	0.5
Illinois	1847	6.4	2.5	0.4
Georgia	74	1.4	2.7	6.8
Oklahoma	502	1.0	2.4	2.6
Maryland	345	2.3	9.3	1.2
California	350	4.0	1.1	2.9
Total	4237	5.4	2.7	1.1

In the past year, investigators from CDC, in cooperation with state health departments, have investigated five outbreaks of camplylobacter infection (Table 3). Outbreaks ranged in size from 11 to 2000 cases. Using case-control analysis, vehicles for transmission were implicated in all five outbreaks including stream water, tap water, raw clams, processed turkey meats and cake icing.

Table 3 Five outbreaks of campylobacter enteritis in the United States. Investigated by CDC Personnel, 1980

State	No. persons affected	Vehicle*
Connecticut	41	cake icing
Wyoming	21	stream water
California	11	processed turkey
Connecticut	1500	municipal water
New Jersey	18	raw clams

* Identified by case-control analysis

DISCUSSION

Dr Blazer replying to Dr Sutton said that they had not been able to isolate camplylobacter from any of the suspected vehicles involved in the outbreaks. The median age for diarrhoea cases (26.5 years) was calculated on those patients from whom the organism was cultured.

2
Campylobacter enteritis in Tokyo

T. ITOH, K. SAITO, Y. YANAGAWA, S. SAKAI and M. OHASHI

Tokyo Metropolitan Research Laboratory of Public Health, Tokyo, Japan

Recent findings suggest that the thermophilic campylobacters are a cause of human enteritis. We report some epidemiological, bacteriological and serological studies of human and animal strains isolated by us since 1979.

(1) STUDIES OF SPORADIC CASES OF ENTERITIS DUE TO CAMPYLOBACTER

Table 1 presents the results of bacteriological studies on 1686 patients with diarrhoea seen either as in-patients or out-patients at the Tokyo Metropolitan

Table 1 Detection of thermophilic campylobacter in sporadic cases of diarrhoea at Tokyo Metropolitan Bokuto Hospital (April, 1979–April, 1980)

Subjects	Number of cases examined	Thermophilic campylobacter	V. parahaemolyticus	Salmonella	Y. enterocolitica	E. coli, enteropathogenic serotype	Shigella	Others
Children	846 (100%)	76 (9.0%)	5	65	9	8	—	17
Adults	840 (100%)	39 (4.6%)	91	23	3	2	1	17
Total	1686 (100%)	115 (6.8%)	96	88	12	10	1	34

Bokuto Hospital, between April 1979 and April 1980. It is clear that *C. jejuni* is an important cause of enteritis in Japan, particularly amongst children.

Little seasonal variation was found throughout the year.

(2) DIARRHOEA IN TRAVELLERS FROM OVERSEAS

C. jejuni was isolated from 3.1% of the patients who had recently travelled overseas (Table 2). Most were probably infected in southeast Asian countries such as Thailand and the Philippines though some may have been infected in Korea, Taiwan or Mainland China, which indicates the extensive distribution of the organism throughout Asia.

(3) CLINICAL

The main clinical symptoms encountered in the sporadic cases observed are summarized in Figure 1. Children had a much higher incidence of bloody stools, vomiting and of fever, and had a generally more severe illness.

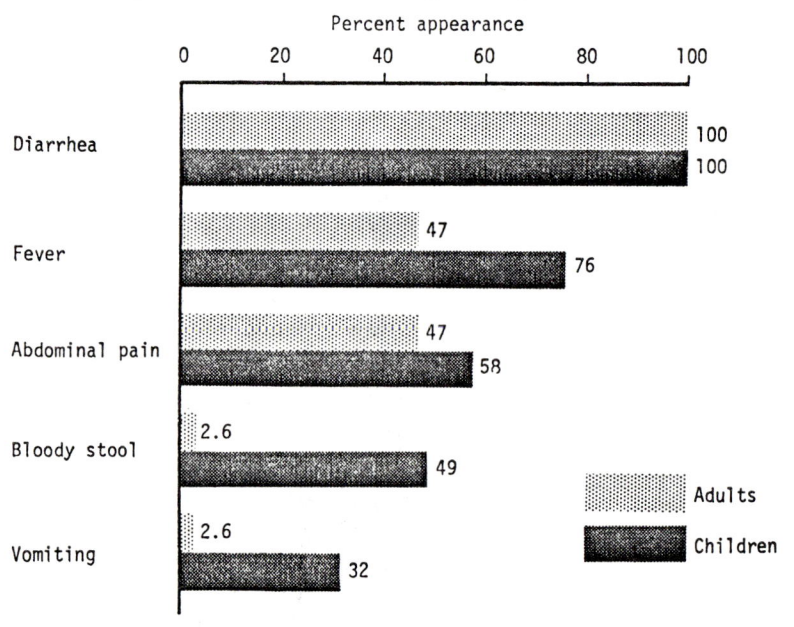

Symptom	Adults (%)	Children (%)
Diarrhea	100	100
Fever	47	76
Abdominal pain	47	58
Bloody stool	2.6	49
Vomiting	2.6	32

Figure 1 Major symptoms in 76 children and 39 adults with campylobacter enteritis at Tokyo Metropolitan Bokuto Hospital, between April, 1979 and April, 1980

(4) EPIDEMIOLOGICAL STUDIES ON OUTBREAKS OF ENTERITIS DUE TO CAMPYLOBACTER

Between January 1979 and December 1980, 222 outbreaks of food poisoning involving 6327 cases occurred in Tokyo, of which 9 (4.1%) were attributable to *C. jejuni*.

The main features of these outbreaks are presented in Table 3. In only two outbreaks was there evidence to suggest the nature of the vehicle of

Table 2 Detection of thermophilic campylobacter and other enteropathogens in overseas travellers' diarrhoeal cases (1980)

Subjects	Number of cases examined	Number of pathogen positives	Total	Thermophilic campylobacter	V. cholerae, 0-1	V. cholerae, other than 0-1	V. parahaemolyticus	Shigella	Salmonella	E. coli, enterotoxigenic	E. coli, invasive type	E. coli, enteropathogenic serotype	Y. enterocolitica	F-group vibrio
Acute cases	375 (100%)	221 (58.9%)	260	12	2	5	40	21	37	130	3	6	1	3
Convalescent cases	1817 (100%)	451 (24.8%)	495	56	2	39	122	34	235	*	1	3	1	3
Total	2192 (100%)	672 (30.7%)	755	68 (3.1%)	4	44	162	55	272	130	4	9	2	6

* = Not tested

Table 3 Outbreaks of enteritis due to *Campylobacter jejuni* in Tokyo (1979–1980)

	Outbreak 1	Outbreak 2	Outbreak 3	Outbreak 4	Outbreak 5	Outbreak 6	Outbreak 7	Outbreak 8	Outbreak 9
Date	14–20 Jan., 1979	13–16 May, 1979	8–14 Aug., 1979	10–12 Sep., 1979	11–15 Sep., 1979	2–9 Nov., 1979	7–14 May, 1980	12–19 June, 1980	4–8 Nov., 1980
Place	Nursery school	Restaurant	Hotel (students)	Hotel (students)	Dormitory (students)	Hotel (students)	Dormitory (students)	Hotel (students)	Household
Number of persons at risk	93	118	23	42	33	180	736	232	10
Number of patients (%)	36 (38.7)	101 (93.5)	21 (91.3)	21 (50.0)	12 (36.4)	106 (58.9)	107 (14.5)	113 (48.7)	4 (40.0)
Vehicle	un	Clam salad	un	un	un	un	un	un	Chicken meat
Incubation period range (mode)	un	20–60 h (35.6 h)	un	un	un	un	un	un	20–104 h (51.3 h)
Detection of *C. jejuni* in patients faeces (%)	14/35* (40.0)	9/52 (17.3)	3/16 (18.8)	8/18 (44.4)	6/12 (50.0)	38/101 (37.6)	20/50 (40.0)	23/96 (24.0)	2/3 (66.7)
Serotype of isolate	TCK 1**	TCK 18	TCK 2	TCK 3	TCK 4	TCK 5	TCK 6 & 14	TCK 7	TCK 3

*Number of positive cases/Number of cases examined, **Our own serotyping system, un, Unknown

transmission. In outbreak number 2 six different parties ate at a certain restaurant in Tokyo over a 2 day period, and 93.5% of those taking clams developed diarrhoea. The period of incubation time based on the time of consumption of the clams was 20–60 hours (mode 36 hours). In outbreak number 9 left-over chicken meat was found to contain the same serotype of *C. jejuni* as that isolated from affected patients, and the incubation period was 20–104 hours (mode 51 hours).

Major symptoms observed in the patients varied considerably from one outbreak to another, e.g. in the frequency of blood and mucus in the stool (Figure 2) and, inasmuch as different serotypes were involved, it is at least possible that strains vary in pathogenicity.

Antibody response was variable as determined by the agglutination titre against the homologous isolate. In only one of five outbreaks investigated was a response demonstrated (the nursery school).

(5) BACTERIOLOGICAL STUDIES ON ISOLATES OF CAMPYLOBACTER OBTAINED FROM HUMANS AND ANIMALS

For isolation the Skirrow method[1] was used with slight modifications. Isolates after two days incubation were identified according to Véron and Chatelain[2]. Their biological features were further examined by the methods described by Skirrow and Benjamin[3]. The results are presented in Table 4.

The majority of human isolates (86%) were classified as *C. jejuni* biotype 1. The remainder were *C. coli. C. jejuni* biotype 2 isolates were not identified as a cause of enteritis in this population of 90 human cases. Neither was *C. jejuni* biotype 2 identified in any of the animal isolates.

(6) SEROLOGICAL TYPING OF THERMOPHILIC CAMPYLOBACTER

A serotyping scheme has been developed based on 18 serotypes. (TCK 1–TCK 18). The details of the development of this scheme are described in the section on Serology (p. 106). The serological types identified from the outbreaks and other sources are shown in Table 5. Ten serotypes were identified from the nine outbreaks with one outbreak involving two different serotypes. It may be of interest that some of the hippurate hydrolysis negative strains from overseas travellers diarrhoea patients were found to share heat-labile antigens with hippurate positive strains. Similarly some of the *C. coli* strains from swine shared type specificities with *C. jejuni* of human origin.

References
1. Skirrow, M. B. (1977). Campylobacter enteritis: a "new" disease. *Br. Med. J.*, **2**, 9–11
2. Véron, M. and Chatelain, R. (1973). Taxonomic study of the genus *Campylobacter* Sebald and Véron and designation of the meotype strain for the type species *Campylobacter fetus* (Smith and Taylor) Sebald and Veron. *Int. J. Systemat. Bacteriol.*, **23**, 122–134
3. Skirrow, M. S. and Benjamin, J. (1980). Differentiation of enteropathogenic campylobacter. *J. Clin. Pathol.*, **33**, 1122

CAMPYLOBACTER: GEOGRAPHICAL EPIDEMIOLOGY

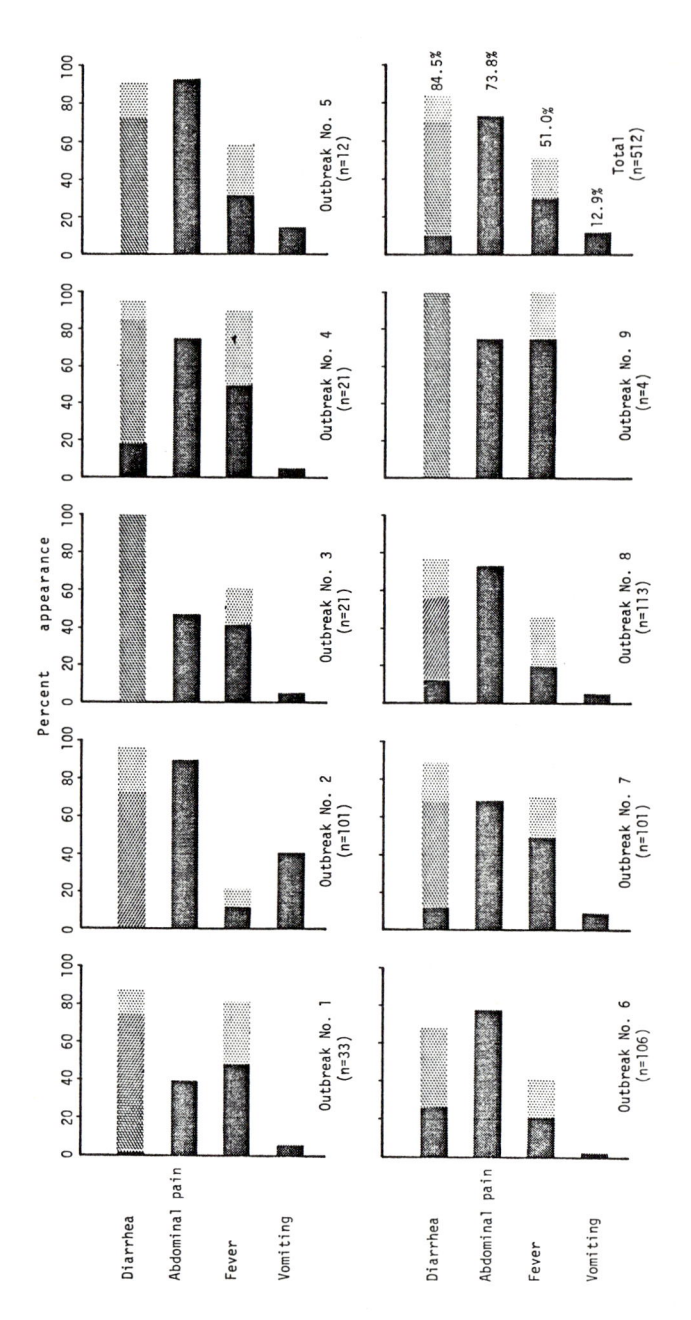

Figure 2 Major symptoms of the patients involved in outbreaks. Diarrhoea: Bloody/mucus ▓ Watery ▒ Loose, Fever: ▓ 38.0 °C or higher ▒ 37.9 °C or lower

10

Table 4 Biochemical characteristics of thermophilic campylobacter isolated from human diarrhoeal cases and animals

	\multicolumn{8}{c}{Source of isolates}
	Human (n = 90)		Poultry (n = 28)		Swine (n = 100)		Cattle (n = 4)	
Characteristics	Sign	%+	Sign	%+	Sign	%+	Sign	%+
Catalase	+	100	+	100	+	100	+	100
Growth at 25 °C	−	0	−	0	−	0	−	0
at 42 °C	+	100	+	100	+	100	+	100
Growth in 1% glycine	+	100	+	100	+	100	+	100
Hippurate hydrolysis	+/−	86	+	100	−	2	+	100
H_2S production								
in sensitive medium	+	100	+	100	+	100	+	100
in iron medium	−	0	−	0	−	0	−	0
Nalidixic acid sensitivity (30 μg disc)	+	99	+	96	+	98	+	100

+ = positive reaction for 90–100% of strains; +/− = positive reaction for 50–89% of strains; − = negative reaction for 90–100% of strains

Table 5 Serotypes of thermophilic campylobacter isolated from human diarrhoeal cases and animals

Sources	Hippurate hydrolysis	Number of strains examined	\multicolumn{18}{c}{Number of strains serotype (TCK):}	Total	Untypable
			1	2	3	4	5	6	7	8	9	10	11	12	13	14	15	16	17	18		
Human diarrhoea outbreaks																						
No. 1	+	15	15	—	—	—	—	—	—	—	—	—	—	—	—	—	—	—	—	—	15	0
No. 2	+	5	—	—	—	—	—	—	—	—	—	—	—	—	—	—	—	—	—	4	4	1
No. 3	+	3	—	3	—	—	—	—	—	—	—	—	—	—	—	—	—	—	—	—	3	0
No. 4	+	14	1	—	12	—	—	1	—	—	—	—	—	—	—	—	—	—	—	—	14	0
No. 5	+	7	—	—	—	7	—	—	—	—	—	—	—	—	—	—	—	—	—	—	7	0
No. 6	+	18	1	—	—	—	14	—	—	—	1	—	—	—	—	—	—	—	—	—	16	2
No. 7	+	10	—	—	—	—	—	4	—	—	—	—	—	—	—	6	—	—	—	—	10	0
No. 8	+	31	1	—	—	—	—	—	30	—	—	—	—	—	—	1	—	—	—	—	31	0
No. 9	+	3	—	—	3	—	—	—	—	—	—	—	—	—	—	—	—	—	—	—	3	0
Sporadic cases {	+	105(100%)	5	3	1	1	—	2	2	6	2	4	1	7	2	2	1	5	1	10	55(52%)	50(48%)
	—	16	—	2	—	—	—	—	—	1	—	—	—	1	—	—	—	1	—	2	7	9
poultry {	+	29(100%)	1	1	—	—	—	4	2	2	1	—	—	—	—	—	—	—	—	1	11(38%)	18(62%)
	+	2	1	1	—	—	—	—	—	—	—	—	—	—	—	—	—	—	—	—	2	0
Swine {	—	69(100%)	—	—	1	—	2	3	7	—	—	—	2	—	1	—	—	—	—	—	15(22%)	54(78%)
	+	4	1	—	—	—	—	—	—	—	—	—	—	—	—	—	—	—	—	—	2	2
Cattle																						
Total		331(100%)	25	9	17	8	14	13	37	16	4	4	1	10	3	9	1	6	1	17	195(59%)	136(41%)

12

3
Campylobacter jejuni: a common cause of diarrhoea in Sweden*

B. KAIJSER and A. SVEDHEM

Institute of Medical Microbiology, University of Göteborg, Sweden

---

Many reports during the last 3 years have shown that *C. jejuni* is one of the most common causes of bacterial diarrhoea in man. The present investigation reports the situation in Sweden.

Campylobacter was the most common cause of bacterial diarrhoea (10.9%) at the Clinic for Infectious Diseases in Göteborg, Sweden. Most patients were between 20 and 34 years of age. Only a few children were diagnosed. A seasonal variation was seen with peaks in July–August and January. About 60% of the individuals were infected abroad. 90% of the cases had no campylobacter in their stools after 5 weeks and the incubation time was 1–6 days. Almost all patients recovered without antibiotic treatment. The disease was often experienced very severely during its, generally, short course. Campylobacter diarrhoea must therefore be considered more frequently as a cause of diarrhoea in Sweden.

DISCUSSION

Dr Butzler noted that campylobacter enteritis appears to be a cause of travellers' diarrhoea in Sweden. This could lead to problems in the described seasonality, since travellers may return in the cooler or warmer months depending on where they travelled.

---

* First published in *Journal of Infectious Diseases*, 142, 353, 1980.

4
Acute enteritis due to campylobacter – an epidemiological study

M. WALDER and A. FORSGREN

Department of Clinical Bacteriology, University of Lund, Sweden

---

Campylobacter jejuni/coli was isolated from 386 patients (6.9%) in samples from 5571 patients with a history of acute diarrhoea, between December 1977 and June 1980. In the same samples salmonella was cultured in 4.1%, shigella in 1.7% and *Yersinia enterocolitica* in 2.1% (Table 1). Only five (0.25%) of 2000 health check up patients had *C. jejuni* in their stools. 53% of the patients had acquired their infection in Sweden. The peak incidence for *C. jejuni* was from July to September (Figure 1). More than 50% of the patients were in the age group 16–35 years. Within 1 month of the acute enteritis, 80% had negative stool cultures for *C. jejuni*. In general, campylobacter enteritis is not a severe disease and only 11% were admitted to hospital. High fever (35%), frequent watery diarrhoea (37%), colics or abdominal pains (87%), and fresh

Table 1 Distribution of bacterial intestinal pathogens: salmonella, shigella, *Yersinia enterocolitica* and *C. jejuni* in stool samples investigated at the bacteriological laboratory in Malmö from December 1977 to June 1980

Pathogens	No. of isolates	No. of isolates from enteritis patients*	\multicolumn{4}{c}{Isolation frequency in enteritis patients %}
			1978	1979	1980	31 months
Salmonella	395	229	4.9	3.2	3.2	4.1
Shigella	130	97	1.9	1.2	1.7	1.7
Yersinia enterocoliticia	158	120	2.3	2.3	1.8	2.1
Campylobacter	435	386	6.2	7.8	6.8	6.9
Total	1118	832				14.8

* From 5571 patients with acute enteritis

ACUTE ENTERITIS DUE TO CAMPYLOBACTER

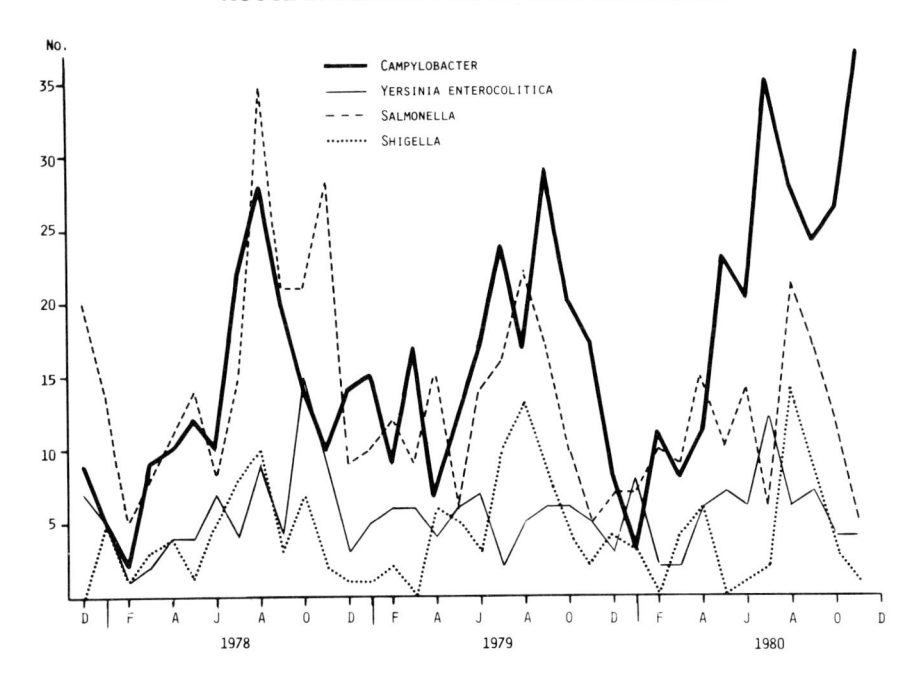

NO. OF PATIENTS IN MALMÖ WITH BACTERIAL INTESTINAL PATHOGENS DURING 36 MONTHS

blood in stools (12%), were the most common symptoms. Antibiotic treatment was given in 13% of patients and was either erythromycin (56%) or doxycycline (26%). If chemotherapy was given to a sensitive strain no relapse occurred within 2 weeks of the treatment. The antibiogram for 435 strains showed that the aminoglycosides, erythromycin, doxycycline, chloramphenicol and nalidixic acid were the most effective drugs. This study implies that *C. jejuni* is a common cause of bacterial diarrhoea in Sweden.

5
Some epidemiological features of campylobacter infections in Oslo

A. MAELAND

Ullevål Hospital, Oslo, Norway

During a $2\frac{1}{2}$ year period approximately 3300 stool samples were cultured for campylobacter using the Skirrow technique. The laboratory serves a 1700 bed general hospital, including a paediatric ward and an infectious disease unit. Campylobacters were found in 46 patients. In the same period 70 salmonella, 25 shigella and four *Yersinia enterocolitica* isolates were cultured, and 142 cases of rotavirus were identified by electron microscopy.

About half of the 46 patients were hospitalized because of acute campylobacter enteritis. Five were hospitalized for other reasons, whilst 13 were outpatients. Five patients had other enteropathogens demonstrated.

Two thirds of the isolates were imported, mostly from the Mediterranean, Asia and Africa. One third of the patients had contracted their campylobacter infections in Norway, including two cases of secondary transmission from one traveller returning from abroad. One indigenous patient had a dog who harboured campylobacter.

Though the laboratory serves a paediatric ward admitting children with diarrhoea, we have only seen five community acquired cases of campylobacter enteritis in children. This is a small number compared to the 142 cases of rotavirus enteritis diagnosed in the same period. We conclude that rotavirus remains the main agent in children and that campylobacter is an infrequent cause of infectious diarrhoea in children in Oslo.

Since the problem of infectious diarrhoea is less frequent in Oslo than in most other places in the world, the culture of stools for campylobacter is most important in cases of enteritis acquired abroad. Community acquired cases of campylobacter are seen more frequently than either salmonellosis or shigellosis, but the numbers reported are few. The nature of the reserve of campylobacter in Oslo is unknown.

6
Human campylobacter infections 1977–80: national data based on routine laboratory reporting

S. E. J. YOUNG

Communicable Disease Surveillance Centre, 61 Colindale Avenue, London NW9

Between March 1977 and December 1980, 25 791 reports of the isolation of campylobacters from humans have been received by the Communicable Disease Surveillance Centre (CDSC). The annual total has increased from 1349 in 1977 to 9506 in 1980 and a peak has occurred each year in summer and early autumn (Figure 1). The number of reporting laboratories increased during the first 18 months but has been fairly constant since mid 1978.

Analysis by age and sex of the 11 941 cases where this information is available shows that the group most affected was aged < 5 years and that the overall male:female ratio was 1.16:1.0 (Figure 2). 57 infections were reported in neonates and 15 of their mothers also had positive faecal cultures.

Campylobacter bacteraemia (excluding *C. fetus*) was reported in 37 patients, aged 4 days–88 years; the organisms being isolated from both the blood and faeces of 21 patients.

Contact with ill dogs or cats was reported for 94 humans and in 56 cases campylobacters were also isolated from the animals.

Data are reported weekly to CDSC for the Communicable Disease Report by laboratories of the Public Health Laboratory Service and hospitals in England, Wales and Ireland.

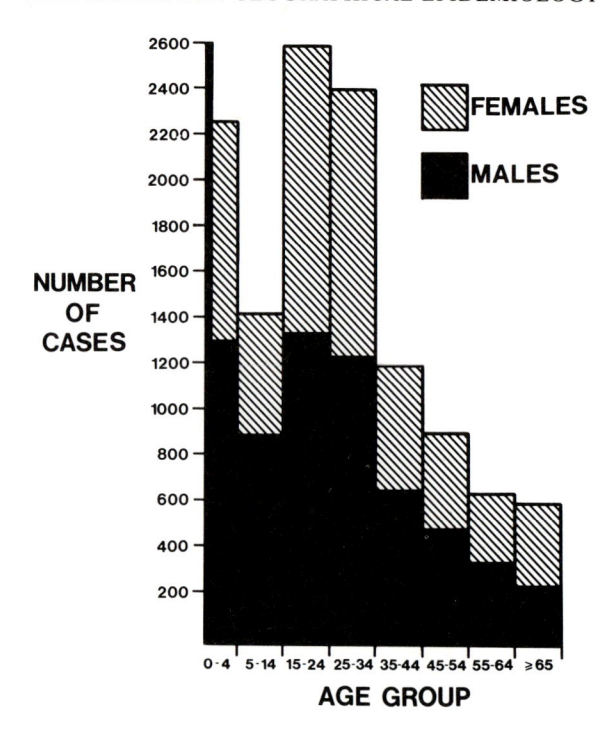

Figure 1

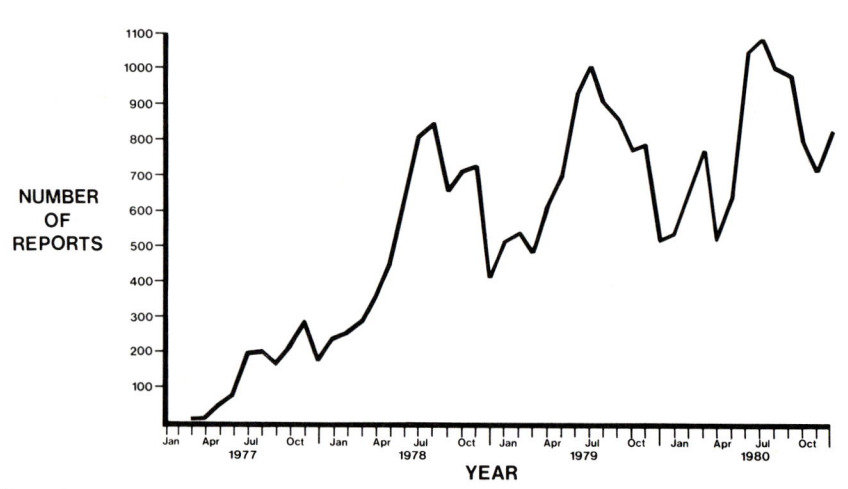

Figure 2

7
Campylobacter enteritis in Hong Kong and Western Australia

D. B. McGECHIE*, T. B. TEOH†, and V. W. BAMFORD‡

Fremantle Hospital, † State Health Laboratories, Western Australia and ‡ Government Institute of Pathology, Hong Kong

HONG KONG

841 faecal specimens from 587 patients attending an 1800 bed hospital were examined for *C. jejuni* for a 4 week period commencing March 1978. *C. jejuni* was isolated from 27 patients and salmonellas from 42 of them. There were two deaths among the campylobacter patients. *C. jejuni* was isolated from bile from a case of acute-on-chronic cholecystitis and *Campylobacter intestinalis* from a specimen of pus from a tubo-ovarian abscess. It was clear that campylobacter infections were sufficiently common and serious to justify the inclusion of suitable selective media as part of the routine examination of faecal specimens. An analysis of the isolations made in 1978 and 1980 is presented in Table 1. A comparison of the seasonal variation in salmonella and campylobacter isolations in 1980 (Figure 1) indicates that campylobacter infections are more common in the cooler months in Hong Kong. This is contrary to the summer

Table 1 Bacterial analysis of faecal specimens in Hong Kong in March/April 1978 and during 1980

Hong Kong	March/April 1978	1980
Faecal specimens	841	11 017
Pathogens	*No. of patients positive*	
Salmonellas	42	513
Campylobacters	27	201
Campylobacter + salmonella	1	19
Campylobacter + pathogenic *E. coli*	—	7
Campylobacter + shigella	—	3
Pathogenic *E. coli*	5	144
Shigella	2	157

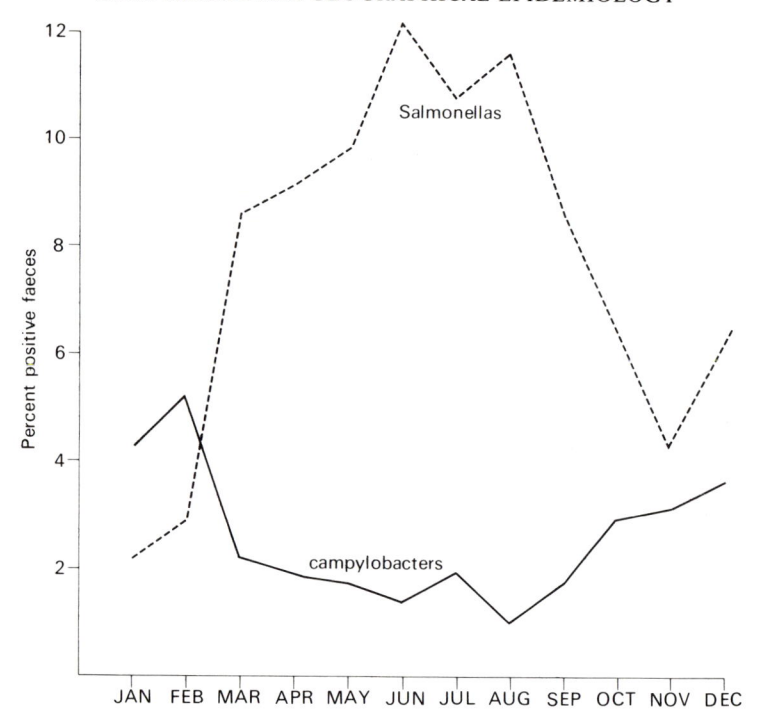

Figure 1 Seasonal isolation of salmonellas/campylobacters in 1980 in Hong Kong

prevalence observed in other countries and may reflect a different epidemiology between tropical and subtropical climates. A similar trend was seen in the variations for 1979.

WESTERN AUSTRALIA

At Fremantle Hospital, a 435-bed teaching hospital, the Microbiology Laboratory examines 95 faecal specimens per month. Since December 1978 campylobacters have been found in 38 patients. Ten were from domiciliary practice. Seven out of 13 outpatients recovered without treatment. Of 15 inpatients, three had initial diagnosis of ulcerative colitis, one each of diverticular disease, aortic aneurysm and Meckel's diverticulum. The State Health Laboratories examined 2905 diarrhoeal stools in 1980. Campylobacters were isolated in 196 (6.75%) specimens from 167 patients (Table 2). Chickens from three processors in Perth have been examined. 40 out of 40 cloacal swabs taken from live animals grew campylobacter, and 12 out of 20 carcass swabs were positive.

C. jejuni commonly caused mild infection.

Table 2 Isolation of campylobacter from country areas from diarrhoeal specimens by the State Health Laboratories, Western Australia

Region	Population	Campylobacter cases	Salmonella cases
Kimberley	17 500	44	211
Pilbara	43 000	18	135
Central	52 500	23	63
South east	43 000	4	33
South west	207 500	59	125

The Kimberley region accounts for 4.8% of the country population and 30% of the campylobacter cases. The population of the Kimberley is largely Aboriginal

8
Campylobacter jejuni as an aetiological agent of diarrhoeal disease in Israel

M. SHMILOVITZ and B. KRETZER

W. Hirsch Regional Microbiology Laboratory, Kupat Holim Haifa and Western Galilee, Israel

During a 17 month period starting 22nd July 1979, *C. jejuni* was isolated from 2024 stool cultures from 1649 persons. These included 1635 (4.3%) out of 38 226 patients with acute gastroenteritis and 14 of 165 asymptomatic household contacts. Table 1 presents the comparison of the bacterial isolates in cases of enteritis for the period January to December 1980 only. No isolates of *C. jejuni* were obtained from any of a control group of 222 made up of healthy subjects and patients without gastrointestinal disorders. A selective medium combining Skirrow's and Butzler's inhibitors was used and proved to be effective. A GasPak system without catalyst was in use for microaerophilic incubation at 43 °C. In 73 patients *C. jejuni* was associated with salmonella, in 55 with shigella and only in three were there both. *C. jejuni* occupies the second place in the bacterial aetiology of acute enteritis following shigella. The illness was mild to severe with positive blood culture in one patient only. All patients, including 51 requiring hospitalization recovered uneventfully. The age of the patients ranged from 2 weeks to 88 years, with infants and children comprising 83% of the total (Table 2). 387 patients came from 16 family and 58 institutional outbreaks which extended up to a period of 5 months. Except in one case, related to a *C. jejuni* infected dog, no source or route of transmission

Table 1 *C. jejuni* in comparison with other bacterial agents in the aetiology of 36.199 enteritis patients (January–December 1980)*

Aetiological agent	No. of patients	Percentage
Shigella	3818	10.6
Campylobacter jejuni	1418	3.9
Salmonella	1022	2.8
Total	6258	17.3

* Mixed infections excluded

Table 2 Distribution of 1635 *C. jejuni* enteritis patients according to age, sex and location (22 July 1979–21 December 1980)

Data	No. of cases	Percentage
Age group*		
from 2 weeks to 11 months	310	24.3
from 1 year to 4 years	556	43.6
from 5 years to 14 years	189	14.8
from 15 years to 64 years	191	15
over 65 years	28	2.2
Males	1007	61.5
Females	628	38.4
Urban†	1014	62
Rural‡	621	38

* In 1274 patients data were available
† 18 localities (towns and cities)
‡ 115 settlements (kibbutzim and villages)

had been established. 62% of the patients came from 18 urban localities and 38% from 115 rural settlements widely dispersed throughout Northern Israel. Lastly, *C. jejuni* was isolated from 183 patients in nine other laboratories throughout the country. This stressed further the importance of *C. jejuni* as a frequent aetiological agent of acute enteritis in Israel.

COMMENT

The selective medium employed was a Heart Infusion Agar, containing 6% human blood and a supplement of antibacterials which provides the following concentration per ml medium: vancomycin (10 µg), bacitracin (25 µg), trimethoprim (5 µg), novobiocin (5 µg), polymyxin B(5U) and amphotericin B(2U). This medium was found to be more inhibitory than others, mainly towards proteus, pseudomonas, streptococcus and candida species, which may be found in stool samples and appears to be nontoxic to campylobacters.

In some patients *C. jejuni* was excreted for a period up to 80 days and the percentage of *C. jejuni* infected patients ranged from 2.7% to 10.3% in certain months.

It should be noted that during the first 8 months of the study, the patients tested for *C. jejuni* were selected on the pathological nature of their stools. Afterwards, all patients regardless of the nature of their stools were tested for *C. jejuni*. Thereafter, *C. jejuni* was isolated from 187 patients whose stools appeared to be normal when sent to the laboratory.

In spite of occupying second place overall in the aetiology of bacterial enteritis, *C. jejuni* leads for a period of 5 months (January–May 1980), exceeding the incidence of shigella during March and May by three and two fold respectively.

As previously reported by other workers, all local isolates tested were resistant to beta-lactam antibiotics, and a third of these isolates were also resistant to co-trimoxazole. No resistance was observed toward erythromycin.

9
Campylobacter enteritis in Northern Greece

V. DANIELIDES, P. AUGOUSTIDOU-SAVVOPOULOU,
S. MANIOS, G. SIDIRA and A. KANZOUZIDOU

Infectious Disease Hospital, Thessaloniki, Greece

During a 2-year period stool cultures for Campylobacter and the common enteropathogens were carried out.

Campylobacter jejuni was found in 89 out of 1512 (6%) patients with diarrhoea admitted to our hospital, in one out of 97 patients with diseases other than diarrhoea, in none of 72 healthy controls and in 8 out of 115 (7%) family contacts.

C. jejuni was also found in the stools of 23 out of 247 (9%) dogs and on the carcasses of 300 out of 433 (69%) oven-ready chickens.

The chief clinical symptoms of the patients with campylobacter enteritis studied were, in order of frequency, diarrhoea, fever, vomiting, anorexia and abdominal pain. Stools were watery, extremely foul-smelling and occasionally bloody. In most patients the gastroenteritis was of slight to moderate severity, but in adult patients the illness was more severe. Diarrhoea was chronic in 12 of our cases.

All campylobacter strains isolated were sensitive to gentamicin, nalidixic acid, furazolidone, chloramphenicol, tetracycline, amicacin and tobramycin. Four out of 89 strains (6%) were resistant to erythromycin.

In the present study most of the patients (71%) were under the age of 1 year and the cases occurred both in the cold and warm months.

The role played by animals, birds, food or water in the cases of campylobacter enteritis could not be established.

Salmonella and shigella were isolated from 5% and 7% of diarrhoeal stools respectively.

It is concluded that *C. jejuni* is a common bacterial cause of gastro-enteritis in our area and probably the commonest bacterial cause of sporadic cases of gastroenteritis.

10
Campylobacter enteritis in developing countries

P. DE MOL

Department of Microbiology, Saint Pierre Hospital, Brussels

Campylobacter has been isolated in faeces from human beings from all over the world.

In developed countries, the presence of campylobacter seems to be associated with diarrhoeal disease.

In developing countries, the role of these bacteria, mainly in children over 1 year old is controversial. The results of a study performed in Zaire in 1979 are presented.

In this study the isolation rate of campylobacter was 13% among 271 children presenting with diarrhoea; at the same time campylobacter were isolated in 3% of the cases in a control group of 200 children of the same origin. They were investigated during a vaccination campaign. The highest frequency of isolation occurred in children under 2 years old (Table 1).

Clinical features were characterized by fever and watery or, more rarely, mucous stools.

The antimicrobial susceptibility was the same as found in Europe.

Table 1   Isolation rate (%) of *C. jejuni* from outpatients by age. (Lwiro, Zaïre, 1979)

Age group (yr)	Diarrhoeic patients No.	Diarrhoeic patients I.R.	Non-diarrhoeic patients No.	Non-diarrhoeic patients I.R.
0–1	145	19.9	55	5.4
2–3	49	4.1	47	0.0
4–14	77	7.7	98	3.1
Total	271	13.4	200	3.0

DISCUSSION

Dr Watson considered that the clinical presentation of 52% of patients with watery diarrhoea and only 14% with blood in the stool was contrary to current teaching, but Dr de Mol replied that the same pattern was seen in migrant workers in Belgium. Dr Butzler and Dr Feldman both emphasized that patient selection could, and did, affect figures of this kind, i.e. patients attending hospital as opposed to those who did not. In reply to a question by Dr Bokkenhouser, Dr Price stated that the gut pathology was not different between patients with watery and those with bloody diarrhoea.

11
Epidemiologic features of campylobacter enteritis in Bangladesh

R. I. GLASS*, I. HUQ, P. J. STOLL*, G. KIBRIYA* and
M. J. BLASER†

*International Centre for Diarrhoeal Disease Research,
Bangladesh
† Centers for Disease Control, Atlanta, GA, U.S.A.

Preliminary reports suggest minor differences in the epidemiology and the clinical consequences of *Campylobacter jejuni* infection in developed and less developed countries. To determine whether campylobacter is an enteropathogen in Bangladesh, we began monitoring campylobacter infections and disease symptoms in three Bangladeshi populations in February 1980. The selected groups were a 4% sample of patients with diarrhoea attending the cholera hospital in Dacca, family contacts of patients with diarrhoea (40 cases caused by campylobacter and 40 caused by other agents), who have had culture specimens taken every other day for at least 2 weeks, and a cohort of 180 village children aged 6 months to 6 years who have had culture specimens taken during every diarrhoeal episode as well as on routine monthly examination.

C. jejuni is commonly isolated in Bangladesh, but its role in the pathogenesis of diarrhoeal disease remains unclear. Although the organism was isolated from 475 to 3392 (14%) patients at hospitals in Dacca, the isolation rates for family contacts of diarrhoeal patients with and without campylobacter infection were the same; neither differed significantly from the rate for hospital patients when adjustment was made for age.

Campylobacter was isolated more frequently ($p < 0.01$) from village children who had culture specimens taken each month during an examination (135/1465) than from those whose culture specimens were taken because they had diarrhoea (16/360). With repeated monthly cultures, 60% of all these children and 75% of those under 3 years old had campylobacter isolated at least once. No characteristic set of signs and symptoms for campylobacter enteritis could be defined for any group.

Because of this difficulty in linking campylobacter with disease, we are examining paired serum specimens from patients, serotyping isolates, and trying to identify microbiological markers of pathogenicity that might help explain our results in the light of those observed in more developed areas.

DISCUSSION

Dr Butzler said that in Belgium there was a marked quantitative difference in the number of organisms in stools between patients who had diarrhoea and those who were not ill. Dr Glass, however, found no such differences in the groups he studied. Dr Karmali quoted Dr Bokkenhouser's study in children, 9–24 months of age, in which salmonellas and shigellas were found equally frequently in children with and without diarrhoea. Because of the relatively high prevalence of enteric infection in developing countries, it may be difficult to choose a control group. Dr Blazer pointed out that the duration of excretion studies following campylobacter infection have all been done in developed countries and may not be relevant to developing countries in which the epidemiology is quite different. Dr Glass found a mean duration of excretion overall, of 5 days both in the overall population and in children and agreed with Dr Blazer that, in choosing a control group, the people should not have had a diarrhoeal illness for at least the previous 2 weeks. Dr Skirrow enquired about events following a baby encountering its first campylobacter and whether immunity was acquired from the mother. Dr Glass had some data on this subject but it had not yet been analysed.

12
Campylobacter enteritis in Zaria

A. M. YAKUBU and C. S. BELLO

Ahmadu Bello University Hospital, Zaria, Nigeria

INTRODUCTION

The mortality and morbidity of gastroenteritis are highest in the developing countries. In spite of our understanding of the pathophysiological mechanism of this condition, our knowledge of the aetiological agents is still incomplete. In Zaria, we are able to isolate pathogenic agents in one third of diarrhoeal diseases in children.

The aim of this study was to look for campylobacter in diarrhoeal stools of both children and adults in Zaria and to compare our findings with those reported from elsewhere.

MATERIALS AND METHODS

297 diarrhoeal stool specimens, comprising 213 from adults and 84 from children under 5 years, were screened for campylobacter in addition to other routine pathogens like salmonella, shigella and enteropathogenic *E. coli* (EPEC).

The stool specimens were plated out on Butzler's selective medium and incubated in a metal anaerobic jar with hydrogen/CO_2 generating pack and incubated at 42 °C for 48–72 hours, after which the plates were examined for typical campylobacter colonies. Screening for other bacterial pathogens were carried out using conventional methods.

RESULTS

The results are given in Table 1. None of the 297 stool specimens yielded any campylobacter species.

Table 1 Bacterial pathogens from 297 stool specimens (Yakubu and Bello)

	Salmonella sp.		Shigella sp.		EPEC		C. jejuni
	No.	%	No.	%	No.	%	No.
Adults	14	14.7	4	1.4	0	0	0
Children under 5 yrs	5	1.7	2	0.7	12	4.0	0

DISCUSSION

We present here our limited experience in an attempt to isolate *C. jejuni* from routine stool specimens, in Zaria.

Our failure to isolate campylobacter from 297 diarrhoeal stools may be due to one of the following reasons:

(1) faulty technique
(2) wrong season
(3) unusual strains in Zaria
(4) other reasons
(5) their genuine absence.

COMMENT

Dr Fleming suggested that stool specimens should be examined under phase contrast microscopy. If campylobacter were observed but still not grown then the problem was in the culturing technique. Such a quality control technique is simple, inexpensive and fast.

13 Editorial discussion

This first workshop was concerned primarily with the global distribution of campylobacter enteritis, as compared with the relationships between epidemiology and the environment which was the subject of discussion in a later workshop.

The importance of diarrhoeal disease in the developing world is irrefutable. The significance and magnitude of campylobacter enteritis has, however, yet to be appreciated. It is apparent from the data presented that studies of the disease in developed countries may not reflect the disease in undeveloped areas; for example the age distribution, seasonality and clinical consequences all appear to depend on geographical location. Studies in developing countries are further complicated by the difficulties in providing adequate controls from populations where asymptomatic infection can occur and the superimposition of campylobacter infections with other potential enteric pathogens. Additionally the relevance of immunity, from previous infections, in susceptible populations has yet to be established.

Epidemiological studies in the developed world need to focus on the evaluation of outbreaks in order to identify the source of infection. To this end techniques for the recovery of campylobacters from probable vehicles, such as water, universally acceptable serotyping and/or biotyping methods of identification and laboratory procedures for the demonstration of pathogenic organisms must be established.

The significance of travellers diarrhoea should not be overlooked in those countries where travel is frequent and may confuse seasonal distributions. Furthermore the role of person to person transmission has not yet been established especially in those cases where chronic infection and long term excretion can occur.

The ubiquitous nature of campylobacter infections was emphasized, throughout this workshop, and is known to occur in all parts of the world and in all age groups. The control of such infections is essential, especially in the developing world, but considerably more investigations must be undertaken, into the nature of the disease, before advice on adequate control measures can be given.

SECTION II
TAXONOMY AND TYPING

Chairmen: M. B. Skirrow and M. Véron

---

14 Identification, nomenclature and taxonomy of catalase-positive campylobacters
M. A. Karmali, S. A. De Grandis, A. K. Allen and P. C. Fleming — 35

15 The classification of 'thermophilic' campylobacters and their distribution in man and domestic animals
M. B. Skirrow and J. Benjamin — 40

16 Are the *Campylobacter jejuni* strains from different species similar?
T. U. Kosunen, S. Pollanen, M. L Hanninen and D. Danielsson — 45

17 Biotype characteristics of *Campylobacter* species, with emphasis on strains isolated in North America
R. E. Weaver, D. G. Hollis, G. A. Hebert and M. J. Blaser — 50

18 Techniques for phage typing *Campylobacter jejuni*
John H. Bryner, A. E. Ritchie and J. W. Foley — 52

19 Anaerobic respiration of fumarate by catalase-positive campylobacters
Michel Véron and Annie Lenvoisé-Furet — 57

20 Some simple tests for differentiating between campylobacters
M. H. H. Razi and R. W. A. Park — 59

21 The use of *Pseudomonas aeruginosa* for the typing of thermophilic campylobacters
W. A. Telfer Brunton and A. Moyes — 60

22 The characteristics of type and reference cultures of *Campylobacter* species held in the National Collection of Type Cultures (NCTC)
R. J. Owen and S. Leaper 62

23 General discussion and editorial comment 65

14
Identification, nomenclature, and taxonomy of catalase-positive campylobacters

M. A. KARMALI, S. A. DE GRANDIS, A. K. ALLEN and P. C. FLEMING

Department of Bacteriology, The Hospital for Sick Children, Toronto, Canada M5G 1X8

Currently, available tests for differentiating catalase-positive campylobacters are inadequate and it has become clear that they need to be extended. We have therefore evaluated a number of additional characteristics for their ability to distinguish catalase-positive campylobacters. These characteristics include cell size, swarming ability and coccal degeneration[1,2] and the susceptibility of strains to various cephalosporins[3].

CELL SIZE, SWARMING ABILITY, AND COCCAL DEGENERATION

The 32 catalase-positive campylobacter strains studied consisted of 16 strains of *C. jejuni* (corresponding to the *C. jejuni/C. coli* group of Véron and Chatelain[4]), 12 strains of *C. fetus* ssp. *fetus*, and four strains of *C. fetus* ssp. *venerealis*. Included in the strains studied were all the ATCC catalase-positive campylobacter reference strains. The species or subspecies identification of each strain was based on tests outlined in Table 1.

Table 1 Differentiation of catalase-positive campylobacters

	Growth at 25°C	Growth at 42°C	Growth in 1% glycine	Nalidixic acid sensitivity (40 mg/l)
C. jejuni	−	+	+	S
C. fetus ssp. *fetus*	+	−	+	R
C. fetus ssp. *venerealis*	+	−	−	R

S = sensitive; R = resistant

For studies on cell size, suspensions of colonies from 48-hour blood agar cultures of each strain were examined by phase-contrast microscopy under oil immersion. High-power fields containing spiral forms were photographed and prints were made at a final magnification of ×7200 for each strain. The dimensions of between 2–4 wavelengths of the spiral forms of each strain were measured, and hence the average wavelength (λ) and average amplitude (α) of the waveforms could be determined. The range of wavelengths and amplitude as well as the mean wavelength and amplitude of each species are recorded in Table 2. The differences in wavelength between the groups were highly

Table 2 Morphological differentiation of catalase-positive campylobacters: wavelength and amplitude of 'spirals'

	C. jejuni	C. fetus ssp. fetus	C. fetus ssp. venerealis
Wavelength			
Range (μm)	0.89–1.31	1.36–2.13	2.25–2.56
Mean (μm)	1.12	1.80	2.43
Amplitude			
Range (μm)	0.35–0.63	0.49–0.68	0.69–0.79
Mean (μm)	0.48	0.55	0.73

significant ($p < 0.001$). It should be noted that there was no overlap at all between the ranges of wavelengths of each of the three groups. The differences in amplitude between *C. fetus* ssp. *venerealis* and the other two groups were also significant ($p < 0.01$). Organisms belonging to the different groups could be distinguished visually on the basis of size alone without actual measurement.

For studies on swarming, each strain was spotted onto a quadrant of a moist blood agar plate. The plates were incubated for 48 hours at 37 °C under reduced oxygen tension. Under these experimental conditions, swarming was found to be a feature only of *C. jejuni* and not of the other two groups.

For studies on coccal transformation, 48-hour blood agar cultures of each strain were left on the bench in room air. Colonies from each culture were subsequently examined for cellular morphology by phase-contrast microscopy at daily intervals. All cultures of *C. jejuni* so examined showed coccal transformation after one day, and this was virtually complete after 2 days. All cultures of *C. fetus* ssp. *fetus* and *C. fetus* ssp. *venerealis* retained predominantly normal cellular morphology at 48 hours (<5% coccal forms) and in many cases even at 4 days.

Duplicate 48-hour blood agar cultures of *C. jejuni* left on the bench for 2 days in closed jars containing a reduced oxygen tension failed to undergo rapid coccal transformation, indicating that exposure to room air was an important factor leading to coccal degeneration.

SUSCEPTIBILITY OF CATALASE-POSITIVE CAMPYLOBACTERS TO EIGHT CEPHALOSPORINS

Table 3 shows the ranges of MICs of eight cephalosporins for *C. fetus* ssp. *fetus* (8 strains), and *C. jejuni* (60 strains)[3]. *C. jejuni* was significantly more resistant than *C. fetus* ssp. *fetus* to cephalosporin 'C', cephaloridine, cephalothin, cefazolin and cefamandole. No species differences in susceptibility were noted with cephalexin, cefotaxime and cefoxitin. Rapid species differentiation on the basis of an antibiogram could be attained by the disc diffusion method. *C. jejuni* failed to produce a zone of inhibition around a 30 μg cephalothin disc, but produced a significant zone size ranging from 21–38 mm (mean, 31 mm) in diameter around a 30 μg nalidixic acid disc. *C. fetus* ssp. *fetus*, on the other hand, produced no zone around a 30 μg nalidixic acid disc, but produced a significant zone size ranging from 16–25 mm (mean, 21 mm) around the 30 μg cephalothin disc.

Table 3 Range of MICs (mg/l) of eight cephalosporins for *C. fetus* ssp. *fetus* and *C. jejuni*

Antibiotic	C. fetus *ssp.* fetus	C. jejuni
Cephalosporin C	≤0.5–2	4–32
Cephaloridine	≤0.5–1	8–128
Cephalothin	16–32	128–≥512
Cefazolin	8–32	128–≥512
Cefamandole	16–64	128–≥512
Cephalexin	32–128	16–≥512
Cefotaxime	4–16	2–32
Cefoxitin	32–64	32–≥512

The disc diffusion method is not suitable for testing the susceptibility of strains of *C. fetus* ssp. *venerealis* to cephalothin and nalidixic acid, because of the relatively slow growth of these organisms. However, we found that all five strains of *C. fetus* ssp. *venerealis* in our collection were resistant to 40 mg/l of nalidixic acid and susceptible to 32 mg/l of cephalothin when tested by the agar dilution method.

A list of differential characteristics incorporating our findings is shown in Table 4.

Table 4 Differentiation of catalase-positive campylobacters

	Size	Swarming on moist media	Rapid coccal transformation	Cephalothin 32 mg/l
C. jejuni	'small'	+	+	R
C. fetus ssp. *fetus*	'medium'	–	–	S
C. fetus ssp. *venerealis*	'large'	–	–	S

S = sensitive;   R = resistant

NOMENCLATURE OF CATALASE-POSITIVE CAMPYLOBACTERS

The nomenclature of catalase-positive campylobacters has been clarified to a great extent by the publication of the *Approved Lists of Bacterial Names*[5]. This list regards as valid the nomenclature used by Véron and Chatelain[4] for catalase-positive campylobacters. *C. fetus* ssp. *fetus* (corresponding to '*Vibrio fetus intestinalis*' of Florent[6]) was designated as type species of the genus campylobacter by Véron and Chatelain on the presumption that it was this subspecies and not *C. fetus* ssp. *venerealis* that corresponded to the strains originally designated '*Vibrio fetus*' by Smith and Taylor[7] in 1919. The exact nature of Smith and Taylor's strains will never be known because their strains of '*Vibrio fetus*' were not preserved. Smith's original report[8] however does have a clue that might indicate the subspecies that corresponds to the original strains of '*Vibrio fetus*'. Smith recorded the average wavelength and amplitude of his strains to be about 2.0 and 0.5 µm respectively. From the results obtained in our study on cell size, these dimensions conform closest to those of Véron and Chatelain's *C. fetus* ssp. *fetus* ('*V. fetus intestinalis*' of Florent[6]), and therefore support the designation of the latter subspecies as the type species of the genus *Campylobacter*.

The taxonomic basis (as opposed to historical basis) for separating thermophilic catalase-positive campylobacters into two species *C. jejuni* and *C. coli* remains to be established. Listed in Table 5 are the original strains of *C. jejuni* (one strain) and *C. coli* (nine strains) used by Véron and Chatelain in their taxonomic study. An examination of the hippurate reactions and Penner serotypes[9] of the strains emphasizes the limitations of the physiological and biochemical tests originally used to separate the two groups. A more satisfactory scheme for separating thermophilic campylobacters may well become possible now that an effective serotyping system[9] is available.

Table 5 Correlation of the collection Institut Pasteur strains of *C. jejuni* and *C. coli* with Penner serotype and ability to hydrolyse hippurate

CIP no.	'Species'	Hippurate	Serotype
702	*C. jejuni*	+ve	23, 36
7077	*C. coli*	−ve	34
7086	*C. coli*	+ve	37
7078	*C. coli*	−ve	24
7079	*C. coli*	−ve	34
6825	*C. coli*	+ve	23, 36
7081	*C. coli*	+ve	31
7054	*C. coli*	−ve	34
715	*C. coli*	−ve	24
7080	*C. coli*	−ve	NT

References

1. Karmali, M. A., Allen A. K. and Fleming P. C. (1980). Rapid differentiation of catalase-positive campylobacters. *Can. J. Public Health*, **71**, 204
2. Karmali, M. A., Allen A. K. and Fleming P. C. (1981). Differentiation of catalase-positive campylobacters with special reference to morphology. *Int. J. Syst. Bacteriol.*, **31**, 64–71

3. Karmali, M. A., De Grandis, S. A. and Fleming, P. C. (1980). Antimicrobial susceptibility of *Campylobacter jejuni* and *Campylobacter fetus* subsp. *fetus* to eight cephalosporins with special reference to species differentiation. *Antimicrobial Agents and Chemotherapy*, **18**, 948–51
4. Véron, M. and Chatelain, R. (1973). Taxonomic study of the genus *Campylobacter* Sebald and Véron and designation of the neotype strain for the type species *Campylobacter fetus* (Smith and Taylor) Sebald and Véron. *Int. J. Syst. Bacteriol.*, **23**, 122–34
5. Skerman, V. B. D., McGowan, V. and Sneath, P. H. A. (1980). Approved Lists of Bacterial Names. *Int. J. Syst. Bacteriol.*, **30**, 270–1
6. Florent A. (1959). Les deux vibrioses génitales: la vibriose due à *V. fetus venerealis* et la vibriose d'origine intestinale due à *V. fetus intestinalis*. *Mededlingen der Vecartsenijschool van de Rijksuniversiteit te Gent*, **3**, 1–60
7. Smith, T. and Taylor, M. S. (1919). Some morphological and biological characters of the spirilla (*Vibrio fetus*, n. sp.) associated with disease of the fetal membranes in cattle. *J. Exp.* **30**, 299–312
8. Smith, T. (1918). Spirilla associated with disease of the fetal membranes in cattle. *J. Exp. Med.*, **28**, 701–19
9. Penner, J. L. and Hennessy, J. N. (1980). Passive haemagglutination technique for serotyping *Campylobacter fetus* subsp. *jejuni* on the basis of soluble heat-stable antigens. *J. Clin. Microbiol.*, **12**, 732–7

DISCUSSION

Table 5 caused some confusion. Dr C. E. Park was puzzled by the fact that *C. coli* strains were shown to be hippurate positive, but according to Skirrow and Benjamin (see below) this feature identifies them as *C. jejuni*. Dr Karmali explained that they were merely quoting the CIP names, which Professor Véron confirmed were already allocated when he did his 1973 work. The implication was that these strains should be re-designated, and Dr. Skirrow said that this had already happened with the first strain he deposited with the NCTC in 1977 (NCTC 11168) provisionally named *C. coli*, but which, in the light of later work, proved to be a typical strain of *C. jejuni*. Further discussion, which included the status of *C. coli* is reported later (p. 66).

Dr Wilson asked whether anything akin to the Dienes phenomenon had been observed between the swarming growths of different strains of *C. jejuni*. Dr Lior said that he had not found it – swarming growths merged imperceptibly together. Dr Skirrow and Dr Telfer Brunton both confirmed this observation.

15
The classification of 'thermophilic' campylobacters and their distribution in man and domestic animals

M. B. SKIRROW and J. BENJAMIN

Worcester Royal Infirmary, Worcester WR1 3AS, U.K.

In a previous communication[1] we described tests that helped to differentiate *Campylobacter* strains belonging to the 'thermophilic' group (*C. jejuni*, *C. coli* – Véron and Chatelain[2]; *C. fetus* ssp. *jejuni* – Smibert[3]). The most useful tests were then found to be sensitivity to nalidixic acid, tolerance to 2,3,5-triphenyltetrazolium chloride (TTC), and growth at 30.5 and 45.5 °C. Nalidixic acid resistant strains (NARTC) formed a distinct group, but orthodox sensitive strains could be divided into nine categories according to the results of the TTC and temperature tests: strains in low-number categories resembled the Institut Pasteur *C. jejuni* type strain (category 1), and in high-number categories the *C. coli* type strain (category 8); but the existence of strains with intermediate characteristics prevented clear demarcation of the two 'species'. We now describe two simple tests – hippurate hydrolysis and production of H_2S in an iron-containing medium — that clarify these groupings and form a basis for distinguishing *C. jejuni* from *C. coli* and for dividing *C. jejuni* into two biotypes.

MATERIALS AND METHODS

A total of 457 campylobacter strains (Table 1), that had been identified and categorized according to earlier tests[1], were tested for their ability to hydrolyse hippurate and to produce H_2S in an iron-containing medium.

Hippurate hydrolysis test

The hippurate hydrolysis test was modified from Hwang and Edlerer[4]. Growth from a blood agar culture, which had been incubated overnight at 37 °C, was suspended in 2 ml of sterile distilled water to an optical density of 1.0 measured

Table 1 Identity and source of 457 campylobacter strains studied

No. of strains	Identity	Source
18	C. fetus ssp fetus	Man, sheep, cattle, pig
15	NARTC*	Various animals other than man
382	C. jejuni/C. coli	Field strains from man and other animals (see Table 3).
37	C. jejuni/C. coli	Penner serotype strains†
5	C. jejuni/C. coli (see Table 2)	Reference strains
457		

* Nalidixic acid-resistant 'thermophilic' campylobacter (Skirrow and Benjamin[1])
† Penner, Hennessy and Goodbody p. 89

at a wavelength of 540 nm in a 1 cm cell. 0.5 ml of a 5% aqueous solution of sodium hippurate was added to the suspension which was thoroughly mixed and placed in a water bath at 37 °C for 2 h. 1 ml of ninhydrin solution (ninhydrin 3.5 g, acetone 50 ml, butanol 50 ml) was then added and the test left for a further 2 hours at 37 °C. The development of a deep purple colour resembling gentian violet was taken to indicate a positive reaction; no colour, or a pale mauve tint, were regarded as negative. Negative and weak-positive control strains were included in every test run.

H_2S production in iron-containing medium – H_2S(FBP)

A portion of growth about the size of a small pea taken from an overnight blood agar culture (37 °C) was inoculated as a lump into a tube of broth containing the FBP supplement of Hoffman et al.[5] (Oxoid Nutrient Broth No. 2, 25 g/l; Oxoid Technical Agar No. 3, 1.2 g/l; $FeSO_4 \cdot 7H_2O$, 0.5 g/l; sodium metabisulphite, 0.5 g/l; and sodium pyruvate, 0.5 g/l). The test was left at room temperature for 4 hours and then examined for blackening around the lump of growth (positive).*

RESULTS

All 18 strains of C. fetus ssp. fetus gave negative results in both tests ($-/-$). All 15 NARTC strains were negative in the hippurate test and positive in the H_2S(FBP) test ($-/+$) although some were only weakly positive in the latter test.

C. jejuni/C. coli strains (nalidixic acid sensitive) gave one of three combinations of results: $+/-$, $+/+$, or $-/-$. The relationship of each of these groups with our nine formerly described categories is shown in Figure 1 (categories 4,5 and 6,7 have been transposed because this gives a clearer

* Some workers have found it necessary to leave the test overnight before reading

division of the three groups; this is equivalent to reversing the priority of the TTC tolerance test over the 30.5 °C test as shown in our original schema). In general, the hippurate positive strains filled the low-number categories and the hippurate negative strains the high-number categories. $H_2S(FBP)$ positive strains, all of which were also hippurate positive, occupied a more intermediate position but overlapped the other (H_2S negative) hippurate positive strains. Thus we regard hippurate positive strains as *C. jejuni*, hippurate negative strains as *C. coli*, and divide *C. jejuni* into two biotypes according to their ability to produce H_2S in the FBP medium. The position is summarized in Table 2 which also includes NARTC and *C. fetus* ssp. *fetus*.

The distribution of our proposed *C. jejuni* biotypes 1 and 2, and *C. coli*, in indigenous human infections and in various domestic animals is shown in Table 3, and their relationship to the Penner serotype strains is shown in Table 4.

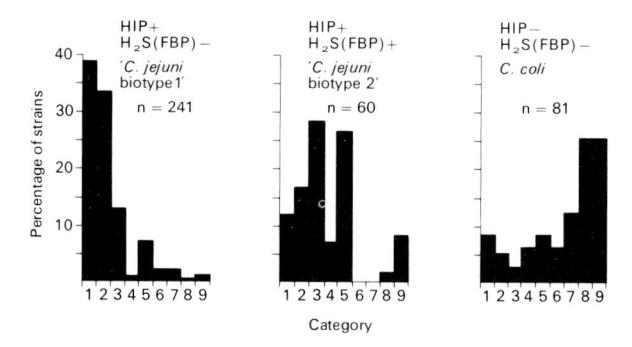

Figure 1 Relationship of strain category (Skirrow and Benjamin, 1980) to hippurate hydrolysis (HIP) and $H_2S(FBP)$ tests for strains of *C. jejuni/C. coli*

Table 2 Identification chart for intestinal campylobacters

	C. fetus*	NARTC**	C. jejuni biotype 1†	C. jejuni biotype 2‡	C. coli§
Growth at: 25.0 °C	+	−	−	−	−
43.0 °C	−	+	+	+	+
Nalidixic acid (30 µg disc)	R	R	S	S	S
Hippurate hydrolysis	−	−	+	+	−
H_2S production (FBP)	−	+	−	+	−

\+ = growth; − = no growth; R = resistant (0 mm); S = sensitive (≧ 6 mm from edge of disc)
Reference strains
* Includes NCTC 5850
** Includes NCTC 11352
† Includes CIP 702 (type strain) and NCTC 11168
‡ Includes NCTC 11392
§ Includes CIP 7080 (type strain) and NCTC 11353

Table 3 Distribution of *C. jejuni* biotypes 1 and 2 and *C. coli* in man and domestic animals

	Number of strains (%)			
	C. jejuni biotype 1	C. jejuni biotype 2	C. coli	Total
Man*	70 (77)	16 (18)	5 (5)	91 (100)
Cattle	70 (88)	5 (6)	5 (6)	80 (100)
Sheep	36 (72)	5 (10)	9 (18)	50 (100)
Dogs	39 (72)	13 (24)	2 (4)	54 (100)
Poultry	23 (41)	21 (38)	12 (21)	56 (100)
Pigs	3 (6)	0 (0)	48 (94)	51 (100)
Total	241 (63)	60 (16)	81 (21)	382 (100)

* Indigenous infections diagnosed at Worcester Royal Infirmary during 14 months

Table 4 Relationship of *C. jejuni* biotypes and *C. coli* to Penner serotype strains

Biotypes	Penner Serotype strains ('T' Nos.)	No. of strains
C. jejuni biotype 1	1–4, 7, 8, 10, 11, 13, 15–19, 22, 23, 31, 35–37, 40	21
C. jejuni biotype 2	9, 21, 27, 32, 33, 38, 41	7
C. coli	5, 20, 24–26, 28, 30, 34, 39	9
		37

DISCUSSION

Harvey[6] observed that *C. fetus* ssp. *fetus* and *C. fetus* ssp. *venerealis* failed to hydrolyse hippurate, whereas most strains of *C. jejuni* did so. Two of the *jejuni*-like strains in her collection were exceptional in failing to hydrolyse hippurate. One of them was known to us as a strain closely similar to the Institut Pasteur *C. coli* type strain, and this provided the clue to the possibility that the test might be used to differentiate the two species.

The chemistry of the production of H_2S from the FBP broth is unknown. It is independent of the presence of bisulphite in the medium, although stronger reactions are obtained when bisulphite is included (unpublished observations). We have also observed that H_2S(TSI) positive *Proteus* ssp. are negative in the H_2S(FBP) test. Moreover, the performance of campylobacters in the latter test bears little or no relationship to their performance in the orthodox 'standard' and 'sensitive' (cysteine) media of Véron and Chatelain[2]. For example, *C. coli* strains scored high in the orthodox tests yet they are negative in the H_2S(FBP) test.

The two tests now described largely replace the growth temperature (30.5 and 45.5 °C) and TTC tolerance tests, but the finer differentiation that can be attained by the latter may still have a place in epidemiological investigations pending the development of serotyping methods. The distribution of the two biotypes of *C. jejuni* and *C. coli* in man and domestic animals follows the pattern already described in Skirrow and Benjamin[1] except that an even sharper polarization of *C. jejuni* biotype 1 in cattle (88%) and *C. coli* in pigs (94%) is evident. The highest proportion of *C. jejuni* biotype 2 strains was found in poultry (38%).

References

1. Skirrow, M. B. and Benjamin, J. (1980). '1001' Campylobacters: cultural characteristics of intestinal campylobacters from man and animals. *J. Hyg. (Cambridge)*, **85**, 427–42
2. Véron, M. and Chatelain R. (1973). Taxonomic study of the genus Campylobacter Sebald and Véron and designation of the neotype strain for the type species *Campylobacter fetus* (Smith and Taylor) Sebald and Véron. *Int. J. Syst. Bacteriol.*, **23**, 122–34
3. Smibert, R. M. (1974). Campylobacter. In: Bergey's Manual of Determinative Bacteriology, 8th edn. Williams & Wilkins, Baltimore, 207–11
4. Hwang, M. and Ederer, G. M. (1975). Rapid hippurate hydrolysis method for presumptive identification of group B streptococci. *J. Clin. Microbiol.*, **1**, 114–5
5. Hoffman, P., Krieg, N. R. and Smibert, R. M. (1979). Studies of the microaerophilic nature of *Campylobacter fetus* subsp. *jejuni*. I Physiological aspects of enhanced aerotolerance. *Canad. J. Microbiol.*, **25**, 1–7
6. Harvey, S. M. (1980). Hippurate hydrolysis by *Campylobacter fetus*. *J. Clin. Microbiol.*, **11**, 435–7

16
Are the *Campylobacter jejuni* strains from different species similar?

T. U. KOSUNEN,* S. PÖLLÄNEN,* M. L. HÄNNINEN†
and D. DANIELSSON‡

* Department of Bacteriology and Immunology, University of Helsinki, Helsinki, Finland

† Department of Food Hygiene, College of Veterinary Medicine, Helsinki, Finland

‡ Central County Hospital, Örebro, Sweden

INTRODUCTION

Heterogeneity of the *Campylobacter jejuni* group has been demonstrated recently by the use of tests for the hydrolysis of hippurate[1], H_2S production[1], and tolerance to triphenyltetrazolium chloride[2], as well as by the detection of antigenic differences by hemagglutination[3] and co-agglutination tests[4]. Since these tests offer new markers for strain identification, they promised to be of epidemiological value, so we applied some of them, together with antibiotic sensitivity tests, to compare campylobacter isolates from patients and various domestic animals.

MATERIALS AND METHODS

Campylobacter strains

Eighty-seven field strains were studied of which 30 were human strains isolated from stool cultures of enteritis patients and 57 were animal strains cultured from faecal samples obtained from slaughter houses and farms (Table 1). The latter included seven farms which were investigated following the isolation of a campylobacter strain from a patient at the farm. The strains were isolated on the medium described by Skirrow[5] to which actinomycin B (2 mg/l) had been added[6]. Organisms that grew at 43 °C, produced oxidase and catalase, were sensitive to nalidixic acid, and showed the typical curved and spiral

Table 1 Co-agglutination reaction patterns of 87 strains of *C. jejuni* showing their relationship to source, ability to hydrolyse hippurate (HIP), tolerance to triphenyltetrazolium chloride (TTC), and sensitivity to metronidazole (MET) and erythromycin (ERY)

| Antigenic group | Co-agglutination reactions |||||| No. of strains | Source of strains |||||| HIP +/− | TTC S/I/R* | MET S/R* | ERY S/R* |
	VTP67	372	113	441	341		Man	Cattle	Swine	Chicken	Dog	Sheep				
A	−	+	−	+	−	43	17	18	5	2	1		43/0	37/3/3	37/6	42/1
B	−	+	+	−	−	14	4		3	1		6	0/14	4/3/7	14/0	13/1
C	−	+	+	+	−	7	1	2	1	3			7/0	4/1/2	7/0	7/0
D	−	−	−	+	−	4	1	1	2				4/0	2/2/0	3/1	4/0
E	−	+	−	−	+	2		1		1			1/1	1/0/1	2/0	2/0
F	−	+	+	−	−	1	1						0/1	0/0/1	1/0	1/0
G	−	−	−	−	−	1	1						1/0	1/0/0	1/0	1/0
H	+	+	−	+	−	6	3	3					5/1	5/0/1	3/3	6/0
I	+	+	+	+	−	1	1						1/0	1/0/0	0/1	1/0
J	+	+	+	−	−	2			1	1			0/2	0/0/2	1/0	0/1
K	+	+	−	−	−	1		1					0/1	0/0/1	1/0	1/0
L	+	−	−	−	−	3	1		2				1/2	1/0/2	3/0	3/0
M	+	+	+	−	−	2				2			2/0	2/0/0	2/0	2/0
Total (groups A–M)						87	30	26	14	10	1	6	65/22	58/9/20	75/11	83/3

* S = sensitive, I = intermediate, R = resistant

morphology of campylobacters were regarded as members of the *C. coli/C. jejuni* group.

Co-agglutination tests

Eleven co-agglutination reagents were prepared by sensitizing Cowan I-staphylococci with rabbit antisera produced against formalinized campylobacter suspensions. These reagents and testing methods have been described previously[4]. The following strains were used for the production of antisera: one strain of *C. fetus* ssp. *venerealis* (strain 13823), two strains of *C. fetus* ssp. *fetus* (strains 13014, 14865) and eight strains of *C. jejuni* (strains VTP 67, 372, 113, 105, 441, 341, ATCC 29428 and ST8). When each sensitized staphylococcal reagent was tested against its homologous and heterologous campylobacter strains (1 % suspension of living bacteria harvested from blood agar plates incubated at 43 °C for 48 hours), the strongest reaction was always with the homologous pair. The suspensions of *C. fetus* ssp. *venerealis* and *C. fetus* ssp. *fetus* cross-reacted with two of the *C. jejuni* reagents, but the *C. jejuni* suspensions showed several interstrain cross-reactions.

Hydrolysis of hippurate (HIP) and tolerance to triphenyltetrazolium chloride (TTC)

These tests were carried out and interpreted as described by Skirrow and Benjamin[1,2]. In the TTC tests (strip diffusion) inhibition zones of 0–2 mm were graded as resistant, 3–4 mm as intermediate, and $\geq$ 5 mm as sensitive.

Antimicrobial sensitivity tests

Disc diffusion tests were carried out on blood agar plates incubated at 43 °C for 24 hours to give semi-confluent growth. Discs of nalidixic acid (130 µg), metronidazole (16 µg) and erythromycin (78 µg) were used (A/S Rosco, Taastrup, Denmark); inhibition zones of $\geq$ 23 mm diameter were regarded as sensitive and anything less as resistant.

RESULTS

General findings

Co-agglutination reactions of all but one of the 87 *C. jejuni* strains studied were negative with the reagents of *C. fetus* ssp. *venerealis* and *C. fetus* ssp. *fetus*. All 87 strains reacted with three of the *C. jejuni* reagents (105, ATCC29428 and ST8), but a variety of reactions were found with the remaining five reagents, which permitted the formation of 13 antigenic groups (Table 1). Also shown in Table 1 are the relationships of these groups to strain source and performance in the biochemical and sensitivity tests. About half of the strains gave the same co-agglutination pattern (antigenic group A) and all of these strains were hippurate positive. Neither the few strains tolerant to TTC, nor those resistant to metronidazole appeared to be associated with any particular group or source. The six sheep strains reacted in the same way in all except the TTC test, but since they were obtained from only two farms, they might have represented only one or two strains.

Most of the smaller antigenic groups consisted of strains that were either all hippurate positive or all negative, but in three groups there was a mixture of positive and negative strains. In general, the TTC tolerant strains were hippurate negative and the TTC sensitive ones hippurate positive.

Findings in individual farms

In the seven farms investigated because of the diagnosis of a human enteritis patient, comparison of each index strain with strains obtained from various domestic animals showed both similarities and differences (Table 2). In six cases differences of antigenic group or resistance to antibiotics excluded certain animals as the source of the infection of the human index patient, but in five farms the human and animal isolates were indistinguishable. In one such case the index patient had acquired a puppy a few days before she developed enteritis. The dog had diarrhoea on its arrival, it was not eating well, and a campylobacter strain was isolated from its faeces. It had lived only indoors due to the cold winter and eaten only commercial pellets. The only contact with cattle were via the boots of its original owner, which it used to lick. She wore the boots when working with about 40 calves that she was raising. Faecal samples from four of 15 calves were positive for campylobacter, and three of them were still positive 4 months later.

Table 2 Comparison of *C. jejuni* strains isolated from animals associated with human index patients

Index patient	Age	Similar strains	Different strains	Criterion for exclusion
1. Woman	51		1 bovine	antigens
2. Boy	1	1 bovine 1 chicken	2 bovine	metronidazole
3. Boy	10	4 bovine	1 bovine	antigens
4. Man	30		1 bovine	metronidazole, erythromycin
5. Boy	11	1 swine	2 chicken 1 swine	antigens erythromycin
6. Boy	12	1 bovine		
7. Woman	25	1 canine 3 bovine	1 bovine	metronidazole

DISCUSSION AND CONCLUSIONS

The grouping of strains according to their reactions in co-agglutination tests, even with a limited number of reagents, was of value in epidemiological studies, although 74 of the 87 strains studied belonged to only five of the 13 antigenic groups and there was a predominance of group A strains. As an example of the potential value of this serotyping scheme we are able to show that six strains from an unusually large family outbreak of campylobacter enteritis, in which six of the eight family members were affected, were antigenically indistinguishable (unpublished data), and that nine strains from the large suspected waterborne epidemic in central Sweden in 1980 described by Mentzing (p. 278) were also indistinguishable.

Most of the groups were homogenous in relation to the ability to hydrolyse hippurate, a property that has been shown to divide the *C. jejuni* strains into two distinct groups[1].

It is clear from the present study that many strains from cattle, swine, chicken, sheep, and dogs are indistinguishable from those found in human campylobacter enteritis and that it is possible that these animals are, directly or indirectly, sources of human infection.

Acknowledgements

This study was aided by grants from the Sigrid Jusélius Foundation, Helsinki, Finland and the Research Foundation of the Örebro County, Örebro, Sweden. The skillful technical assistance of Mrs Maire Laakso and Tuula Nykänen is gratefully acknowledged.

References

1. Skirrow, M. B. and Benjamin, J. (1980). Differentiation of enteropathogenic campylobacter. *J. Clin. Pathol.*, **33**, 1122
2. Skirrow, M. B. and Benjamin, J. (1980). '1001' Campylobacters: cultural characteristics of intestinal campylobacters from man and animals. *J. Hyg. Camb.*, **85**, 427–42
3. Penner, J. L. and Hennessy, J. N. (1980). Passive haemagglutination technique for serotyping *Campylobacter fetus* subsp. *jejuni* on the basis of soluble heat-stable antigens. *J. Clin. Microbiol.*, **12**, 732–7
4. Kosunen, T. U., Danielsson, D. and Kjellander, J. (1980). Serology of *Campylobacter fetus* ssp. *jejuni* ('Related' campylobacters). *Acta. Pathol. Microbiol. Scand.* (B), **88**, 207–18
5. Skirrow, M. B. (1977). Campylobacter enteritis: a 'new' disease. *Br. Med. J.*, **2**, 9–11
6. Wang, W. L., Blaser, M. and Cravens, J. (1978). Isolation of campylobacter. *Br. Med. J.*, **2**, 57

DISCUSSION

In answer to a question from Dr Skirrow, Dr Kosunen said that he did not know what antigens were involved in the co-agglutination reaction.

17
Biotype characteristics of campylobacter species, with emphasis on strains isolated in North America

R. E. WEAVER, D. G. HOLLIS, G. A. HÉBERT and M. J. BLASER

Centers for Disease Control, Atlanta, Georgia, U.S.A.

Seventy-three strains of *Campylobacter jejuni* (50 from blood or stool cultures from sporadic cases in the U.S.A. and the 23 serotype strains of Penner) were placed in eight biotypes on the basis of three test reactions: hippurate hydrolysis, alkaline phosphatase activity, and deoxyribonuclease (DNAase) activity. The results are shown in Table 1.

Table 1 Division of 73 strains of *C. jejuni* into eight biotypes

Biotype	Hippurate hydrolysis	Alkaline phosphatase	DNAse	No. of strains
1	+	+	+	34
2	+	+	−	18
3	+	−	+	4
4	+	−	−	7
5	−	+	+	4
6	−	+	−	3
7	−	−	+	1
8	−	−	−	2
				73

Sixty-six (88%) of 75 strains of *C. jejuni* isolated in the U.S.A. were found to hydrolyse hippurate. All of the 28 strains of *C. fetus* ssp. *fetus*, three strains of *C. fetus* ssp. *venerealis*, two strains each of *C. sputorum* ssp. *bubulus* and *C. fecalis*, and one strain each of *C. sputorum* ssp. *sputorum* and *C. sputorum* subsp. *mucosalis* were negative. Eighteen (78%) of the 23 Penner serotype strains of *C. jejuni* hydrolysed hippurate.

By the use of gas–liquid chromatography, we examined the cellular fatty acids of the 14 hippurate negative strains of *C. jejuni* [ostensibly *C. coli* – ed.]. In 11 strains, a 19-carbon cyclopropane acid was present, but in three strains it was absent.

Editorial note

Since the workshop took place it has been confirmed that Dr Weaver's and Dr Skirrow's results of hippurate hydrolysis tests on the Penner serotype strains agree. Thus Skirrow and Benjamin's *C. jejuni* biotypes 1 and 2 are represented by Weaver biotypes 1–4 and *C. coli* is represented by Weaver biotypes 5–8. The relationship of the $H_2S(FBP)$ test – which distinguishes Skirrow and Benjamin's *C. jejuni* biotypes 1 and 2 – to the Weaver system has yet to be determined.

DISCUSSION

In answer to Dr Ferguson, Dr Weaver confirmed that the three exceptional hippurate negative strains of '*C. jejuni*' that did not have 19-carbon cyclopropane acid were nalidixic acid sensitive, i.e. they were what Skirrow and Benjamin regard as *C. coli* and not NARTC strains which Curtis (p. 234) found to lack this fatty acid.

Dr Lawson questioned the wisdom of giving equal credence to the results of inductive and non-inductive tests, and as an example he asked whether a hippurate negative strain could be made hippurate positive if pre-grown on hippurate agar. Mr Razi said that he had not been able to convert the hippurate reaction from negative to positive in this way.

In answer to a question as to whether anyone had tested campylobacters in the API–ZYM system, Dr Karmali stated that he had tested about 40 strains of *C. jejuni* and found very little activity; the maximum score in any test was '2' and this was in the alkaline phosphatase test (*Staphylococcus* scored '5'). Mr Lander and Mr Benjamin agreed with Dr Karmali about a general lack of activity in API–ZYM tests.

18
Techniques for phage typing *Campylobacter jejuni*

JOHN H. BRYNER, A. E. RITCHIE and J. W. FOLEY

National Animal Disease Center, P.O. Box 70, Ames, Iowa, U.S.A.

Fletcher and Bertschinger[1] first reported the association of phages in '*Vibrio coli*' in studies on the role of this organism in swine dysentery. They detected '*V. coli*'-active phage in 24% of the infected swine. Morphology of the phages appears to be similar to phages we have obtained from *C. jejuni* isolates from aborted sheep fetuses. Fletcher[2] reported '*V. coli*' phages were not active on *C. fetus* ssp. *venerealis*. Firehammer and Border[3], Ritchie[4] and Bryner et al.[5,6] described phages from *C. fetus* ssp. *venerealis* and ssp. *fetus* and showed that *C. jejuni* strains were not lysed by these phages. Chang and Ogg[7-9] reported transduction of glycine tolerance, streptomycin resistance and serotype conversion mediated by phage in '*V. fetus*'.

In work reported here *C. jejuni* phages were propagated in thioglycollate cross-cultures and detected by modification of the lawn-spot technique of Bryner et al.[5]). The modifications were: incubation at 42 °C rather than 37 °C; replacement of Albimi brucella agar by Mueller Hinton agar; use of log-phase shaker cultures grown for 5 hours at 42 °C and adjusted to an optical density of 0.2 rather than 0.4 for lawn inocula; and induction of phage in lawns of suspect lysogenic strains of *C. jejuni* with discs of mitomycin C (1 µg).

Plaques at the periphery of zones of inhibition were picked to isolate phages (Figure 1).

The protocol for testing phage activity on host lawns and for phage typing *C. jejuni* isolates from various animals is as follows:

(1) Culture strain on Mueller Hinton agar for 24 hours at 42 °C.
(2) Harvest loopful of cells into 5 ml Albimi broth.
(3) Incubate broth for 2 hours at 42 °C.
(4) Inoculate 50 ml Albimi broth with the broth culture.
(5) Shake culture for 2 hours at 42 °C (OD 0.2 at 540 nm).
(6) Mix 0.3 ml of culture into 2.7 ml soft overlay agar (50 °C).
(7) Pour overlay agar onto Mueller Hinton agar.
(8) Spot 0.001 ml phage suspension on host lawn.
(9) Incubate culture for 24 hours at 42 °C.

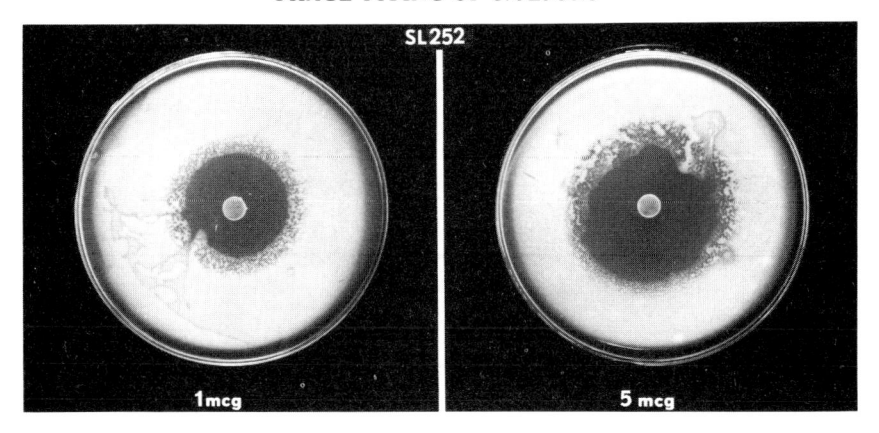

Figure 1 Lawns of *C. jejuni* host strain SL 252 with mitomycin C discs of 1 μg and 5 μg. Phase plaques appear at the periphery of the zones of inhibition, and phages were isolated from them

Figure 2 illustrates the lytic activity of type-C phage on NADC strain 958.

Six type-C phages were isolated from presumed lysogenic strains of *C. jejuni*. Table 1 shows the lytic activity of these phages on 15 *C. jejuni* isolates from aborted sheep fetuses. A phage lysate (M) prepared from a mixture of three pools of *C. jejuni* strains in broth had more lytic activity than any of phages 1–6 alone, a phenomenon that may represent the synergistic or additive effect of multiple phages.

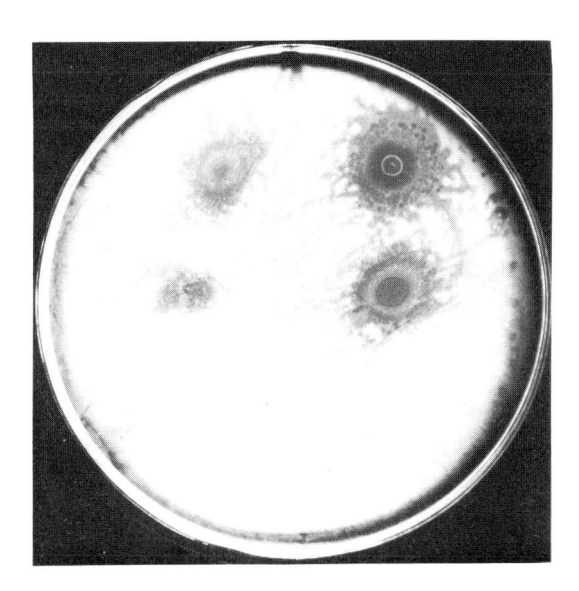

Figure 2 Lawn of *C. jejuni* host strain 958 spotted with type-C phage showing lysis of the lawn around the phage spot

CAMPYLOBACTER: TAXONOMY AND TYPING

Table 1 Lysis of ovine strains of *C. jejuni* by type-C phages. Lytic activity is scored as follows: — = no lysis; 1 = 1–49 plaques; 2 = 50 or more plaques; 3 = partial lysis; 4 = complete lysis

C. jejuni *strain*	\multicolumn{7}{c}{Type-C Bacteriophage}
	1	2	3	4	5	6	M*
495	4	4	4	4	—	—	4
652	—	3	1	1	3	—	1
655	4	3	—	3	—	—	—
657	—	—	4	4	4	4	—
958	4	4	4	4	4	4	4
1114	2	2	2	3	—	3	4
1115	4	3	3	3	2	—	4
1116	—	—	—	—	—	—	4
1117	—	2	—	1	4	1	4
1119	2	2	2	3	3	3	4
1122	2	2	2	1	1	2	2
1217	2	—	1	1	—	—	1
1220	4	—	—	4	—	—	4
1269	4	2	2	4	2	1	4
1272	—	—	—	—	—	—	—

* Phage lysate from pooled strains (see text)

Table 2 shows the lytic activity of type-C phages on *C. jejuni* isolates from seven animal species. Activity was observed in 85% of the sheep isolates and 71% of the human isolates. The number of strains tested from the remaining five species was too small to draw conclusions.

Table 2 Lysis of *C. jejuni* by type-C phages

Source	No. of strains	\multicolumn{4}{c}{No. of strains showing lytic activity}
		None	1–49 plaques	>50 plaques	Complete lysis
Man	49	14	18	10	7
Sheep	15	1	2	1	11
Chicken	8	3	2	1	2
Pig	7	6	0	0	1
Primate	4	0	3	0	1
Dog	2	0	2	0	0
Goat	1	0	0	0	1

It was shown by electron microscopy that type-C phages have a contractile protein sheathed tail with a characteristic fuzzy surface (Figures 3 and 4). They are morphologically distinct from phages of *C. fetus* ssp. *venerealis* which have a long flexuous 'kitetail' (Figure 5).

PHAGE TYPING OF *C. JEJUNI*

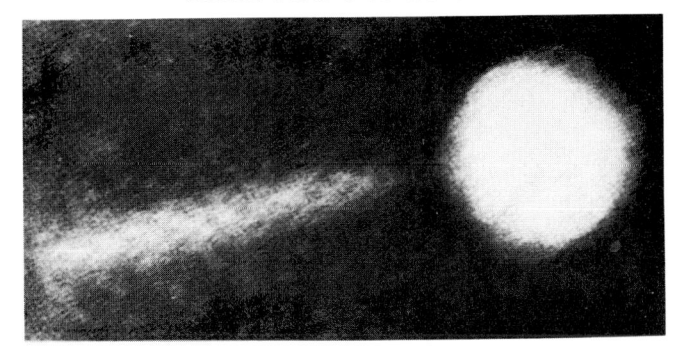

Figure 3 Type-C phage with contractile protein sheath

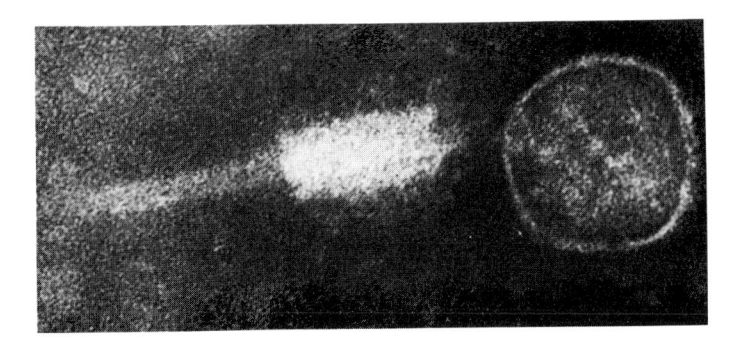

Figure 4 Type-C phage with needle exposed

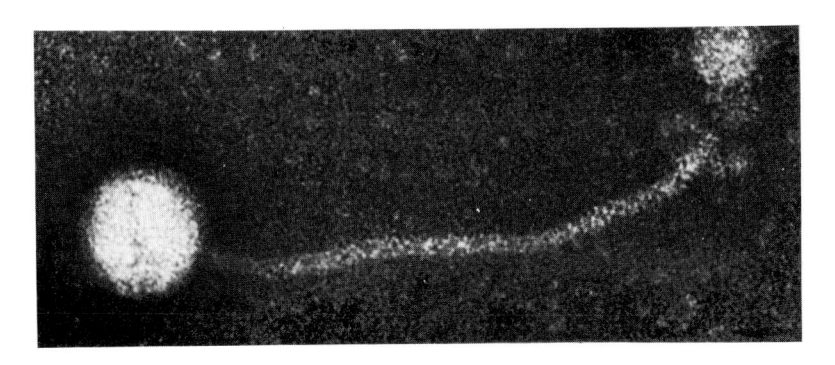

Figure 5 Phage of *C. fetus* ssp. *venerealis* with long flexuous non-sheathed tail

References

1. Fletcher, R. D. and Bertschinger, H. (1964). A method of isolation of *Vibrio coli* from swine fecal material by selective filtration. *Zentralblatt für Veterinaeromed Reiche B.*, **11**, 469–74
2. Fletcher, R. D. (1965). Activity and morphology of *Vibrio coli* phages. *Am. J. Vet. Res.*, **26**, 361–4
3. Firehammer, B. D. and Border, M. (1968). Isolation of temperate bacteriophages from *Vibrio fetus*. *Am. J. Vet. Res.*, **29**, 2229–35
4. Ritchie, A. E. and Bryner, J. H. (1968). A structural element in the envelope system of *Vibrio fetus*. In: Arceneaux, C. J., ed. Proceedings 26th Annual Meeting of Electron Microscopists Society of America, 878–79
5. Bryner, J. H., Ritchie, A. E., Foley, J. W. and Berman, D. T. (1970). Isolation and characterization of bacteriophage for *Vibrio fetus*. *J. Virol.*, **6**, 94–9
6. Bryner, J. H., Ritchie, A. E., Booth, G. D. and Foley, J. W. (1973). Lytic activity of vibrio phages on strains of *Vibrio fetus* isolated from man and animals. *Appl. Microbiol.*, **26**, 404–9
7. Chang, W. and Ogg, J. E. (1970). Transduction of streptomycin resistance in *Vibrio fetus*. *Am. J. Vet. Res.*, **31**, 919–24
8. Chang, W. and Ogg, J. E. (1971). Transduction and mutation to glycine tolerance in *Vibrio fetus*. *Am. J. Vet. Res.*, **32**, 649–53
9. Ogg, J. E. and Chang, W. (1972). Phage conversion of serotypes in *Vibrio fetus*. *Am. J. Vet. Res.*, **33**, 1023–9

19
Anaerobic respiration of fumarate by catalase-positive campylobacter

MICHEL VÉRON and ANNIE LENVOISÉ-FURET

Bacteriology Laboratory, Faculty of Medicine, Necker-Enfants, Malades, Paris

---

The effect of fumarate on the growth of catalase-positive campylobacter strains was compared under aerobic (5% oxygen, 10% carbon dioxide and 85% nitrogen) and anaerobic (10% carbon dioxide and 90% nitrogen) conditions. On Albimi medium (Brucella Broth and Pfizer) growth is much poorer under anaerobic than aerobic conditions and fumarate is inhibitory. Therefore, a semi-synthetic medium was used consisting of a base TGF (inorganic salts and yeast extract, as described by Wolin et al.[1] for the cultivation of *Vibrio succinogenes*) supplemented with sodium thioglycollate (0.05%) and sodium formate (0.25%). In the presence of 1% fumarate, formate enhances growth greatly, except in the case of *C. jejuni* incubated under anaerobic conditions. The maximum growth obtained within 72 hours incubation with plain TGF, and TGF + 1% fumarate, media was measured for nine strains of *C. fetus* ssp. *fetus* (14 tests), two strains of *C. fetus* ssp. *venerealis* (three tests), and 22 strains of *C. jejuni* (33 tests). In the presence of fumarate, the ratio of maximum anaerobic growth over maximum aerobic growth was 1.14 ± 0.28 for *C. fetus* ssp. *fetus*, 1.17 ± 0.09 for *C. fetus* ssp. *venerealis*, and 0.23 ± 0.17 for *C. jejuni*. Therefore, unlike *C. jejuni*, the two *C. fetus* subspecies are able to respire fumarate anaerobically in the above conditions. These results have been substantiated by gas–liquid chromatographic identification of the relevant metabolites.

Reference

1. Wolin, M. J., Wolin, E. A. and Jacobs, N. J. (1961). Cytochrome producing anaerobic *Vibrio succinogenes*. *J. Bacteriol.*, **81**, 911–7

DISCUSSION

Dr Park drew attention to the paper by Razi and Park (p. 59) which reported results similar to those of Professor Véron, namely that the addition of nitrate, aspartate or fumarate does not enable strains of *C. jejuni* to grow anaerobically as they do for the subspecies of *C. fetus*, yet all are capable of reducing nitrate. Dr Hollander (Osnabruck) reported that *C. jejuni* produces menaquinones in the same manner as bacteria capable of respiring nitrate or fumarate. Yet this species is unable to use this electron carrier to transfer electrons to nitrate or fumarate under anaerobic conditions. So these results are in agreement with those of Véron, but the reasons for this anomaly are unknown, and Dr Hollander said he knew of no parallel among other bacteria.

20
Some simple tests for differentiating between campylobacters

M. H. H. RAZI and R. W. A. PARK

Department of Microbiology, University of Reading, London Road, Reading RG1 5AQ

Campylobacters are generally regarded as microaerophilic bacteria but there are reports of anaerobic growth with nitrate, or aspartate, or fumarate. The ability of campylobacters to grow anaerobically in the presence of various substances can readily be assessed by inoculation into semi-solid agar and looking for growth throughout the medium as opposed to growth restricted to near the surface. By the use of this procedure it has been found that, in general, *C. fetus* grows anaerobically in the presence of nitrate, aspartate or fumarate, but *C. jejuni* does not[1]. NARTC strains[2] differ in that they are able to grow anaerobically in the presence of aspartate, fumarate, and also trimethylamine N-oxide[1].

C. fetus strains can be differentiated from *C. jejuni* and NARTC strains by paper strip tests to detect their greater resistance to toluidine blue and methylene blue and their greater sensitivity to azide.

We confirm that the ability to hydrolyse hippurate distinguishes *C. jejuni sensu strictu* from *C. coli* strains.

References
1. Razi, M. H. H., Park, R. W. A. and Skirrow, M. B. (1981). Two new tests for differentiating between strains of campylobacter. *J. Appl. Bacteriol.*, **50**, 55–7
2. Skirrow, M. B. and Benjamin, J. (1980). '1001' Campylobacters: cultural characteristics of intestinal campylobacters from man and animals. *J. Hyg. (Cambridge)*, **85**, 427–2

21
The use of *Pseudomonas aeruginosa* for the typing of thermophilic campylobacters

W. A. TELFER BRUNTON and A. MOYES

University of Edinburgh, Department of Bacteriology, University Medical School, Teviot Place, Edinburgh EH8 9A

We set out to determine whether pyocine producing strains of *Pseudomonas aeruginosa* could be used to type campylobacters. Initial studies involving partially purified extracts made from strains of *Ps. aeruginosa* and known to contain R-type pyocines, indicated that some campylobacters were sensitive to these extracts. As the preparation of partially purified extracts containing R-type pyocines is tedious and time consuming, and their stability is limited, a simpler and more readily acceptable technique was sought.

We report the results of a study examining the application of a pyocine typing method[1] for the typing of campylobacters of human origin. Sixty-nine pyocine producing strains of *Ps. aeruginosa* and 125 campylobacters were examined. Fifty-six of the *Ps. aeruginosa* strains inhibited growth of all campylobacters tested, seven produced no inhibition of any campylobacter, and six strains produced reproducibly different degrees of inhibition with different campylobacters.

In this preliminary study pyocine typing did not distinguish well between strains from different outbreaks and work is in progress to relate pyocine typing to other methods of identifying campylobacters.

Reference

1. Gillies, R. R. and Govan, J. R. W. (1966). Typing of *Pseudomonas pycocyanea*. J. Pathol. Bacteriol., **91**, 339–45

DISCUSSION

Dr Telfer Brunton said that there was good evidence that pyocine attaches to sensitive campylobacters. He had been unable to detect bacteriocine production by campylobacters.

PS. AERUGINOSA IN CAMPYLOBACTER TYPING

Dr Sticht-Groh described how she had tried the classical Abbott method for colicine typing, at various temperatures, but with negative results. She had also induced R-type pyocines with mitomycin C, concentrated the crude extract by ultracentrifugation at 100 000 g, and dissolved it in TRIS buffer. This partically purified extract was then applied to lawns of campylobacters in log-phase growth and although there was some activity, the results had not been reproducible.

22
The characteristics of type and reference cultures of *Campylobacter* species held in the National Collection of Type Cultures (NCTC)

R. J. OWEN and S. LEAPER

National Collection of Type Cultures, Central Public Health Laboratory, London NW9 5HT, U.K.

At present 18 strains of campylobacter are maintained as freeze-dried cultures in the NCTC (Table 1). The first deposition was made in 1939[1]. The cultures now include the strains accorded the status of nomenclatural types in the *Approved Lists of Bacterial Names*[2], and the various strains recommended as biochemical test controls by Skirrow and Benjamin[3].

In the present study, type strains of *C. coli*, *C. jejuni* and *C. fetus*, a reference strain of the nalidixic acid resistant thermophilic group (NARTC), and various 'thermophilic' campylobacters from cases of human enteritis and gull cloacal swabs were characterized by 17 bacteriological tests and by gas–liquid chromatographic analysis of their cellular fatty acids. The tests most useful in species differentiation were: growth at 25 and 42 °C; H_2S production; tolerance to nalidixic acid and 2,3,5-triphenyltetrazolium chloride; and hippurate hydrolysis. Differences between *C. fetus* and the *C. jejuni* group were confirmed by cellular fatty acid compositions[4]. A numerical analysis of the bacteriological results indicated that *C. fetus* and *C. jejuni* were distinct species and that the NARTC strains were intermediate between them but linked to *C. jejuni* at a slightly higher level of similarity. The results support the use of the classification of Véron and Chatelain[5] adopted in the *Approved Lists*. In the future, combination of the bacteriological and fatty acid data might provide the basis for a simple computer assisted probabilistic identification scheme for campylobacters.

Table 1 Campylobacters maintained as freeze-dried cultures in the NCTC (March 1981)

Campylobacter Sebald and Véron 1963

Campylobacter coli (Doyle 1948) Véron and Chatelain 1973

11366	1407 (CIP 7080) ←CIP in 1980 ←A. Florent, Brussels Pig faeces	Type strain
11349	Tan (CIP 7086) ←CIP in 1980 Human blood culture, 1970	
11350	P875 (CIP 715) ←CIP in 1980 ←A. Florent, Brussels in 1971 Pig faeces, 1971	
11353	4620/78 ←M. B. Skirrow in 1980 ←MAFF, Cardiff Pig placenta, 1978	

Campylobacter fetus ss. *fetus* (Smith and Taylor, 1919) Véron and Chatelain, 1973

10842	Mouton 1 (CIP 5396, ATCC 27374) ←R. Chatelain, Paris in 1972 ←R. Vincent Sheep fetus brain	Type strain
	Véron, M. and Chatelain, R. (1973). *Int. J. Syst. Bact.*, **23**, 122–134	
5850	Milton ←T. Dalling, Cambridge in 1939 Contagious abortion, sheep	
10348	192/3 ←R. W. A. Park, Reading in 1962 Vaginal mucus of heifer	
	Park, R. W. A. *et al.* (1962). *Br. Vet. J.* **118**, 411	

Campylobacter fetus ss. *venerealis* (Florent, 1959) Véron and Chatelain, 1973

10354	X/161/5 (ATCC 19438) ←R. W. A. Park, Reading in 1962 Vaginal mucus of heifer	Type strain
	Lawson, J. R. and MacKinnon, D. J. (1952). *Vet. Rec.*, **64**, 763	

Campylobacter jejuni (Jones, Orcutt and Little, 1931) Véron and Chatelain, 1973

11351	Uccle 91 F.B. (CIP 702) ←CIP in 1980 ←A. Florent, Brussels Bovine faeces	Type strain
11322	VPI H840 (ATCC 29428) ←ATCC in 1979 ←N. R. Krieg, VPI Blacksburg ←P. Dekeyser, Brussels Diarrhoeic stool of child, 1972	
11168	5936/77 Lucitt ←M. B. Skirrow, Worcester in 1977 Faeces	Biotype 1
	Butzler, J. P. *et al.* (1973). *J. Pediat.*, **82**, 493 Skirrow, M. B. (1977). *Br. Med. J.*, **ii**, 9	

Table 1

11392	852/79 ←M. B. Skirrow, Worcester in 1980	Biotype 2
10983	McCallum 89067 ←A. M. M. Wilson in 1975 Blood culture	

Campylobacter sputorum ss. *bubulus* (Florent, 1953) Véron and Chatelain, 1973

11367	Wat. (CIP 53103) ←CIP in 1980 ←A. Florent, Brussels Bull sperm	Type strain
	Thouvenot, H. and Florent, A. (1954). *Ann. Inst. Pasteur.*, **88**, 237	
10355	G14 ←R. W. A. Park, Reading in 1962 Semen of normal bull	
	Park, R. W. A. et al. (1962). *Br. Vet. J.*, **118**, 411	

Campylobacter sputorum ss. *mucosalis* (Lawson et al. 1975)

11000	253/72 ←G. H. K. Lawson, Edinburgh in 1975 Porcine small intestine	
	Lawson, G. H. K. et al. (1975). *Res. Vet. Sci.*, **18**, 121	
11001	302/72 ←G. H. K. Lawson, Edinburgh in 1975 Porcine intestinal mucosa	

Campylobacter sp.

11352	3034/77 ←M. B. Skirrow, Worcester in 1980 Cloacal swab of herring gull (*Larus argentatus*), 1976	Nalidixic acid resistant thermophilic group NARTC

References

1. Catalogue of the National Collection of Type Cultures. (1972). HMSO, London
2. Skerman, V. B. D., McGowan, V. and Sneath, P. H. A. (eds.) (1980). Approved Lists of Bacterial Names. *Int. J. Syst. Bacteriol.*, **30**, 225–420
3. Skirrow, M. B. and Benjamin, J. (1980). '1001' Campylobacters: cultural characteristics of intestinal campylobacters from man and animals. *J. Hyg. Camb.*, **85**, 427–42
4. Leaper, S. and Owen, R. J. (1981). Identification of catalase producing campylobacter species based on biochemical characteristics and cellular fatty acid composition. *Curr. Microbiol.*, **6**, 31–35
5. Véron, M. and Chatelain, R. (1973). Taxonomic study of the genus campylobacter Sebald and Véron and designation of the neotype strain for the type species *Campylobacter fetus* (Smith and Taylor) Sebald and Véron. *Int. J. Syst. Bacteriol.*, **23**, 122–34

23
General discussion and editorial comment

(1) DESIGNATION OF TYPE SPECIES FOR THE GENUS CAMPYLOBACTER

Dr Karmali has adequately dealt with this point in his paper (p. 35). By comparing Smith's original data on morphology with his own, he produced evidence to support the adoption of Florent's '*Vibrio fetus intestinalis*' as the type strain (*C. fetus* ssp. *fetus*) by Véron and Chatelain, which in turn was included in the *Approved Lists of Bacterial Names* (*1980*). Thus the approved nomenclature for the subspecies of *C. fetus* is: *C. fetus* ssp. *fetus* and *C. fetus* ssp. *venerealis*. *C. fetus* ssp. *intestinalis* is no longer an acceptable name.

(2) STATUS OF THE THERMOPHILIC CAMPYLOBACTER GROUP

It is considered that since these organisms differ in as many ways from the two subspecies of *C. fetus*, they must constitute a separate species or group of species. The cultural differences originally described by Véron and Chatelain[1] have recently been confirmed by Skirrow and Benjamin[2]. Additional differences in morphology such as size, wavelength and the tendency to coccal transformation (Karmali *et al.* p. 36), bacteriophage morphology and specificity (Bryner *et al.* p. 52), modes of anaerobic respiration (Véron *et al.* p. 57; Razi and Park, p. 59), cellular fatty acid composition, particularly in the possession of C19-cyclopropanic acid (Blaser *et al.*[3]; Johnsson *et al.*, p. 233; Curtis, p. 234; Owen and Leaper, p. 62) and antigenicity, suggest that there are two distinct groups of organisms. Thus it was deemed that the term *C. fetus* ssp. *jejuni* should be abandoned in favour of *C. jejuni* – as in the *Approved Lists of Bacterial Names* (*1980*).

The status of *C. coli* has then to be questioned. Professor Véron explained in the general discussion that the strains studied in his 1973 work[1] came from the Institut Pasteur collection and were already named. His view was that *C. jejuni* and *C. coli* strains were sufficiently similar to be included in a single species. *C. jejuni* was the more appropriate name since there is a difficulty concerning the adoption of Doyle's name '*Vibrio coli*'[4], which was given to strains isolated from pigs suffering from swine dysentery. Doyle stated that *V. coli* did not reduce nitrate, whereas the Institut Pasteur strains designated *C. coli* did so (as do the great majority of 'thermophilic' campylobacters isolated from pigs and other animals). It is possible that Doyle's nitrate reduction tests were at fault, but as none of his strains survive we shall never know. Professor Véron proposed therefore that the name *C. coli* be considered as a *nomen nodum* until someone described the nitrate negative strains that might fit Doyle's description. This opinion was well received and participants were reminded by Dr Karmali that Neill *et al.*[5] had described nitrate negative campylobacters from aborted pig fetuses, although these organisms had other characteristics – such as a maximum growth temperature of 36° C – that placed them apart.

Professor Véron's proposal that the name *C. coli* should be suspended from its present use means that the hippurate negative strains described as *C. coli* by Dr Skirrow (p. 40) might be termed *C. jejuni* biotype 3. To group these organisms under one species (*C. jejuni*) would certainly simplify clinical reporting. However as no results are yet available from DNA hybridization studies, though several laboratories are currently engaged in such studies, these taxonomic decisions should await their results.

While the subject of catalase-negative campylobacters such as *C. sputorum* and certain atypical strains was discussed briefly, almost all of the discussion centred on the catalase-positive species.

Sincere regret was expressed by the Chairmen at the absence of Dr Robert Smibert since it was felt that his experience and knowledge would have been most valuable in the clarification of the nomenclature of the campylobacters.

Summary

The consensus was that the nomenclature for the catalase-positive campylobacters in the *Approved Lists of Bacterial Names* (*1980*) was essentially correct and that it should be generally adhered to, but that the status and nomenclature of *C. coli* is in doubt pending the results of DNA hybridization studies.

References

1. Véron, M. and Chatelain, R. (1973). Taxonomic study of the genus campylobacter (Sebald and Véron) and designation of the neotype strain for the type species *Campylobacter fetus* (Smith and Taylor) Sebald and Véron. *Int. J. Syst. Bacteriol.*, **23**, 122–34
2. Skirrow, M. B. and Benjamin, J. (1980). '1001' Campylobacters: cultural characteristics of intestinal campylobacters from man and animals. *J. Hyg.* (Cambridge), **85**, 427–42
3. Blaser, M. J., Moss, C. W. and Weaver, R. E. (1980). Cellular fatty acid composition of *Campylobacter fetus. J. Clin. Microbiol.*, **11**, 448–51
4. Doyle, L. P. (1948). The etiology of swine dysentery. *Amer. J. Vet. Res.*, **9**, 50–1
5. Neill, S. D., Ellis, W. A. and O'Brien J. J. (1979). Designation of aerotolerant campylobacter-like organisms from porcine and bovine abortions to the genus Campylobacter. *Res. Vet. Sci.*, **27**, 180–6

SECTION III
GROWTH REQUIREMENTS AND CULTURE MEDIA

Chairmen: M. Skirrow ⎫ Growth requirements
M. Véron ⎭

J. Wells ⎫ Discussion group on culture media
K. Lander ⎭

24	The effect of incubation atmosphere and temperature on the isolation of *Campylobacter jejuni* from human stools W. L. Wang, L. B. Reller, M. J. Blaser and N. W. Luechtefeld	69
25	Simplified isolation techniques for *Campylobacter jejuni* M. de Boeck	71
26	Clinical observations on the microaerophilic requirements of campylobacter organisms especially *Campylobacter fetus* ssp. *venerealis* J. M. Carter and P. J. Seamon	73
27	The occurrence of *Campylobacter jejuni* in fresh food and its survival under different conditions B. Kaijser and Å. Svedhem	74
28	A selective medium for isolating *Campylobacter jejuni* F. J. Bolton and L. Robertson	75
29	A selective, enrichment and transport medium for campylobacters K. P. Lander	77
30	A selective enrichment procedure for the isolation of *Campylobacter jejuni* from foods C. E. Park and Z. K. Stankiewicz	79
31	Evaluation of selective media for the isolation of *Campylobacter jejuni* J. G. Wells, C. A. Bopp and M. J. Blaser	80

CAMPYLOBACTER: GROWTH REQUIREMENTS AND CULTURE MEDIA

32 General discussion on culture media   83
33 Editorial discussion   85

24
The effect of incubation atmosphere and temperature on the isolation of *Campylobacter jejuni* from human stools

W. L. WANG, L. B. RELLER, M. J. BLASER and N. W. LUECHTEFELD

VA Medical Center, University of Colorado Health Sciences Center, Denver, CO, U.S.A.

Campylobacter jejuni requires a microaerobic atmosphere for optimum growth. The purpose of this study was to compare growth in 5%, 10% and 15% oxygen, BBL CampyPak II gas generating kit, and candle jar, each at 42 °C and 37 °C. The plating medium used was Campy-BAP.

In a preliminary quantitative study, ten positive human stool samples were cultured in 5%, 10% and 15% oxygen and candle jar. Best growth was obtained in 5% or 10% oxygen at 42 °C.

In a further comparison between CampyPak II, 5% oxygen, and candle jar, with six human isolates, similar rates of recovery were obtained at 42 °C and 37 °C, but larger colonies were observed in the CampyPak II system and in 5% oxygen than in the candle jar; in addition it was found that where CampyPak II was used with 12 plates per jar, colonies were reduced in size compared with their use with six plates per jar. Growth in all three systems, especially the candle jar, was much poorer at 37 °C.

Further studies on 19 positive human stools showed that at 42 °C all three systems gave similar yields of *C. jejuni* (median 10^6 colony forming units/g), but CampyPak II (12 plates) missed two positives and the candle jar missed one. Similarly, colony sizes with CampyPak II (6 plates) were similar to those with 5% oxygen but larger than with CampyPak II (12 plates) ($p = <0.05$) or candle jar ($p = <0.005$). (Wilcoxson sign-rank test for matched pairs.) At 37 °C all three systems gave similar median colony counts, but CampyPak II (12 plates) missed one of 16 positive samples and the candle jar missed four. Colony sizes in the candle jar were smaller than those from CampyPak II (6 plates) ($p = <0.006$) or 5% oxygen ($p = <0.003$).

We conclude that CampyPak II (6 plates per jar), 5% and 10% oxygen at 42 °C are most satisfactory for culturing *C. jejuni* from human stools.

Editorial note
In her presentation Dr Wang stated that the actual oxygen concentrations were measured and they were as follows: '5%' was 7.5%, '10%' was 12.6%, '15%' was 16.1%, and the candle jar was 17.2%. The method used to obtain reduced oxygen concentrations was to evacuate a jar to a predetermined pressure and refill with a 90% nitrogen/10% carbon dioxide mixture.

References

1. Skirrow, M. B., Benjamin, J., Razi, M. H. H. and Waterman, S. Isolation, cultivation, and identification of *Campylobacter jejuni* and *C. coli. J. Appl. Bacteriol.* (in press)
2. Ware, D. A., Colley, P. J. and Park, R. W. A. (1977). Oxygen requirement and sensitivity of *Campylobacter* spp. *Proceed. Soc. Microbiol.*, **5**, 19

DISCUSSION

Dr Park pointed out that, for campylobacters, almost anaerobic conditions were best for the initiation of growth, but once growth had begun they needed more oxygen; this had been shown by Skirrow *et al*[1]. Dr Park also referred to work by Ware *et al.*[2] which showed that in continuous cultures oxygen concentrations above 12–13% inhibited growth. But it was agreed that under clinical conditions the sequential use of two gas mixtures was impracticable and that one had to strike a balance. Yet Dr Park's point was a valid one when reasons for culture failure were considered. For example the failures of the CampyPak-12 plates system presumably resulted from lack of oxygen, because the volume of gas in the jar was too small for the amount of hydrogen generated. In this case the campylobacters were probably beginning to grow but the colonies were too small to see; further incubation might have yielded growth. In contrast, the failures of the candle jar system probably resulted in death of the organisms through too high oxygen concentrations. Dr Blaser pointed out that CampyPaks were designed to work in a specific volume of air and that they had to be used correctly if they were to perform well.

25
Simplified isolation techniques for *Campylobacter jejuni*

M. DE BOECK

Microbiology Department, St. Pieters Hospital, Brussels

Two simple methods for reducing oxygen tension in the culture atmosphere were compared with our normal incubator atmosphere of 6% oxygen, 6% carbon dioxide and 88% nitrogen. The first utilized the Fortner principle as used by Karmali and Fleming[1]: four campylobacter culture plates were sealed in a plastic bag together with a fifth blood agar plate inoculated with a proteus strain. The second method utilized a candle jar (BBL). Butzler's selective medium[2] (15 g/l agar) was used in each system both with and without FBP supplement (Oxoid).

All cultures were incubated at 42 °C. The results of culturing faeces samples from 516 human patients and 100 chickens are shown in Table 1. In a second study only the candle jar system with the FBP supplemented medium was compared with the standard incubator conditions (Table 1). Failure to isolate *C. jejuni* in one or the other system was always associated with samples yielding only a few colonies.

It is concluded that the candle jar method is a reliable and easy method for the isolation of *C. jejuni* provided supplemented selective medium is used.

References

1. Karmali, M. A. and Fleming, P. C. (1979). Application of the Fortner principle to isolation of campylobacter from stools. *J. Clin. Microbiol.*, **10**, 245–7
2. Lauwers, S., De Boeck, M. and Butzler, J. P. (1978). Campylobacter enteritis in Brussels. *Lancet*, **1**, 604–5

Questions and comments
Dr Van Landuyt (Bruges) reported preliminary results with a commercially available medium (Oxoid) containing the antimicrobials used in Butzler's medium, but with a Columbia agar base (1% agar) and FBP supplement. It performed as well as Butzler's medium in 5% oxygen and in a candle jar at 42 °C, but less well (74% of positive samples detected) in a candle jar at 37 °C (Butzler's medium was not tested at 37 °C).

Editorial note
A further discussion on the use of candle jars is reported in an account of the Media Session (p. 83).

Table 1 Results of parallel cultures in three atmospheric systems with plain and FBP supplemented medium

	Origin of stools	No. of samples	Butzler medium			Butzler medium + FBP	
			Incubator (6% O_2)	Plastic bag (Fortner)	Candle jar	Plastic bag (Fortner)	Candle jar
1st study	Human patients	516	32 (6.2)	29 (5.6)	30 (5.8)	30 (5.8)	30 (5.8)
	chickens	100	93	86	91	95	96
2nd study	Human patients	2194	159 (7.2)	NT	NT	NT	156 (7.1)

Figures in parentheses indicate percentages. NT = not tested

26
Clinical observations on the microaerophilic requirements of campylobacter organisms especially *Campylobacter fetus* ssp. *venerealis*

J. M. CARTER and P. J. SEAMON

Veterinary Investigation Centre, Sutton Bonington, Loughborough, Leicester, U.K.

In this laboratory the isolation rate of campylobacters, in particular *Campylobacter fetus* ssp. *venerealis*, decreased after the introduction of controlled environment incubators. The growth rates of ten campylobacter strains were found to be better in jars containing 6% oxygen, 10% carbon dioxide and 84% nitrogen than in the controlled incubators (10% carbon dioxide in air). Differences were most pronounced with strains of *C. fetus* ssp. *venerealis*.

It was observed that some strains of *C. fetus* ssp. *venerealis* failed to grow on either Skirrow's or Butzler's selective agar. Such strains were found to be sensitive to polymyxin B sulphate and cephazolin sodium at the concentrations used in these media. The culture of clinical material for *C. fetus* ssp. *venerealis* should therefore include culture on a non-inhibitory medium after filtration through a 0.65 µm membrane filter. For optimum results plates should be incubated in an atmosphere containing oxygen at a concentration near to 6%.

27
The occurrence of *Campylobacter jejuni* in fresh food and its survival under different conditions

B. KAIJSER and Å. SVEDHEM

Department of Clinical Bacteriology, Institute of Medical Microbiology, University of Göteborg, Göteborg, Sweden

---

The present investigation was undertaken to study the occurrence of campylobacter in fresh foods and the survival of the bacteria under different conditions. *C. jejuni* was found in 60% of chickens analysed. These had been purchased in foodstores and prepared for consumption. Campylobacter was also found in all of the samples of minced meat (mainly pork) that were tested. The bacteria remained viable in the food for at least 1 week when stored at about 4°C, and there was 80% survival in chickens frozen for 3 months.

Studies on heat sensitivity were performed on 13 strains: none survived 60°C for more than 15 minutes and most were killed by less heat.

The results showed that domestic animals are the most probable origin of human diarrhoea caused by *C. jejuni*. The bacteria can survive for several days in food products from animals, but they are killed by moderate heat.

28
A selective medium for isolating *Campylobacter jejuni*

F. J. BOLTON and L. ROBERTSON

Public Health Laboratory, Royal Infirmary, Meadow Street, Preston, U.K.

The Preston medium described in this paper shows a high degree of selectivity and has been successfully used for the isolation of *C. jejuni* from environmental specimens, and human, animal and avian faeces.

The Blood Agar Base No. 2 (Oxoid CM 271), used in Skirrow's medium, contains yeast extract, which we found greatly reduced trimethoprim activity despite the addition of lysed horse blood. This was presumed to account for the high level of contamination on Skirrow's medium. Therefore a nutrient base that contained fewer trimethoprim antagonists was adopted for the Preston medium. Also, rifampicin proved to be more successful than vancomycin and less expensive than bacitracin for the inhibition of *Bacillus* spp. that swarm on culture media and are common contaminants of abattoir and cattle specimens.

The Preston medium formula is as follows: Nutrient Broth No. 2 (Oxoid CM67) containing 1.2% New Zealand agar, 5% saponin lysed horse blood, 5000 iu/l polymyxin B, 10 mg/l rifampicin, 10 mg/l trimethoprim and 100 mg/l actidione.

This medium, when compared with Skirrow's, proved to be more selective and is more successful for the isolation of campylobacters from environmental, animal, poultry and human sources. The FBP supplement of George et al.[1] was found to improve qualitative growth of *Campylobacter* spp. on primary isolation.

When made up in the form of a broth (i.e. without agar) this medium was used successfully as an 'enrichment' medium. It gave a greater isolation rate for all types of specimen examined and it proved to be essential for non-human specimens, which may contain few campylobacters.

The results of an abattoir and butchers shop survey indicated that *Campylobacter* spp. are common organisms in the abattoir environment but that butchered meat is not a likely source of human infection. A detailed assessment of these media has been reported elsewhere[2].

References

1. George, H. A., Hoffman, P. S., Smibert, R. M. and Krieg, N. R. (1978). Improved media for growth and aerotolerance of *Campylobacter fetus*. *J. Clin. Microbiol.*, **8**, 36–41
2. Bolton, F. J. and Robertson, L. A selective medium for isolating *Campylobacter jejuni/coli*. *J. Clin. Path.*, (in press)

29
A selective, enrichment and transport medium for campylobacters

K. P. LANDER

Ministry of Agriculture, Fisheries & Food, Central Veterinary Laboratory, New Haw, Weybridge, Surrey KT15 3NB, U.K.

Various aspects of a new selective, enrichment and transport medium for catalase-positive campylobacters are described.

Method of use: the inoculated medium is incubated according to the species of campylobacter expected (37 °C or 42 °C for 2 or 3 days) and then subcultured on a selective and non-selective agar plates which are incubated in microaerobic conditions (approximately 7% oxygen, 10% carbon dioxide and 83% nitrogen).

The medium has been in use for 18 months and the following properties have been investigated:

(1) *Transport:* the medium has been shown to maintain the viability of campylobacters in both pure and contaminated milieux at room temperature for up to 7 days before incubation.

(2) *Selectivity:* many successful isolations have been made from contaminated sources such as bovine preputial washings and bovine, feline, canine, avian and simian faeces.

(3) *Sensitivity:* campylobacters have been isolated in large numbers from initial inocula of six organisms of *C. jejuni* (suspended in bovine faeces), 25 of *C. fetus* ssp. *fetus* (in bovine faeces) and 25 of *C. fetus* ssp. *venerealis* (in bovine preputial washings).

(4) *Shelf life:* media stored at room temperature in the dark for up to 90 days have shown no deterioration in properties.

The medium does not require a microaerobic atmosphere for incubation. As a liquid it can be subjected to a wide range of laboratory procedures, for example, centrifugation (for immunofluorescence) and filtration (for further selectivity).

Formula
Veal Infusion Broth (DIFCO Laboratories) containing:

Lysed horse blood	7%
Bacteriological charcoal (Oxoid, Ltd)	0.5%
Vancomycin	40 mg/l
Trimethoprim	10 mg/l
Polymyxin B	50 000 iu/l
Actidione	100 mg/l
5-Fluorouracil	100 mg/l

The Veal Infusion Broth and charcoal are made up and autoclaved at 120 °C for 15 minutes. After cooling, the other ingredients (sterile) are added aseptically. The medium can be dispensed in 5 ml volumes in $\frac{1}{4}$ oz Bijou bottles, or 10 ml in $\frac{1}{2}$ oz McCartney bottles.

30
A selective enrichment procedure for the isolation of *Campylobacter jejuni* from foods

C. E. PARK and Z. K. STANKIEWICZ

Microbiology Research Division, Bureau of Microbial Hazards, Food Directorate, Health Protection Branch, Health and Welfare Canada, Ottawa, Canada K1A OL2

A new enrichment system has been developed for the isolation of small numbers of campylobacters in foods in the presence of large numbers of other contaminating bacteria.

About 1 kg of food was massaged with 250 ml of nutrient broth in a plastic bag and the contents filtered through a double layer of cheese cloth. The filtrate was centrifuged at 16 300 g for 15 minutes and the resulting sediment suspended in 100 ml of enrichment broth: Brucella Broth buffered with 0.1 M TRIS at pH 8.3 and containing vancomycin (8 mg/l), trimethoprim (4 mg/l), cephalothin (30 mg/l), colistin (3 mg/l), $FeSO_4 \cdot 7H_2O$ (0.2%), sodium metabisulphite (0.025%), sodium pyruvate (0.05%) and calf serum (3%). Incubation was at 42 °C for 1–2 days under reduced oxygen tension which was obtained by one of three methods: (i) replacing the air of an anaerobic jar with mixed gases (5% O_2, 10% CO_2 and 85% N_2); (ii) maintaining a constant flow of the same gas mixture into the broth culture at a rate of 5–10 ml/min; and (iii) evacuating two-thirds of the air and replacing with CO_2. The enrichment culture (5–10 ml) was then filtered through a membrane filter (0.65 μm) and the filtrate plated in parallel on Skirrow's agar and on Skirrow's agar supplemented with a ten-fold concentration of polymyxin B.

Maximum recovery was obtained under conditions of continuous flow of the mixed gases through the enrichment medium. For optimum recovery both Skirrow's agar and modified Skirrow's agar had to be used. The system recovered as few as one organism in 10 g in the presence of 10^4–10^6 competitors per gram.

31
Evaluation of selective media for the isolation of *Campylobacter jejuni*

J. G. WELLS, C. A. BOPP and M. J. BLASER

Centers for Disease Control, Atlanta, Georgia, U.S.A.

Three selective plating media, Skirrow's medium[1], Butzler's medium[2] and Campy-BAP[3], are the plating media most widely used today for isolation of *Campylobacter jejuni*. Patton *et al.* have developed a fourth selective medium, BU40, which is a modification of Butzler's medium in which the level of colistin is increased[4]. The purpose of this study was to evaluate the efficiency of these media for isolating *C. jejuni* from human faecal specimens. It was conducted in conjunction with a continuing one-year study to determine the frequency and the clinical and epidemiologic characteristics of campylobacter infection in eight hospitals in different parts of the United States. Two separate comparative studies were done.

In the first study, faecal specimens from 1391 patients were examined at six hospital laboratories. The primary specimens, either stools or rectal swabs, were cultured on three plating media: Skirrow's medium (Blood Agar Base No. 2 (Oxoid), 7% lysed horse blood, 10 mg/l vancomycin, 2500 iu/l polymyxin B and 5 mg/l trimethoprim); Butzler's medium (fluid thioglycollate medium (Difco), 3% agar (Difco), 10% sheep blood, 2500 iu/l bacitracin, 5 mg/l novobiocin, 10 000 iu/l colistin, 15 mg/l cephalothin and 50 mg/l Actidione); and Campy-BAP (Brucella Agar Base (BBL), 10% sheep blood, 10 mg/l vancomycin, 5 mg/l trimethoprim, 2500 iu/l polymyxin B, 15 mg/l cephalothin and 2 mg/l amphotericin B). All plates were incubated at 42°C in atmosphere of 5% oxygen, 10% carbon dioxide and 85% nitrogen. Plates were examined after 48 hours incubation and all isolates were identified by standard procedures. Isolation rates were highest with Campy-BAP followed by Skirrow's and Butzler's medium (Table 1). The differences were statistically significant between Campy-BAP and Skirrow's ($p < 0.05$), Skirrow's and Butzler's ($p < 0.001$) and Campy-BAP and Butzler's ($p < 0.001$) media.

In the second study, faecal specimens from 592 patients obtained by two hospital laboratories were sent to the CDC laboratory for analysis. Swabs coated with faeces were transported in Cary–Blair medium at 4°C, and the interval between the time of collection and examination of specimens ranged

Table 1 Performance of plating media in relation to testing laboratory and period of incubation

Agar medium	Number of C. jejuni isolation (%)		
	Hospital laboratories	CDC laboratory 48 h	CDC laboratory 24, 48 and 72 h
Skirrow	80 (78)	36 (80)	38 (84)
Campy-BAP	93 (90)	39 (87)	40 (89)
Butzler	58 (56)	30 (67)	35 (78)
All three media	103 (100)	45 (100)	45 (100)

from 3–11 days. Transported specimens were inoculated on to four plating media: Skirrow's, Campy-BAP, Butzler's and BU40 (Butzler's medium with colistin increased from 10 000 to 40 000 units per litre). Plates were examined after 24, 48 and 72 hours. The results are also shown in Table 1 and although the same trend was observed, in that more isolations were obtained on Campy-BAP than the other three media, the differences were not statistically significant. Thus the performances of the three media were more similar when used at the CDC laboratory than at the hospital laboratories.

The differences in technique which largely accounted for these results was that the plates at the hospital laboratories were read only at 48 hours, whereas the plates at CDC were examined at 24, 48 and 72 hours. If only the 48-hour plate readings performed at CDC are included in the analysis, the results are much nearer to those of the hospital laboratories (Table 1). Thus for optimum results plates should be read at all three time intervals, but if plates can be read only at 48 hours Campy-BAP would be the medium of choice.

Higher isolation rates were obtained by the use of more than one plating medium (Table 2). Combinations of Campy-BAP and Skirrow's, or Skirrow's

Table 2 Comparison of four plating media used alone or in combination for the isolation of C. jejuni

Agar medium	No. positive	Percentage* positive
Campy-BAP	40	89
Skirrow	38	84
BU40	36	80
Butzler	35	78
Skirrow + Campy-BAP	44	98
Skirrow + BU40	44	98
Campy-BAP + BU40	42	93
Campy-BAP + Butzler	41	91
Skirrow + Butzler	41	91
Butzler + BU40	41	91
Skirrow + Campy-BAP + Butzler	45	100

* Percentage of total number positive on all media examined

and BU40 media detected 98% of the positive specimens, 9% more than the figure for the best single plating medium (Campy-BAP).

Unlike Patton *et al.*, who found BU40 to be superior to Butzler's and Skirrow's media, we did not find this to be the case. We found Butzler's and BU40 media to be similar in performance and both inferior to Skirrow's. Patton's work, however, was with faecal specimens from both ill and well dogs and cats, whereas our specimens were from ill people. Human and animal strains may differ in antibiotic susceptibilities and thus be more likely to be isolated on one plating medium than another; or proportionally more competing organisms may be present in animal specimens, for which a more selective medium such as Butzler's or BU40 might be more effective. Thus the optimal medium probably depends on the type of specimen to be examined.

In our experience of reading these plates we found Campy-BAP to be easier to read than Skirrow's or Butzler's media. There were more contaminating organisms on Skirrow's medium and although we could ultimately isolate the organism, the presence of competitors made isolation more difficult. Butzler's medium was much more inhibitory and although there were fewer competitors on the plate, the colonies were frequently more difficult to see because of their small size (but see discussion below about agar concentration – ed.).

To summarize, plates should ideally be read at 24, 48 and 72 hours, but if plates can only be read once, 48 hours would be the time of choice. The four media in this study (Skirrow's, Campy-BAP, Butzler's and BU40) are comparable in performance provided they are examined at all three time intervals, but for maximum sensitivity more than one type of selective medium must be used.

References

1. Skirrow, M. B. (1977). Campylobacter enteritis: a 'new' disease. *Br. Med. J.*, **2**, 9–11
2. Lauwers, S., De Boeck, M. and Butzler, J. P. (1978). Campylobacter enteritis in Brussels. *Lancet*, **(i)**, 604–5
3. Blaser, M. J., Berkowitz, I. D., LaForce, F. M., Cravens, J., Reller, L. B. and Wang, W. L. (1979). Campylobacter enteritis: Clinical and epidemiologic features. *Ann. Intern. Med.*, **91**, 179–85
4. Patton, C. M., Mitchell, S. W., Potter, M. E. and Kaufmann, A. F. (1981). Comparison of selective media for primary isolation of *Campylobacter fetus* subsp. *jejuni*. *J. Clin. Microbiol.*, **13**, 326–30

32
General discussion on culture media

Professor Butzler suggested that the smaller colonies seen by Mrs Wells on Butzler's medium could be explained by the high level (3%) of agar used. He said that since reducing the agar concentration to 1.5% he did not have a problem with small colonies. He also recommended that Butzler's medium should be read after 48 hours incubation.

Dr N. Luechtefeld and others had obtained better results from animal specimens by using a more inhibitory medium such as Butzler's, particularly when such media contained a fungistat or a fungicide such as cycloheximide or amphotericin B. Dr Sutton thought that media containing antifungals might be more effective in vegetarian communities. Some workers replaced the brucella agar in Campy-BAP with tryptose agar and reported better results.

Dr Oosterom obtained good results with a broth medium containing the antibiotics found in Skirrow's medium but with the addition of cycloheximide and ox-bile (1.5%). He recommended that for better standardization a compound such as lauryl sulphate could be used in place of ox-bile.

Professor Bokkenheuser obtained 10–15% more isolations by the use of a double filtration technique rather than selective media. His method employed prefilters of pore size 8.0 μm and 1.2 μm connected to a 0.65 μm filter. The plating medium was chocolate agar.

Dr Prescott suggested the use of a technique whereby the sample was simply placed on top of a 0.45 μm membrane filter lying on an agar plate. This was incubated overnight, the filter and sample removed, and the growth underneath streaked out. Dr Pearson had used a similar technique successfully for water samples.

Mr Bolton replaced the vancomycin in Skirrow's medium with rifampicin and added cycloheximide. He used this formulation in the form of broth and agar media and reported that he obtained better inhibition of contaminants, particularly *Bacillus* species (see p. 75).

Mr Bolton and Mrs Wells both suggested that the thymidine content of rich media was such that the 7% lysed horse blood would not be able to antagonize it, and that the trimethoprim would thus be prevented from exerting its full action. But Professor Butzler said that without lysed horse blood Skirrow's medium failed to control *Proteus* species.

Mr Bolton and others questioned the need for blood as a growth stimulant for campylobacters and suggested that its concentration could be reduced to as low as 1% or it could be replaced by blood components such as haematin.

Regarding the use of candle jars, Dr Wang said that their use for the incubation of plates from clinical samples gave a slightly lower isolation rate than conventional microaerobic incubation. Dr Leuchtefeld cited the work of colleagues who had achieved equally good isolation rates with candle jars but she added that specimens transported in Cary–Blair transport medium were often cultured less successfully in candle jars and suggested that this might be due either to smaller numbers of campylobacters surviving the transport or to the survivors being less hardy than in fresh specimens. This may mean that growth is initiated less easily in candle jars than in conventional systems. The Belgian workers recommended the use of FBP supplement if plates are to be incubated in candle jars. Several people emphasized that candle jars incubated at 42 °C gave significantly better results than those incubated at 37 °C. (It is difficult to standardize the preparation of candle jars. The differences in results reported here may be explained by differences in preparation of the jars – ed.)

Dr Fleming said that polymyxin was less active at 42 °C than at 37 °C.

In discussions on the isolation of *C. fetus* ssp. *venerealis* Dr Stovell reported very good results using the transport and enrichment medium of Clark (an Australian medium based on coagulated serum with the addition of brilliant green, bacitracin, polymyxin, cycloheximide and 5-fluorouracil). Dr Bryner has developed a transport and enrichment medium based on the Blacksburg Anaerobic Meat medium with added polymyxin, cycloheximide, 5-fluorouracil, cystein hydrochloride and brilliant green. This is a broth medium which is easy to prepare and use and it has a long shelf-life. It was suggested that both of these should be assessed for the ability to isolate *C. jejuni*.

Mrs Wells and Professor Butzler suggested that the main requirements for developing new isolation methods were:

(1) Non-antibiotic based selective media.
(2) Broth enrichment media.
(3) Cheaper media.
(4) Cheaper incubation techniques.

The last two would be of particular value in developing countries.

33
Editorial discussion

For completeness the workshop presentations on growth conditions have been grouped with a discussion-group session organized on culture media. It was apparent from these presentations, and the discussion which followed, that the major cultural requirements for the isolation of campylobacters from a variety of clinical and environmental sources are (i) selectivity of the campylobacters, concomitant with inhibition of contaminants, and (ii) sensitivity to allow the culture of very low numbers of organisms.

Several media formulations are now available as selective media containing a variety of antibiotics to suppress contamination and the relative efficiency of some of these media have been the subject of several recent publications. Nonetheless, choice of media still appears to be quite subjective. Unfortunately the sensitivity of campylobacter species to many of the antibiotics is variable, i.e. cephalothin may inhibit *C. fetus* ssp. *fetus* (Taylor, Pathogenesis, p. 163) whilst polymyxin B sulphate and cephazolin sodium are apparently inhibitory to *C. fetus* ssp. *venerealis* (Carter *et al.*, Growth conditions and media, p. 73). As these differential sensitivities may account for some of the reported differences in isolation rates from animals, selective culture techniques independent of antibiotics should be developed. Few practical suggestions are however available. Filtration techniques may be suitable but these may also be selective, i.e. against *C. fetus* ssp. *fetus* (Firehammer *et al.*, Pathogenesis, p. 168). In the meantime additional antibiotics and/or antifungal agents may be relevant in particular cases like animal faeces or for use in vegetarian populations.

Purification of isolates may provide problems in samples with high levels of contamination and higher concentrations of agar, although producing smaller colonies, allow easier isolation by restricting campylobacter mobility.

Sensitivity is undoubtedly the larger problem. The very low numbers of campylobacters contaminating food and water indicate a need for concentration techniques such as enrichment media, several of which have been described and evaluated (Lander, Growth conditions and media, p. 77 and Park and Stankiewicz, Growth conditions and media, p. 79).

The sensitivity of the isolation techniques for human faecal specimens improves with the freshness of the specimen, reading the plates at 24, 48 and 72 hours, the use of two or more media and the correct microaerophilic conditions. As the initiation of campylobacter growth appears to require near anaerobic conditions whilst maintenance of growth is dependent on microaerophilic conditions, such demanding conditions probably account for the difficulties in isolating campylobacters encountered in underdeveloped countries (Yakubu *et al*. Geographical epidemiology, p. 30). The requirement for easier and cheaper incubation techniques is obvious and perhaps combinations of improved media and simple candle jars will provide the answer.

SECTION IV
SEROLOGY AND SEROTYPING

Chairmen: B. D. Firehammer and J. Davies

34	Development of a scheme for serotyping *Campylobacter jejuni* J. L. Penner, J. N. Hennessy and M. M. Goodbody	89
35	A serotyping scheme for *Campylobacter jejuni* H. Lior, J. A. Edgar and D. L. Woodward	92
36	Serotyping of *C. jejuni*: A useful tool in the epidemiology of campylobacter diarrhoea S. Lauwers	96
37	Provisional antigenic scheme for *Campylobacter jejuni* M. Rogol, I. Sechter, I. Braunstein and Ch. B. Gerichter	98
38	Serotyping of *Campylobacter jejuni* J. D. Abbott, J. Eldridge, D. M. Jones and E. M. Sutcliffe	104
39	Serological typing of thermophilic campylobacter isolates in Tokyo T. Itoh, K. Saito, Y. Yanagawa, S. Sakai and M. Ohashi	106
40	Some serological aspects of the diagnosis of campylobacter infections K. C. Watson and E. J. C. Kerr	111
41	Serology of *Campylobacter jejuni* by tube agglutination and fluorescent antibody methods D. W. Lambe and D. A. Ferguson	113
42	Technique for serotyping *Campylobacter jejuni* J. H. Bryner, A. E. Ritchie and J. W. Foley	117
43	Serological diagnosis of *Campylobacter jejuni* infections by using the enzyme-linked immunosorbent assay principle A. Svedhem, H. Gunnarsson and R. Kaijser	118

CAMPYLOBACTER: SEROLOGY AND SEROTYPING

44 General discussion and editorial comment 122

45 Report of a round table discussion on antigen typing 124

34
Development of a scheme for serotyping *Campylobacter jejuni*

J. L. PENNER, J. N. HENNESSY and M. M. GOODBODY

University of Toronto, Ontario, Canada

We elected to use the passive haemagglutination (PHA) technique (indirect haemagglutination) for titrating antisera because of the advantages it offered over the tube agglutination (tube dilution) technique. Furthermore, some assurance of success was promised as the work of earlier investigators on closely-related *C. fetus* ssp. *fetus* indicated that the bacteria possessed somatic (O) antigens that could be extracted by well-known procedures and that antisera directed against them could be titrated by PHA[1,3,4,6–8].

Titration of antisera by PHA requires soluble antigens that are capable of modifying mammalian erythrocytes to make them agglutinable in antisera containing antibodies directed against the antigens. Antigens that are readily extractable from gram-negative bacteria and have this homosensitizing property for untreated erythrocytes belong, for the most part, to the class known as the somatic (O) antigens. It should be pointed out that Naess and Hofstad (Molecular Biology, p. 242) described phenol-water extracted lipopolysaccharide from *C. jejuni* that sensitized sheep erythrocytes causing them to become agglutinable in homologous, but not in heterologous, antisera. Although some capsular (K) antigens such as the Vi antigen of salmonella also sensitize erythrocytes, they are generally few in number among the strains of a species and, in many cases, are readily differentiated from O antigens by their lack of stability under rigorous heat treatment (120 °C for 1 hour). Therefore, one distinct advantage of PHA over tube agglutination or slide agglutination is that the phenomenon of O-agglutination inhibition caused by the interference of the superficial K antigens in bacterial suspensions is circumvented.

Because extracted antigens are used in PHA, the problem of auto-agglutinability is avoided. In some strains of *C. jejuni*, apparent auto-agglutinability has been ascribed to release from the cells of nucleic acids (Lior *et al.*, Serology, p. 92; and Bryner *et al.*, Serology, p. 117).

In most systems, for serotyping bacteria, there occur reactions known as unilateral, non-reciprocal, one-way or one-sided crosses. Their occurrence in schemes derived from tube agglutination are difficult to explain. With PHA, such unilateral reactions point to mechanisms that can be accounted for on a molecular basis. A hapten (or antigenic determinant) may be covalently linked on some strains or it may not be covalently bound to a carrier but may be more loosely attached, perhaps through hydrophobic bonding, and thus be non-immunogenic on other strains. Antibodies elicited by the former and the lack of stimulation of antibody production by the latter can account, at least in some cases, for the occurrence of unilateral reactions. Another advantage of PHA is that the extracted antigens can also be examined by other immunological techniques such as immunodiffusion, immunoelectrophoresis and polyacrylamide gel electrophoresis to explore further the basis for these complex reactions.

PHA titres are higher than tube agglutination titres and this allows for a more precise definition of the O specificities. Titrations by PHA are readily automated and microtitre plates may be used. Thus, larger numbers of titrations per technologist per day can be performed and smaller volumes of antisera are needed than would be required for titrations by the tube agglutination procedure.

In assembling a set of antisera for the primary purpose of O-serotyping, it is essential that the antisera are selected so that each identifies O-specificity not identified by other antisera of the set. To accomplish this, antisera against selected *C. jejuni* strains were included as typing antisera if they had no reciprocal cross-reactions with previously-defined serotypes. An antiserum included according to this condition may, at a later time, be classified as an O grouping antiserum if the specificity it defines is subsequently shown to be an antigenic complex composed of two or more O factors. In an earlier report, 21 of 23 antisera were selected in this way but two antisera, against serotypes 13 and 16 that were related by reciprocal cross-reactions to a third (serotype 4), were also included because they differentiated among strains that were being frequently isolated[5]. Currently, serotyping is accomplished on the basis of 36 antisera, each of which has been provisionally assigned a number.

A total of 609 *C. jejuni* isolates from human, animal and environmental sources have been serotyped. It was found that isolates generally react in only one antiserum but some react in two or more antisera. The distribution of the isolates according to serotype is shown in Table 1. Serotypes 1, 2 and 4 were the most common and included, respectively, 12.1%, 14.4% and 12.4% of the isolates. Forty-two isolates (6.9%) were untypable and will be examined for new serotypes. Since the 609 isolates include a number that are duplicates of strains obtained from epidemiologically-linked cases, the percentage distribution presented in Table 1 is an approximation. The degree to which it reflects the distribution in nature must await the examination of more isolates.

Before a scheme becomes widely adopted for routine typing it should be demonstrated that its application provides not only effective discrimination among strains of the same species, but also that it identifies linked strains from outbreaks or cross-infections as belonging to the same serotype. To test the latter aspect, isolates were requested from different outbreaks. These were sent to our laboratories along with isolates unrelated to the outbreaks so that the serotyping of the isolates was a blind study. The results showed that the linked

Table 1 Distribution of serotypes among 609 *C. jejuni* isolates

Serotype	No. of isolates	%
2	88	14.4
4	76	12.4
1	74	12.1
3	47	7.7
8	45	7.4
13, 16	41	6.7
13	4	0.7
16	6	1.0
5	36	6.0
23	24	4.0
18	21	3.0
21	12	2.0
7	8	1.3
11	8	1.3
31	8	1.3 (81.3)
Multiple agglutinable (other than 13, 16)	16	2.6
Untypable	42	6.9 (90.3)

isolates were separated from the other isolates and that isolates involved in different outbreaks belonged to serotypes 1, 2, 3, 5, 10, 18 or 22. This indicated that the antigenic specificities were reliable markers for epidemiological studies. These findings and those reported by other workers[2] provided high levels of confidence in recommending the PHA technique for serotyping *C. jejuni*.

References

1. Bokkenheuser, V. (1972). *Vibrio fetus* infection in man: a serological test. *Infect. and Immun.*, 5, 222–226
2. Lauwers, S., Vlaes, L. and Butzler, J. P. (1981). Campylobacter serotyping and epidemiology. *Lancet (Letter)*, 1, 158–159
3. McCoy, E. C., Doyle, D., Burda, K., Corbeil, L. B. and Winter, A. J. (1975). Superficial antigens of *Campylobacter (Vibrio) fetus*: characterisation of an antiphagocytic component. *Infect. and Immun.*, 11, 517–525
4. Newsam, I. D. B. and St George, T. D. (1967). Diagnosis of bovine vibriosis. 3. Indirect haemagglutination using untanned sheep erythrocytes. *Aust. Vet. J.*, 43, 283–285
5. Penner, J. L. and Hennessy, J. N. (1980). Passive haemagglutination technique for serotyping *Campylobacter fetus* subsp. *jejuni* on the basis of soluble heat stable antigens. *J. Clin. Microbiol.*, 12, 732–737
6. Ristic, M. and Brandly, C. A. (1959). Characterisation of *Vibrio fetus* antigens. I. Chemical properties and serological activities of a soluble antigen. *Am. J. Vet. Res.*, 20, 148–153
7. Ristic, M. and Brandly, C. A. (1959). Characterisation of *Vibrio fetus* antigens. II. Agglutination of polysaccharide-sensitised sheep erythrocytes of specific antiserums. *Am. J. Vet. Res.*, 20, 154–161
8. Winter, A. J. (1966). An antigenic analysis of *Vibrio fetus*. III. Chemical, biologic and antigenic properties of endotoxin. *Am. J. Vet. Res.*, 27, 653–658

35
A serotyping scheme for *Campylobacter jejuni*

H. LIOR, J. A. EDGAR and D. L. WOODWARD

National Enteric Reference Centre, Ottawa, Canada

In recent years, improved techniques for isolation have focussed attention on the importance of *C. jejuni* in human gastrointestinal disease. The increasing number of isolates from non-human sources, especially chickens, has questioned the role of these organisms in human disease and emphasized the need for classification. Very few markers are available for the separation of *C. jejuni* for clinical or epidemiological purposes. Serotyping, biotyping phagetyping and antimicrobial resistance patterns, all established techniques in the epidemiology of enteric pathogens, may become useful in the study of *C. jejuni* disease.

A serotyping system has been developed, based on slide agglutination of live bacteria with antisera prepared with formalinized whole-cell antigens. Fifteen type antisera were prepared in rabbits given intravenous injections at 4–5 day intervals, of bacterial suspensions containing about 10^{10} organisms/ml. Homologous and heterologous titres were determined by tube titrations, incubated at 50 °C for 4 hours.

All antisera were absorbed with the homologous heated bacterial suspensions so that they would contain only agglutinins directed against heat-labile factors. Further absorptions with cross-reactive heat-labile factors resulted in the preparation of 15 type specific antisera.

Slide agglutinations were performed using antisera diluted 1/5 with phosphate buffered saline. Presence or absence of agglutinations were determined 45–60 seconds after mixing a drop of antisera with a loopful of bacterial culture which had been grown at 37 °C for 48 hours. Some *C. jejuni* strains, which appeared mucoid and stringy, became smooth after treatment with a nuclease solution containing 0.1 % DNAase.

Six hundred and two isolates from both human sources (462 strains) and non-human sources (140 strains) were investigated. 86 % of human isolates and 66 % of the non-human isolates were found to be typable.

Serotype I was most common among human isolates with 79 strains (Table 1), followed by serotype 4 with 55 isolates, serogroup 7 with 41 and serogroup 2 with 38 isolates.

Among non-human isolates, serogroup 4 was common with chicken isolates, while serogroup 11 appeared most common among swine isolates.

SEROTYPING SCHEME FOR *CAMPYLOBACTER JEJUNI*

Table 1 Serotyping of *C. jejuni* in single antisera

Provisional serogroup	Human source	Nonhuman source					Total
		Chickens	Swine	Pets	Others	Sub-total	
1	79	1	—	—	2[c]	3	82
2	38	4	—	—		4	42
3	19	3	—	1[a]		4	23
4	55	19	2	—	2[e]	23	78
5	22	—	4	—		4	26
6	6	1	1	—		2	8
7	41	3	1	—	1[f]	5	46
8	16	2	—	4[b]		6	22
9	14	3	—	—	1[f]	4	18
10	10	—	—	—		—	10
11	28	2	8	—	3[d]	13	41
12	5	2	5	2[c]		9	14
13	7	—	5	—		5	12
15	10	1	—	—		1	11
Total	350	41	26	7	9	83	433
% of typable	87.2%	82%	100%	100%	100%	90.2%	88%

[a] 1 cat
[b] 3 dogs and 1 cat
[c] 4 ducks
[d] 2 rabbits and 1 goat
[e] 2 bovine
[f] 2 ovine

Fifty of the human isolates and nine chicken isolates, which agglutinated in various pairs of antisera (Table 2), allowed further subdivision of some serogroups into subserogroups. Subserogroup 3, 7 was most common among human isolates. Four subserogroups, found among chicken isolates only, suggests the possibility that some serotypes found in non-human sources only, may not be associated with human disease. Very good serological correlation was seen in 11 family outbreaks and three larger community outbreaks.

Additional epidemiological information has been obtained by the introduction of the rapid hippurate hydrolysis test[1], which allowed the separation of the *C. jejuni* isolates from human sources into two groups: one group comprising 95% of the isolates was hippurate-hydrolysis positive and a second group with 5% of the isolates was hippurate-hydrolysis negative.

The hippurate-hydrolysis positive group could be divided into 2 biotypes by the rapid H_2S test[2]: biotype 1 – H_2S negative after 4 hours incubation – was most common in the human isolates (93%), while biotype 2 – H_2S positive – comprised only 7% of the human isolates.

In the hippurate-hydrolysis negative group, presumably the *C. coli* group[2], 67% of the isolates were from swine and chickens and only 33% were from

Table 2 Serotyping of *C. jejuni* in pairs of antisera

Provisional sub-serogroup	Human source	Non-human source chickens	Total
1, 2	3	—	3
1, 4	8	—	8
1, 6	3	—	3
1, 8	1	—	1
1, 9	4	—	4
1, 10	—	2	2
2, 3	3	—	3
2, 4	1	—	1
2, 7	1	1	2
2, 9	1	—	1
2, 11	2	2	4
3, 4	—	1	1
3, 7	10	—	10
3, 10	1	—	1
4, 7	1	—	1
4, 8	1	—	1
4, 10	2	—	2
4, 11	—	1	1
5, 7	1	—	1
5, 10	1	—	1
5, 14	1	—	1
6, 7	1	—	1
6, 8	1	—	1
6, 11	1	—	1
8, 9	1	—	1
9, 11	2	—	2
12, 14	—	2	2
Total	51	9	60

human cases of gastroenteritis, indicating the association of *C. coli* with human disease.

Biotyping, in conjunction with serotyping, provides additional epidemiological information and we were able to show that isolates from the common serogroup 1, and serogroups 7, 8 and 11 could be further subdivided into biotypes 1 and 2. Serotyping of *C. jejuni* by slide agglutination is easy to perform and together with biotyping are excellent tools in the epidemiology of *C. jejuni* disease.

References

1. Harvey, S. M. (1980). Hippurate hydrolysis by *Camplyobacter fetus*, *J. Clin. Microbiol.*, **11**, 435–437
2. Skirrow, M. B. and Benjamin, J. (1980). Differentiation of enteropathogenic campylobacter. *J. Clin. Pathol.*, **33**, 1122

DISCUSSION

Dr Lior found that repeated subculture on Mueller–Hinton agar generally produces smooth colonies which overcome problems of auto-agglutinability. He also found that 24-hour cultures did not always give reproducible results but that 48-hour cultures were satisfactory.

Concerning the preparation of K and H antigens Dr Lior has made a partially pure flagella preparation by mechanical shearing and differential centrifugation. At present an aflagellate mutant, as a source of K antigen, is not available but they have used cell preparations after the flagella had been sheared and heated at 65 °C for 15 minutes to depolymerize any remaining flagella. Sera prepared against such preparations produce quite different agglutination results from the flagella type of agglutination. The degree of specificity obtained is under investigation.

36
Serotyping of *C. jejuni*: a useful tool in the epidemiology of campylobacter diarrhoea

S. LAUWERS

Department of Clinical Microbiology, Free University, Brussels

We have developed an O-serotyping scheme for *C. jejuni* using the passive haemagglutination technique. Using 50 different rabbit-antisera, arranged in five pools, we are able to type about 75% of *C. jejuni* strains isolated from human faeces at the St Pierre hospital in Brussels. It appears that 31% of the typable strains (in a series of 177 patients) belong to serotype 1, 17% to serotype 2 and an additional 18% to serotypes 3, 4 or 6.

Nineteen serotypes occur regularly, the remaining 31 beng extremely rare. From 46 patients a second isolate was available and belonged to the same serotype as the first, except in four cases where a second strain – different from the first – was recovered a few weeks after the initial infection, providing evidence of re-infection with another strain. We found that several of the common Belgian serotypes seem to occur worldwide (in isolates from England, The Netherlands, The USA, Canada, Bangladesh, Peru, Zaire ...).

Since milk-borne outbreaks of campylobacter infection are reported repeatedly, we examined 61 *C. jejuni* strains isolated from the intestines of cows. Forty-three strains (70%) could be typed: eighteen were serotype 1, five serotype 2, four serotype 5, and the remaining 16 strains belonged to five different uncommon serotypes.

We further investigated 23 *C. jejuni* strains from dogs. 12 strains out of 23 were typable: two were serotype 1, four serotype 2, two serotype 3, with the remaining four strains belonging to uncommon serotypes. These preliminary results suggest that dogs and cows may be sources of infection.

O-serotyping should be of great help in the further investigation of campylobacter epidemiology.

DISCUSSION

In reply to a question regarding differences in antigen preparation for the passive haemagglutination technique Dr Lauwers said that Dr Penner used sheep red cells heated for 1 hour while she uses O rhesus-negative red blood cells heated for 2 hours and adsorbs the whole suspension onto the red cells without prior centrifugation. Dr Penner commented that temperature made no difference and antigen autoclaved at 121 °C for 1 hour was satisfactory.

Both workers had exchanged strains and found that there were serotypes common to Canada and Belgium.

37
Provisional antigenic scheme for *Campylobacter jejuni*

M. ROGOL, I. SECHTER, I. BRAUNSTEIN and CH. B. GERICHTER

Central Laboratories, Ministry of Health, Jerusalem, Israel

The role of *Campylobacter jejuni* as one of the main aetiological agents of enteritis, especially in children, is now well established and many laboratories can now isolate the organism. The search for sources of the infection has shown that *C. jejuni* can be isolated from domestic animals[1,2], fowls, birds and various environmental sources including water[3], non-pasteurized milk[4], frozen chicken and other food[5].

The biochemical and cultural characteristics of *C. jejuni* are similar in almost all the isolates. Epidemiological investigation must rely on techniques such as serotyping or phage-typing to differentiate strains.

At the Central Laboratories of the Ministry of Health in Jerusalem, a serotyping scheme for *C. jejuni* has been developed.

THE SEROTYPING METHOD

Fresh cultures of *C. jejuni* on blood agar were suspended in 0.5% formolized physiological saline and adjusted to a density of 0.5% transmittance at 540 nm on a "Spectronic 20" spectrophotometer. These suspensions were used for three intravenous inoculations to rabbits, in doses of 0.25, 0.5 and 1 ml followed by two inoculations (2 and 4 ml) with a live suspension. Bleeding was done at 5–7 days after the last inoculation.

Twenty sera were prepared, using 17 strains of *C. jejuni* isolated in Israel and three strains received from the University of Gottenborg, Sweden. The homologous titre, established by slide-agglutination of fresh cultures, was 1/80 to 1/160. Tube-agglutination (2 hours at 52 °C) gave titres of 1/320 to 1/1280. Cross agglutination by the slide-technique was performed with all the 20 sera at different dilutions, against all the cultures. After eliminating a few sera which gave identical reactions, 14 sera were selected for the serotyping scheme. These sera were prepared using 11 locally-isolated strains and three from Sweden.

Two polyvalent sera were prepared by pooling these 14 sera so that each serum was present in a pool at four times the slide agglutination titre.

RESULTS

The results of cross-testing the 14 sera (at dilutions 1/10 to 1/160) against the 14 antigens, showed that 4 cultures reacted only with their homologous serum. The other 10 cultures reacted at the highest dilution with the homologous serum, but cross-reacted with other sera at 1/2 to 1/8 of the homologous titre (Table 1). Thus, it appears that some cultures possess only the major antigen, but most of them have a major antigen, characteristic of the serogroup, along with one or more minor antigens.

Table 1 Antigenic structure of the 14 cultures used for preparation of sera

No. of strain	Source	Antigenic structure	
2	Israel	1*	(7, 10, 11)†
3	Israel	2	
4	Israel	3	(7, 10, 11)
12	Sweden	5	(7)
78	Sweden	6	(8)
80	Sweden	7	
160	Israel	8	
167	Israel	9	
186	Israel	10	(11)
191	Israel	11	(7, 10)
200	Israel	12	(3, 7, 14)
218	Israel	13	(11)
223	Israel	14	(12, 15)
226	Israel	15	(3, 12)

* Major antigen
† Minor antigens (in brackets)

Using this scheme for serotyping, 67 cultures of *C. jejuni*, comprising 63 isolated from Israel, three from Sweden and one from Montreal, Canada, were tested. Sixty cultures (90%) reacted with one or another of the polyvalent sera and their serogroups were established. The remaining seven cultures were used to prepare a third polyvalent serum.

The 60 cultures which could be serotyped belonged to the 14 serogroups identified (Table 2). The most frequent serogroups were: group 3 with 12 cultures, group 1 with 8 cultures and groups 8 and 11 with 6 cultures each. A total of 41 different serotypes were recognized.

The identification of major and minor antigens demonstrate some aspects of the antigenic structure of *C. jejuni*.

(1) An antigen may appear as a major antigen for one strain but as a minor component in other strains, e.g. antigen 6 is a major antigen in two strains but occurs as a minor antigen in the strains of six other serogroups.
(2) Some minor antigens are frequently associated with a particular major antigen, e.g. antigens 3, 10 and 11 with the major antigen 1, or antigens 5, 6 and 7 with the major antigen 3.

Table 2 Provisional antigenic scheme for 60 cultures of *Campylobacter jejuni* isolated from clinical cases in Israel

Serogroup	Serotype	No. of cultures
1	1*	2
	1 (10, 11)†	1
	1 (3, 10, 11)	2
	1 (11)	2
	1 (3)	
2	2	1
3	3	2
	3 (7)	1
	3 (1, 7)	2
	3 (1)	2
	3 (5, 6)	1
	3 (6, 7, 11)	1
	3 (6, 12)	1
	3 (5)	1
	3 (6, 7)	1
5	5 (11)	2
	5 (6)	1
	5 (10)	1
6	6	2
7	7	2
	7 (3, 6)	1
8	8	2
	8 (12)	3
	8 (12, 7)	1
9	9	3
	9 (2, 6)	1
10	10	1
11	11 (3, 6, 13)	1
	11 (10)	2
	11 (1, 7, 13)	1
	11 (1)	1
	11 (12)	1
12	12	1
	12 (14)	3
13	13	1
14	14 (12)	1
	14 (15)	2
	14 (11)	1
	14 (6, 11, 12)	1
15	15	3
	15 (10)	1
Total 14	41	60

* Major antigen
† Minor antigens (in brackets)

Table 3 Sero-groups and types of *Campylobacter jejuni* isolated from clinical cases in two different hospitals in Israel

Bikur-Cholim Hospital (*Jerusalem*)

Serogroup	Serotype	No. of cultures
3	3*	1
	3 (1, 7)†	1
8	8	1
	8 (12)	4
9	9	1
	9 (2, 6)	1
10	10	1
11	11 (10)	1
13	13	1
15	15	2
	15 (10)	1
Total 7	11	15

Tel-Hashomer Hospital (*near Tel-Aviv*)

Serogroup	Serotype	No. of cultures
1	1	2
	1 (3, 10, 11)	2
	1 (11)	2
	3 (1)	2
	3 (5, 6)	1
	3 (6, 7, 11)	1
	3 (6, 7, 12)	2
	3 (5)	1
6	6	1
7	7 (3, 6)	1
9	9	1
11	11 (10)	1
	11 (1, 7, 13)	1
	11 (12)	1
12	12	1
	12 (14)	2
14	14 (11)	1
	14 (15)	2
	14 (6, 11, 12)	1
Total 8	19	26

* Major antigen
† Minor antigens (in brackets)

(3) To obtain monospecific sera absorption is necessary.

(4) The major antigens 5, 6 and 7 identified by the sera prepared from cultures received from Sweden, were frequently found in strains isolated in Israel, either as major antigens or as minor components of other serogroups. One-third of the 60 cultures reacted with one or more of these three sera.

Regional distribution of serogroups

The serogroups of strains of *C. jejuni*, isolated during the summer period of 1980 in two hospitals were compared (Table 3).

Among the seven serogroups found in B. Cholim Hospital, four (8, 10, 13 and 15) were not found in Tel-Hashomer. Among the eight serogroups found in Tel-Hashomer Hospital, five (1, 6, 7, 12 and 14) were not found in Bikur-Cholim. Of the 12 serogroups identified in these hospitals only three (3, 9 and 11) were common to both hospitals.

These findings suggest a regional distribution of the serogroups of *C. jejuni*.

Some epidemiological aspects

The serotyping scheme may be used to confirm epidemiological observations.

In one case a strain of *C. jejuni* of serotype 14 was isolated from an adult suffering from diarrhoea. A dog in the household also had diarrhoea and was shown to be excreting the same serotype of *C. jejuni*. In another instance serotype 3 of *C. jejuni* was isolated from a mother and from her child, both with diarrhoea.

CONCLUSIONS

The serotyping scheme presented here is provisional. However, these 14 sera allowed us to characterize 60 out of 67 cultures examined. As more cultures are examined from Israel and from abroad, new sera will have to be prepared and new serogroups will be recognized. Since many strains appear to have both major and minor antigens, absorbed sera will be needed for more accurate serotyping.

— The sera used in this scheme were prepared with formolized and live cultures. The preparation of O, K and H sera will naturally lead to a more accurate definition of the serotypes.

— The serological study of strains of *C. jejuni* isolated from fowls, domestic animals, birds and other potential sources, will contribute to the elucidation of the sources of infection and routes of transmission to man.

References

1. Skirrow, M. B. and Benjamin, J. (1980). '1001' Campylobacters: cultural characteristics of intestinal campylobacters from man and animals. *J. Hyg. (Cambridge)*, **85**, 427–441
2. Bruce, D., Zochowski, W. and Fleming, G. A. (1980). Campylobacter species in cats and dogs. *Vet. Rec.*, **107**, 200–201

3. Tiehan, D. and Vogt, R. L. (1978). Waterborne Campylobacter gastroenteritis – Vermont. Morbidity and Mortality Weekly Report. **27,** 207
4. Blaser, M. J., Cravens, J., Powers, B. W., LaForce, F. M. and Wang, W. L. (1979). Campylobacter enteritis associated with unpasteurised milk. *Am. J. Med.,* **67,** 715–718
5. Skirrow, M. B. (1977). Campylobacter enteritis: a 'new' disease. *Br. Med. J.,* **2,** 9–11

38
Serotyping of *Campylobacter jejuni*

J. D. ABBOTT, J. ELDRIDGE, D. M. JONES and
E. M. SUTCLIFFE

Public Health Laboratory, Withington Hospital, Manchester

We have investigated strains of *C. jejuni* isolated from patients in ten outbreaks, many of which were milk-borne.

A representative strain from each outbreak was used to prepare antisera in rabbits by a course of intravenous inoculations. Two types of suspensions were used for raising sera: (a) formolized and (b) heated at 100 °C for 15 minutes.

A comparison was made of different techniques for typing strains:

(1) bactericidal[1],
(2) haemagglutination[2],
(3) tube agglutination with formolized suspensions after incubation at 50 °C for 2 hours[1],
(4) tube agglutination with heated (100 °C for 15 minutes) suspensions after incubation at 50 °C overnight[1].

Using sera raised against formolized suspensions, three methods – bactericidal, haemagglutination and agglutination with formolized suspension – were compared, and gave similar results. There were few cross-reactions and it was not necessary to absorb the sera. It was postulated that the same heat-stable antigens were detected by the three methods, and the agglutination test may also detect 'H' antigens.

Sera raised with heated suspensions were tested by tube agglutination with heated suspensions. These sera showed marked cross-agglutination and most required absorption with a heterologous strain. The specificity of these sera was different to those raised with formolized suspensions.

References

1. Abbott, J. D., Dale, B. A. S., Eldridge, J., Jones, D. M. and Sutcliffe, E. M. (1980). Serotyping of *Campylobacter jejuni/coli. J. Clin. Pathol.,* **33**, 762–766
2. Penner, J. L. and Hennessy, J. N. (1980). Passive haemagglutination technique for serotyping *campylobacter fetus* subsp. *jejuni* on the basis of soluble heat-stable antigens. *J. Clin. Microbiol.,* **12**, 732–737

DISCUSSION

Asked about flagellar antigens, Dr Abbott said he was uncertain how much of the formolized suspension was capsular or flagellar antigens or from the cell envelope. In the passive haemagglutination test the suspension had been boiled for an hour which would destroy the flagellar antigen.

With regard to cross reacting O antigens, it was necessary to absorb sera with one, or occasionally two, heterologous strains.

39
Serological typing of thermophilic campylobacters isolated in Tokyo

T. ITOH, K. SAITO, Y. YANAGAWA, S. SAKAI and M. OHASHI

Tokyo Metropolitan Research Laboratory of Public Health, Tokyo, Japan

---

While serotyping systems for thermophilic campylobacters have been reported by a number of workers, we have established our own methods independently.

Two strains isolated from diarrhoeal cases, CF-1 and CF-256 were treated either by formalin or by heating–121 °C for 2 hours. Antisera to each strain were obtained by immunizing rabbits. Table 1 shows agglutination assay results between corresponding antigens and antisera. These results suggested that the organisms possessed at least two kinds of antigens, heat-stable and heat-labile.

Cross-agglutination experiments were performed to determine the specificity of heat-stable antigens prepared from eight different strains derived from various sources. The results demonstrated no immunological specificity.

On the other hand, tests using formalin-treated heat-labile antigens revealed remarkable specificities among the strains from different sources. Table 2 shows the results of the quantitative cross-agglutination tests on 18 strains and their respective antisera. Each of these antisera showed the highest agglutination titre with its corresponding antigen, and cross reactions with heterologous antigen were rare and weak, even when unabsorbed antisera were examined.

Thus, agglutination tests using antigens prepared by formalin treatment and their corresponding antisera, were found to be a useful method for serological typing of this organism. The slide-agglutination technique was satisfactory for routine use. By means of this system, 18 serotypes have so far been identified among our collection of thermophilic campylobacter strains. They are numbered from TCK 1–TCK 18.

Table 3 summarizes the serological types established by this method for isolates from various sources. Most of the Tokyo outbreaks presented elsewhere in this symposium (Geographical Epidemiology, p. 5 were induced by a single serotype, though one did involve two different serotypes. Sixty-two out of 121 (51%) isolates from sporadic diarrhoeal cases were typable by this system, 17 serotypes being identified.

Table 1 Reactivity in agglutination test of formalin-treated and heat-treated antigens by their antisera

Antigens	Titres of antisera CF-1		Titres of antisera CF-256	
	Anti-formalin-treated cells	Anti-heat-treated cells	Anti-formalin-treated cells	Anti-heat-treated cells
C. jejuni, strain CF-1				
Formalin treated cells	640	20	—	—
Heat treated cells*	80	640	—	—
C. jejuni, strain CF-256				
Formalin treated cells	—	—	2560	20
Heat treated cells	—	—	160	640

* Treated at 121 °C for 120 min. — = Not tested

Table 2 Cross-agglutination reaction of reference strains of each serotype of thermophilic campylobacter

| Reference strains | Serotypes (TCK) | Titre of typing antiserum* ||||||||||||||||||
		1	2	3	4	5	6	7	8	9	10	11	12	13	14	15	16	17	18
CF-1	1	1280	—	—	—	—	—	—	—	—	—	—	—	—	—	—	—	—	—
CF-57	2	—	640	40	—	20	—	—	—	—	—	—	—	—	—	—	—	—	—
CF-60	3	—	—	1280	—	—	—	—	—	—	—	—	—	—	—	—	—	—	—
CF-88	4	—	—	—	1280	—	—	—	—	—	—	—	—	—	—	—	—	—	—
CF-129	5	—	—	—	—	640	20	—	—	80	—	—	—	—	—	—	—	—	—
CF-229	6	—	—	—	—	—	640	—	—	—	—	—	—	—	—	—	—	—	—
CF-256	7	—	—	—	—	—	—	1280	—	—	—	—	—	—	—	—	—	—	—
CF-41	8	—	—	—	—	—	—	—	320	—	—	—	—	—	—	—	—	—	—
CF-17	9	—	—	—	—	—	—	—	—	1280	—	—	—	—	—	—	—	—	—
CF-54	10	—	—	—	—	—	—	—	—	—	5120	—	—	—	—	—	—	—	—
CF-77	11	—	—	—	—	—	—	—	—	—	20	2560	—	—	—	—	—	—	—
CF-181	12	—	—	—	—	—	—	—	—	—	—	—	1280	—	—	—	—	—	—
CF-97	13	—	—	—	—	—	—	—	—	—	—	—	—	1280	—	—	—	—	—
CF-227	14	—	—	—	—	—	—	—	—	—	—	—	—	—	640	—	—	—	—
CF-68	15	—	—	—	—	—	—	160	—	—	—	—	—	—	—	2560	—	—	—
CF-356	16	—	—	—	—	—	—	—	—	—	—	—	—	—	—	—	2560	—	—
CF-314	17	—	—	—	—	—	—	—	—	—	—	—	—	—	—	—	—	640	—
CF-30	18	—	—	—	—	—	—	—	—	—	—	—	—	—	—	—	—	—	320

* Rabbit antisera against formalin-treated cells (unabsorbed)

Table 3 Serotypes of thermophilic campylobacter isolated from human diarrheal cases and animals

Sources	Hippurate hydrolysis	No. of strains examined	1	2	3	4	5	6	7	8	9	10	11	12	13	14	15	16	17	18	Total	Untypable
Human diarrhoea outbreaks																						
No. 1	+	15	15	—	—	—	—	—	—	—	—	—	—	—	—	—	—	—	—	—	15	0
No. 2	+	5	—	—	—	—	—	—	—	—	—	—	—	—	—	—	—	—	4	—	4	1
No. 3	+	3	—	—	3	—	—	—	—	—	—	—	—	—	—	—	—	—	—	—	3	0
No. 4	+	14	1	—	12	—	—	1	—	—	—	—	—	—	—	—	—	—	—	—	14	0
No. 5	+	7	—	—	—	7	—	—	—	—	—	—	—	—	—	—	—	—	—	—	7	0
No. 6	+	18	1	—	—	—	14	—	—	—	1	—	—	—	—	—	—	—	—	—	16	2
No. 7	+	10	—	—	—	—	—	4	—	—	—	—	—	—	—	6	—	—	—	—	10	0
No. 8	+	31	1	—	—	—	—	—	30	—	—	—	—	—	—	—	1	—	—	—	31	0
No. 9	+	3	—	—	3	—	—	—	—	—	—	—	—	—	—	—	—	—	—	—	3	0
Sporadic cases	+	105 (100%)	5	3	1	1	—	2	2	6	2	4	1	7	2	2	1	5	1	10	55 (52%)	50 (48%)
	—	16	—	2	—	—	—	—	—	1	—	—	—	1	—	—	1	—	—	2	7	9
Poultry	+	29 (100%)	1	—	—	—	—	4	2	2	1	—	—	—	—	—	—	—	—	1	11 (38%)	18 (62%)
Swine	{ +	2	1	1	—	—	—	—	—	—	—	—	—	—	—	—	—	—	—	—	2	0
	—	69 (100%)	—	—	1	—	—	2	3	7	—	—	—	2	—	—	—	—	—	—	15 (22%)	54 (78%)
Cattle	+	4	1	—	—	—	—	—	—	—	—	—	—	—	1	—	—	—	—	—	2	2
Total		331 (100%)	25	9	17	8	14	13	37	16	4	4	1	10	3	9	1	6	1	17	195 (59%)	136 (41%)

Some hippurate hydrolysis-negative strains isolated from overseas travellers with diarrhoea were found to share antigens with hippurate hydrolysis-positive strains.

Amongst animal strains 30 out of 104 (29%) have been typed into ten different serotypes. Some of the hippurate-negative, or *C. coli* strains isolated from swine, shared certain type specificities with *C. jejuni* of human origin. In total, 195 strains out of 331 (59%) were typable.

40
Some serological aspects of the diagnosis of campylobacter infections

K. C. WATSON and E. J. C. KERR

Western General Hospital, Edinburgh, Scotland

Infection with *Campylobacter jejuni* is usually characterized by a good antibody response. We have compared the value of agglutination, complement fixation (CFT) and immunofluorescence (IF) tests in a system involving the use of two laboratory reference strains COP and MEL. Formolized suspensions were satisfactory for agglutination and gave classical 'H'-type agglutination. Heat-killed 'O'-type antigens were far less satisfactory, a finding reported by others. CFT antigens were made from saline suspensions heated at 56 °C for 30 minutes but alcohol-killed suspensions proved unsatisfactory. Immunofluorescence preparations were made from live suspensions washed twice in saline and then air dried on slides that were gently fixed by heating. Results are shown in Table 1 below.

Table 1 Examination of 55 sera from 40 culture positive patients

Technique	No. (%) positive		
	COP	MEL	Overall
IF	34 (62)	43 (28)	45 (81)
CF	30 (55)	17 (32)	34 (62)
AGG	13 (24)	15 (27)	21 (39)

Any test positive 35 of 40 patients (87.5)
IF – immunofluorescence test
CF – complement fixation test
AGG – agglutination test

The agglutination test results compare with a positive rate of 69.6% of 66 sera that agglutinated COP reported previously[1] and is attributable to a change in the phenotype of COP. Overall 87.5% of 40 culture-positive patients gave positive serological tests by one or more of the tests employed. Taking both antigens together no sera were negative by IF where one or both of the other two tests were positive. There were five sera that were CFT negative where one or both of the other tests were positive and 11 that were agglutination negative where one or both of the other tests were positive. Fifteen pairs of sera were studied. In six a four-fold, or greater rise in titre, was noted. Two were against MEL by IF; one against MEL by agglutation and against COP by CFT; two against MEL by CFT; and one against COP by agglutination, against COP by CFT and against MEL by CFT. Three other pairs showed marked drops in agglutination titres, one from 5120 against MEL and 320 against COP to less than 20 for both antigens, one from 640 against COP to less than 20 after 17 days and one from 1280 to less than 20 after 11 days.

Results indicate that: (i) suitably chosen reference strains will detect antibody formed against most campylobacter isolates, (ii) that IF gave the highest detection rate, and (iii) that different tests may detect antibodies of different specificities. Attempts to demonstrate incomplete antibody by antiglobulin tests failed due to clumping of organisms on centrifuging.

For reasons to be elucidated 'O'-heated suspensions appear far less satisfactory than formalized suspensions. Again, a number of sera give higher titres against reference strains than against the homologous strain. It is suggested that this may be due to phase variation affecting 'H' antigens.

Reference

1. Watson, K. C., Kerr, E. J. C. and McFadzean, F. M. (1979). Serology of human campylobacter infections. *J. Infect.*, **1,** 151–158

41
Serology of *Campylobacter jejuni* by tube agglutination and fluorescent antibody methods

D. W. LAMBE and D. A. FERGUSON

Department of Microbiology, College of Medicine, East Tennessee State University, Johnson City, Tennessee 37614, U.S.A.

In 1981, Lambe, Ferguson, Wiener and Butzler[1] reported *Campylobacter jejuni* from 18 human cases of acute gastroenteritis in East Tennessee. These 18 cases represented an isolation rate of 8% which is in agreement with isolation rates reported by Skirrow[2], Butzler (personal communication) and others. A sigmoidoscopy on one of our patients revealed a diffusely erythematous and edematous rectal mucous membrane, and a biopsy showed a loss of mucosa, vascular congestion and a small crypt abscess.

The high percentage of our patients who exhibited frank or occult blood in the stool, abdominal pain and severe systemic systems such as chills, high fever, rigours and profuse watery diarrhoea suggests that *C. jejuni* is an invasive organism which may cause mucosal haemorrhage and abscess formation. Because of its severity, we proposed that this disease probably warrants description as an 'acute dysenteric syndrome' rather than simple diarrhoea or gastroenteritis.

In addition to human faecal samples, we also isolated *C. jejuni* from 50% of faecal samples from chickens with no obvious signs of disease.

MATERIALS AND METHODS

Tube agglutination

Berg, Jutila and Firehammer[3] demonstrated three thermostable O antigens and multiple thermolabile antigens. The thermostable antigens provided the basis of Berg's serological classification by slide agglutination. By his scheme, all strains in *C. jejuni* reacted with the same antiserum which he designated as type C.

However, there were no serological differences between strains of *C. jejuni*. Thus, Berg's scheme can be used for identification of campylobacter subspecies but it would not be useful as an epidemiological tool to determine the origin of strains.

Berg also showed that sheep vaccinated with heat-labile *C. jejuni* antigens (formalin-killed cells) were protected against homologous challenge inoculation. However, the heat-stable antigens did not protect sheep against homologous challenge. Because of this evidence that heat-labile antigens are important serologically and immunogenically, we used formalin-killed antigens to immunize rabbits rather than heat-killed cells. Since our antigens for antisera preparation were not denatured by heat, the serological tests that we used detected both group and strain-specific antibodies to *C. jejuni*.

Rabbits were immunized to one of 23 strains of *C. jejuni*. Eighteen of these strains were isolated from humans and five strains were isolated from chickens in East Tennessee. Strains of *C. jejuni* from different sources were tested against the 23 rabbit antisera by tube agglutination.

Cell suspensions for the tube agglutination test were diluted in physiological saline to a density of one-half a McFarland #7 barium-sulphate standard. Equal amounts of cells and the diluted rabbit antiserum were mixed and incubated in a 45 °C waterbath. Agglutination reactions were recorded at 24 and 48 hours as 0–4+.

A 2+ –4+ was considered positive. A significant agglutination titre was 1:80 or greater. Agglutination titres as high as 1:10 240 were recorded.

Direct fluorescent antibody test

Antisera were fractionated and the globulin fraction was conjugated with fluorescein isothiocyanate in a similar manner that I have described in the literature for *Bacteroides fragilis* and the black pigmenting group of *Bacteroides*.

Strains examined by the direct fluorescent antibody method were cultured for 24 hours on an enriched medium. A standardized cellular suspension was prepared and one drop was dispensed on a microscope slide, dried and heat fixed. One drop of FITC conjugate was placed on the bacterial suspension, incubated for 45 minutes, washed with phosphate buffered saline and distilled water, and air dried. The strains tested by the direct fluorescent antibody method included 22 human faecal isolates from East Tennessee and two strains obtained from the Centers for Disease Control (CDC), Atlanta, Georgia. The NCTC strain 11168 is the English type strain. The Belgian strains were supplied by Dr Butzler; the Illinois strains were isolated by Dr Folkens and by Dr Kaplan; and the Colorado strains were isolated by Dr Reller. We also tested 11 strains of *C. jejuni* which were isolated from animals. Five of these strains were isolated from chickens and one strain was isolated from a cow in East Tennessee. The six strains obtained from Dr Bryner's collection were isolated from a pig and five sheep.

Five strains of *C. fetus*, and two strains of *C. fetus* ssp. *fetus* were also examined with both fluorescent antibody conjugates.

Fluorescence of cells was graded from 0–3+. 0– ± was considered negative and 1+ –3+ staining was considered positive. 1+ was considered positive for campylobacter; this grading of fluorescence is different from that we described for the bacteroides conjugates.

RESULTS AND DISCUSSION

The serological classification scheme by tube agglutination was developed as follows. Each of the 23 rabbit antisera was assigned a number from 1–23. If a campylobacter strain reacted with antisera 1 and 17, it was considered to contain antigenic components 1 and 17. This same type of antigenic analysis was used by Edwards and Ewing[4] for serogrouping shigella species, by Pulverer and Ko[5] for serogrouping *Propionibacterium acnes* and by Lambe and Moroz[6] to serogroup *Bacteroides fragilis*.

Our serogroups of *C. jejuni* were constructed by antigenic components which were shared by all strains within the serogroup. For example, serogroup I contained components 1 and 17.

Other antigenic components which were not shared by all strains were called subserogroup components. Therefore, there were three subserogroups in serogroup I. Subserogroup A contained component 8, subserogroup B contained components 2 and 21 and subserogroup C contained components 12, 13, 15 and 21.

Thus, our serogroups were constructed by increased numbers of common components shared by all strains within the group. Serogroup I showed two common antigenic components and serogroup IX showed ten common antigenic components.

There were 26 serological subserogroups that contained strains isolated from human faeces in Tennessee, with other outbreaks in the U.S.A., Belgium and England.

Some serogroups, for example serogroups II, III and IV, contained human strains only, whereas serogroups I and V contained human as well as animal strains. Serogroups VI and VII contained human isolates only, whereas serogroups VIII and IX contained human and animal isolates.

The potential of this serogrouping scheme as an epidemiological tool is illustrated by several examples. Two strains isolated from the mother and the child who suffered from *C. jejuni* gastroenteritis contained components 6, 10 and 11 in common. These strains were serogroup III.

Another example of epidemiological interest occurred in serogroup VIII. A strain isolated from a three-year-old child on a farm and a strain isolated 1 month later from a cow on the same farm shared the same group components. The two strains differed only in subserogroup components 2 and 12. Two additional strains occurred in serogroup VIII. One of these isolates was a chicken isolate from a different farm and the other isolate was NCTC 11168 from Skirrow which we obtained from CDC. Two strains of *C. jejuni* contained a combination of all but one of the 23 antigenic components in our scheme. We selected antisera prepared with these two strains for preparation of fluorescein isothiocyanate conjugates. Our theory was that these two FITC conjugates would give cross-reactive fluorescence with most, or all strains of *C. jejuni*.

All of the human faecal isolates as well as faecal isolates from chickens, cows, pigs and sheep gave positive fluorescence with both conjugates. Therefore, 73 strains of *C. jejuni* gave positive fluorescence with both conjugates.

The five strains of *C. fetus* ssp *venerealis* and the two strains of *C. fetus* ssp. *fetus* that were tested did not react with either conjugate. Additional genera of bacteria which were negative with both FITC conjugates included: *Bacteroides, Escherichia, Enterobacter, Klebsiella, Acinetobacter, Morganella, Proteus, Serratia, Citrobacter, Pseudomonas, Flavobacterium* and *Staphylococcus*.

These results indicated that the two conjugates were specific for *C. jejuni*, and indicated that strains isolated from humans, cows, chickens, sheep and a pig were related to each other antigenically. For example, the two strains of *C. jejuni* isolated from faecal samples from a mother and child with gastroenteritis gave positive fluorescence. Strains isolated from a child and from a cow on the same farm also gave positive fluorescence with both of our conjugates.

We propose that these specific fluorescent antibody conjugates can be used for at least two purposes. Firstly, the FITC conjugates may be used for a rapid identification of *C. jejuni* colonies as soon as they appear on isolation plates in the clinical laboratory. A second use of the specific conjugates to detect serologically similar strains in animals and man.

References

1. Lambe, D. W. Jr., Ferguson, D. A. Jr., Wiener, S. L. and Butzler, J. P. (1981). *Campylobacter fetus* ssp. *jejuni*: Isolation from patients with gastroenteritis. *South. Med. J.*, **74**, 157–161
2. Skirrow, M. B. (1977). *Campylobacter* enteritis: a 'new' disease. *Br. Med. J.*, **2**, 9–11
3. Berg, M. S., Jutila, J. W. and Firehammer, B. D. (1971). A revised classification of *Vibrio* fetus. *Am. J. Vet. Res.*, **32**, 11–22
4. Edwards, P. R. and Ewing, W. H. (1972). Identification of *Enterobacteriaceae*. 3rd edition, Burgess Publishing Company, Minneapolis, Minnesota
5. Pulverer, G. and Ko, H. L. (1973). Fermentative and serological studies on *Propionibacterium acnes*. *Appl. Microbiol.*, **25**, 222–229
6. Lambe, D. W. Jr. and Moroz, D. A. (1976). Serogrouping of *Bacteroides fragilis* subsp. *fragilis* by the agglutination test. *J. Clin. Microbiol.*, **3**, 586–592

42
Techniques for serotyping
Campylobacter jejuni

J. H. BRYNER, A. E. RITCHIE and J. W. FOLEY

National Animal Disease Center, Iowa, USA

Auto-agglutination interferes with sero-testing most strains of *C. jejuni*. When 48-hour cultures of auto-agglutinating strains were examined by electron microscopy, >40% were 'leaky' or disrupted. Many leaky cells had a mantle of closely adhering DNA-like material; disrupted cells also released a kinky, protein-like material that adhered to flagella. DNAase digestion reduced the auto-agglutination, but not completely. Young (18-hour) cultures had few leaky, disrupted cells and minimal auto-agglutination. Two antigens were prepared from 18-hour cultures grown on Mueller–Hinton agar at 43 °C. For a tube agglutination test (heat-labile antigens), cells were harvested in filtered saline containing 3% formaldehyde, fixed 1 hour at 43 °C with shaker agitation, washed three times in saline containing 1:5000 merthiolate, and standardized to 0.5 OD at 540 nm. Tube reactions were read as an OD clearing rather than particulate aggregation, and were useful for endpoint titres to the heat-labile antigens. For a micro-titre bacterial cell agglutination test (heat-labile antigens), cells grown as above were harvested into Albimi Broth and further incubated on a shaker at 43 °C for 5 hours. The broth-shaker cultures were autoclaved 1 hour (121 °C) and, while hot, cells were sedimented at 11 000 g for 20 minutes, and then washed three times in water containing 1% Beckman Buffer (pH 7) and 1:5000 merthiolate. This antigen was standardized to 0.3 OD at 540 nm in the Beckman buffered (pH 7) water containing 1:5000 merthiolate. The microtitre test for heat-stable antigens was read as a shield of agglutinated cells (positive) or as a button (negative). Saline or unbuffered water were improper vehicles for re-suspending the heated antigen cells, i.e. the saline suspension auto-agglutinated and the water suspension failed to react with antibody. The tube-agglutination-test antigen did not function in the microtitre system because the negative controls failed to form a clearly defined button.

43
Serological diagnosis of *Campylobacter jejuni* infections by using the enzyme-linked immunosorbent assay principle

Å. SVEDHEM, H. GUNNARSSON and B. KAIJSER

University of Göteborg, Sweden

Determination of specific antibodies is a valuable complement to cultures in the diagnosis of campylobacter infections. This should be especially efficient in epidemiological studies, as well as in studies of immunity.

Different methods have been employed to detect *C. jejuni* antibodies but only with antigen preparations from the homologous strains. This limits the usefulness of the method.

The aim of the present investigation was to find a serological system for the demonstration of *C. jejuni* antibodies with antigen preparation from heterologous strains covering as many infections as possible.

MATERIALS AND METHODS

Patients

Serum samples were obtained from 71 patients included in an outbreak of *C. jejuni* enterocolitis in Grums, Sweden[1]. The serum samples were collected on two occasions from each patient; the first serum (S_I) 10–12 days and the second serum (S_{II}) 3 months after onset of disease. All patients had *C. jejuni* isolated from a stool sample in the beginning of the disease. Serum samples obtained from 54 healthy blood donors, chosen with the same age distribution as that of the patients, constituted a control group.

Antigen preparations

The *C. jejuni* strains used for preparation of antigens were obtained from ten different patients. These isolates originated from patients who contracted their campylobacter enterocolitis in different parts of the world and without any known connections with each other. The ten patient strains did not originate from the Grums epidemic mentioned above. A separate antigen was prepared from this epidemic strain.

Glycoprotein (GP) antigen, a surface antigen from the bacteria, was produced from the strains by acidification of the cultures with glycine HCl buffer[2]. After neutralization, dialysis and concentration, the antigen was lyophilized. The preparations were tested by gas–liquid chromatography analysis for presence of lipid A from lipopolysaccharide. No lipid A was detected[3].

Antibody production and antigen testing

GP antigen from the ten strains emulsified in Freunds complete adjuvant was used for subcutaneous immunization of rabbits once a week for 5 weeks. The antisera were tested for cross-reacting antibodies against the GP antigen-preparations with diffusion-in-gel *ad mod* Ouchterlony[4,5], crossed immuno-electrophoresis *ad mod* Laurell[6] and DIG-ELISA[7]. GP from two strains were chosen to constitute the antigen pool (GP-pool). These GP antigens expressed strong cross-reactions with all eight heterologous rabbit antisera.

Antibody determination

The diffusion-in-gel enzyme-linked immunosorbent assay, DIG-ELISA, was used to demonstrate antibodies of the IgG and IgM classes to *C. jejuni*[7,8,9]. Two antigen preparations were employed in all tests

(i) GP-pool, as described above,
(ii) GP-epid, which was the antigen prepared from the strain causing the outbreak in Grums.

All serum samples from patients and blood donors were tested against both GP-epid and GP-pool. Horse radish peroxidase-anti-human IgG and IgM were used as conjugates[10]. The reactions were visualized by *p*-phenylenediamine as enzyme-substrate. The diameters of the coloured circular diffusion zones were measured to an accuracy of ± 0.5 mm after 20 minutes.

Statistics

Statistical calculations were performed by using the t-test and deviations were expressed as SEM (standard error of the mean).

RESULTS

Table 1 shows the means of the zone diameters in DIG-ELISA for S_I and S_{II} among the 71 patients tested for IgG and IgM antibodies against GP-pool and GP-epid, respectively. The difference in zone diameters (S_I–S_{II}) for pairs of sera are also indicated. In the IgG tests the zone diameters for S_I and S_{II} are significantly larger when tested against GP-pool than against GP-epid. The

Table 1 Antibody response in 71 patients involved in an epidemic outbreak of *Campylobacter jejuni* enterocolitis

| | DIG-ELISA mean zone diameter (mm) ± SEM ||||
| | IgG || IgM ||
	GP-pool	GP-epid	GP-pool	GP-epid
S_I	10.5 ± 0.8*	8.8 ± 0.7	6.0 ± 0.5	5.5 ± 0.5
S_{II}	8.2 ± 0.8*	6.5 ± 0.7	4.5 ± 0.3	4.3 ± 0.3
S_I–S_{II} pairs	2.1 ± 0.4	2.4 ± 0.4	1.7 ± 0.3	1.3 ± 0.4

SEM – standard error of the mean $p = 0.95$, $n = 71$
* significant difference between GP-pool and GP-epid

decrease between S_I and S_{II} was similar when GP-pool and GP-epid were used. For both IgG and IgM antibodies there were significant differences in the means of zone the diameters of S_I and S_{II} when tested against both antigen preparations. The IgM tests showed no other significant differences.

The blood-donors' tests came out in two groups, one with and one without detectable antibodies against *Campylobacter jejuni*. The former group could be fitted to the normal distribution. The results referring to this group can be seen in Table 2. All these figures are significantly lower and separated from the corresponding ones of the patients' S_I. Regarding the patients' S_{II}, there was a significant difference only for IgG antibodies against GP-epid when compared to the blood donors. Ten (19%) of the 54 blood donors and 15 (28%) of the patients did not react at all with the GP-pool and GP-epid antigen, respectively.

Table 2 Detectable *Campylobacter jejuni* antibodies in 54 blood donors

| | DIG-ELISA, zone diameter (mm) ||
| | IgG | IgM |
	Mean ± SEM	Mean ± SEM
GP-pool	7.5 ± 0.8[76]	4.6 ± 0.4[50]
GP-epid	5.3 ± 0.5[67]	4.5 ± 0.4[26]

( ) per cent of 54 blood donors with detectable antibodies which constitutes the basis for the figures in each system, respectively.

DISCUSSION

In the present study homologous (GP-epid) and heterologous (GP-pool) GP surface antigens were used in the DIG-ELISA to detect *C. jejuni* antibodies in sera from patients within an epidemic outbreak. The immunoglobulin classes IgG and IgM were analysed separately. With both antigen preparations, antibodies were detected at different levels in all patients in at least one of the Ig-classes. The *C. jejuni* strains constituting the heterologous antigen pool, GP-pool, were chosen for their frequent interactions with antisera from other strains. The GP-pool gave significantly stronger reactions in detecting IgG antibodies in the epidemic patient group than did the antigen prepared from the homologous epidemic strain. With the GP-pool there was no significant separation of the blood-donors' sera from the patients' sera, obtained after 3 months, in contrast to the homologous GP-epid antigen. The frequency of blood donors with detectable IgG antibodies was not significantly different from patients. The results show that with the GP-pool a wider range of *C. jejuni* IgG-antibodies was detected and possibly also at lower levels. Regarding IgM-antibodies there were no differences for the two antigens. With both antigens a significant difference was seen in IgG- as well as in IgM-antibodies between the acute 10-day patient sera and the 3-month blood donors' sera.

In conclusion the DIG-ELISA with a surface antigen preparation, GP antigen, from selected strains has been shown to be effective and simple to perform in detecting *C. jejuni* antibodies of both IgG and IgM classes. The technique could be valuable for diagnosis of campylobacter infections as well as for epidemiological studies.

Acknowledgements

These investigations were supported by grants from the Swedish Agency for Research cooperation with Developing Countries, SAREC.

References

1. Mentzing, L. -O. (1981). A water-borne outbreak of campylobacter in central Sweden. In this issue, *Epidemiology*
2. McCoy, E. C., Doyle, D., Burda, K., Corbell, L. B. and Winter, A. J. (1975). Superficial antigen of campylobacter (Vibrio) fetus: Characterization of an antiphagocytic component. *Infection and Immun.*, **11**, 517–525
3. Holdeman, L. V., Cato, E. P. and Moore, W. E. C. (ed.). (1977). *Anaerobic Laboratory Manual*, 4th ed. Virginia Polytechnica Institute and State University, Blacksburg
4. Ouchterlony, Ö. (1958). Diffusion-in-gel methods for immunologic analysis. *Progr. in Allergy*, **5**, 1–78.
5. Wadsworth, C. (1957). A slide microtechnique for the analysis of immune precipitates in gel. *Intern. Arch. Allergy Appl. Immunol.*, **10**, 355–360
6. Laurell, C. B. (1965). Antigen-antibody crossed electrophoresis. *Anal.Biochem.* **10**, 358
7. Elwing, H. and Nygren, H. (1979). Diffusion in gel-enzyme-linked immuno-sorbent assay (DIG-ELISA): A simple method for quantitation of class-specific antibodies. *J. Immunol. Meth.*, **31**, 101–107
8. Engvall, E. and Perlmann, P. (1972). Enzyme-linked immunosorbent assay, ELISA III. Quantitation of specific antibodies by enzyme-labelled anti-immunoglobulin in antigen-coated tubes. *J. Immunol.*, **109**, 129–135
9. Elwing, E., Lange, S. and Nygren, H. (1980). Diffusion-in-gel enzyme-linked immunosorbent assay (DIG-ELISA): Optimal conditions for quantitation of antibodies. *J. Immun. Meth.*, **39**, 247–256
10. Nygren, H., Hansson, H.-A. and Lange, S. (1979). Studies on the conjugation of horseradish peroxidase to immunoglobulin G via glutaraldehyde. *Med. Biol.*, **57**, 187–191

44
General discussion and editorial comment

Dr Kosunen presented two slides showing the reactivity of sera prepared by immunizing rabbits with formolized or with autoclaved bacteria (16 strains). The sera prepared using formolized strains and tested by slide agglutination against live strain gave strong homologous reactions and a few cross reactions – seven sera reacting only with the homologous strain. Sera prepared using autoclaved antigens did not react by slide agglutination and were tested by tube agglutination or by co-agglutination against autoclaved strains. These sera gave extensive cross-reactions and would be unsuitable for serotyping without further treatment.

The serological response of 53 patients with proven campylobacter infection was also described. Using four reference strains, and both formolized and boiled antigens, 39 patients (74%) had serum titres of $> 1/400$ with at least one antigen. A further nine patients showed a four-fold change in titre between two sera. One patient showed a serological response with his own isolate only and did not react with the reference strains.

The general discussion supported the conclusion that effective serotyping procedures using heat-stable and heat-labile antigens, and utilizing various serological tests, had been developed in a number of laboratories. Concern was expressed over the need for co-operation between the different laboratories involved in serotyping. Comments from several individuals indicated that a significant degree of co-operation was developing, with exchanges of strains and typing sera.

There was interest in the geographical distribution of serotypes and evidence was presented indicating that Canada and Belgium have some common serotypes. However, it appeared that the results from international exchange of strains and sera had not produced enough data to make reasonable predictions concerning distribution of serotypes. This point was of concern to those individuals interested in development of a test for diagnosis of campylobacteriosis in human beings. Such a test would also be of value in veterinary medicine for screening populations of animals. The ELISA test using glycoprotein antigen, as presented by Svedhem et al. (Serology, p. 118) was suggested for this purpose. After some discussion it became apparent that it could not meet this need without a truly 'universal' antigen that would detect essentially all of the serotypes likely to be encountered. This test, or other suitably sensitive serological tests, would be of considerable value but more information is required to select an appropriate antigen pool. Some

GENERAL DISCUSSION AND EDITORIAL COMMENT

participants expressed optimism concerning the possibility of eventually developing a polyvalent-test antigen in view of the fact that some isolates of *C. jejuni* contain a relatively high number of antigen factors. Perhaps a small number of selected strains would represent most of the antigens expressed by *C. jejuni*.

A need for more serotyping with adsorbed sera was expressed. There was agreement that the various heat-labile antigen factors had not been adequately identified as to structural source (flagella or capsule). Research on this problem is in progress. Very little information was available concerning the antigenic relationships between *C. jejuni* and *C. coli*.

45
Round table discussion on antigen typing

Chairman: R. A. FELDMAN

In an attempt to establish international collaboration and to coordinate efforts a group of people who were directly involved in the serotyping of campylobacters met to discuss the various antigen typing schemes.

It was apparent that many laboratories were undertaking antigenic typing of medically important campylobacter. In order to allow easier communication it was suggested that a single laboratory should act as a reference centre within each country. The nominated laboratory would then be responsible for the establishment of serotyping schemes, the storage of reference strains and communication with other reference centres.

The following laboratories were identified as reference centres:

Belgium	– Free University, Brussels
Canada	– Laboratory Centre for Disease Control, Ottawa
Israel	– Ministry of Health, Jerusalem
Scandinavia	– Department of Clinical Bacteriology, University of Göteborg, Sweden
United Kingdom	– Public Health Laboratory, Manchester
United States	– Centres for Disease Control, Atlanta.

It was hoped that further laboratories would be identified as reference centres in those countries where laboratories had developed serological competence and which were not represented at the round table.

W. H. O. has designated the Free University, Brussels, as the international centre for campylobacter study.

It was already clear that an exchange of reference strains had considerable value. To facilitate the information obtained from such exchanges Dr Sabine Lauwers (Free University, Brussels) agreed to request a line-listing of reference strains from certain investigators. This list would also include information regarding the source of the strain and its biochemical characteristics. The circulation of this list would then allow interested investigators to request strains for reference purposes, subject to the restrictions imposed by the original investigator. An updated list of reference strains, including cross-typing results would be circulated by Dr Lauwers. Provisionally each investigator will identify their serotypes using as a prescript a series of 3 letters from their last name, i.e. PEN-1, PEN-2, LAU-1 or LAU-2.

ROUND TABLE DISCUSSION ON ANTIGEN TYPING

Finally it was agreed that a small liaison working group should be established and chaired by Dr Penner.

Participants in the round table discussion

Professor D. W. Lambe
Dr M. Rogol
Dr T. U. Kosunen
Dr B. Kaijser
Dr H. Lior
Dr J. L. Penner
Dr S. Lauwers
Professor J. P. Butzler
Dr R. A. Feldman
Dr D. M. Jones
Dr J. D. Abbott
Dr J. H. Bryner
Dr B. R. Merrell
Dr A. Svedhem
Dr R. Weaver

SECTION V
CLINICAL ASPECTS

Chairmen: J. P. Butzler and K. P. Lander

46	Analysis of a small outbreak of campylobacter infections with high morbidity R. P. Mouton, J. J. Veltkamp, S. Lauwers and J. P. Butzler	129
47	Isolation of *C. jejuni* from babies with or without gastroenteritis N. J. Richardson, H. J. Koornhof and V. D. Bokkenheuser	135
48	*Campylobacter fetus* ssp. *fetus* V. D. Bokkenheuser	136
49	Long term infection with *Campylobacter jejuni* V. D. Bokkenheuser and N. J. Richardson	137
50	Campylobacter enteritis: Epidemiological and clinical data from recent isolations in the region of Freiburg/W. Germany M. Kist	138
51	Susceptibility of *Campylobacter jejuni* to 19 antimicrobial agents F. W. Goldstein, T. Lambert, L. Delorme and J. F. Acar	144
52	Colitis and campylobacter infection – a clinico-pathological study B. K. Mandal	145
53	Campylobacter infections in patients presenting with diarrhoea, mesenteric adenitis and appendicitis A. D. Pearson, D. P. Drake, D. Brookfield, W. G. Suckling, S. O'Connel, M. J. Knill, E. Ware and J. R. Knott	147
54	Incidence and clinical features of campylobacter infection in Alsace Y. Piedmont	152
55	Clinical and laboratory aspects of acute campylobacter infections in children M. Rogol, S. Branski and L. Grinberg	154

56 Resistance pattern of different antimicrobial agents in *Campylobacter jejuni* from man and animals
  R. Vanhoof, H. Coignau, G. Stas and J. P. Butzler 155

57 An epidemiological study of campylobacter enteritis in the Bath health district
  D. G. White and P. Gill 156

58 General discussion 158

59 Editorial discussion 159

46
Analysis of a small outbreak of campylobacter infections with high morbidity

R. P. MOUTON*, J. J. VELTKAMP*, S. LAUWERS†
and J. P. BUTZLER

* *University Hospital, Leiden, Netherlands.* † *University Hospital, Brussels, Belgium. St. Pierre Hospital, Brussels, Belgium*

Several outbreaks of infections with *C. jejuni* have been described[1-4]. In some cases the probable source could be traced[2-4] but usually full documentation of the source of the infection, the infection ratio and complete data on the cause of the infection could not be obtained. Non-pasteurized milk[2,3] and contaminated poultry[1,5], especially inadequately cooked chicken and meat juice of thawed deep-frozen chicken have been suspected and evidence obtained that these were the cause of the infection.

We describe here a small outbreak of *C. jejuni*, which could be traced to undercooked chicken livers, which were consumed at a 'Chinese fondue' meal. Collaboration of all 'victims' of this small outbreak, some of whom were working in our hospital, made it possible to collect data on source, incubation time, clinical symptoms and serotyping.

The outbreak

On December 7, 1979, a company of 19 enjoyed a meal at a Chinese restaurant where a 'Chinese fondue' was served. This meal implies the serving of small pieces of raw meat and fish which should be cooked at the table. Each person is supposed to ensure that adequate cooking of each piece of meat or fish takes place, before eating. In this way fish balls, tahoe, chicken liver, pork liver, porkmeat, beef, fillet de sole and two types of shrimps were served. On the 9th of December several of the people attending the meal had fallen ill with gastroenteritis of varying severity and a protocol was established for analysis of this small outbreak.

METHODS

Bacteriological investigations. Faecal samples were obtained from all person's attending the dinner, on the 10th of December (day 3) or shortly after; the last sample arrived on day 13, but most were collected within 3 days. All samples were cultured for salmonella, shigella and *C. jejuni*. For *C. jejuni* isolation a selective blood agar with antibiotics, incubated at 43 °C in an atmosphere with lowered oxygen tension and added CO_2, was used[6]. About 1 month after the outbreak a second faecal sample, from all patients with previous *C. jejuni* isolations, was cultured.

Serotyping of *Campylobacter* ssp. *jejuni*

Antisera. Rabbit hyperimmune sera were prepared against ten campylobacter isolates[7].

Antigens. Suspensions (McFarland 9) of strains to be typed were heated for 2 hours at 100 °C and subsequently mixed 1:1 with a 10% suspension of washed human ORh– RBC in phosphate buffered saline (PBS). The mixture was then washed three times with PBS and a suspension of 0.5% sensitized human RBC's was prepared.

Reaction. A haemagglutination test was performed in microtitre trays with serum dilutions of 1/5–1/1280. The plates were read after 18 hours at 37 °C.

Serological investigations. Blood samples were obtained from all patients attending the dinner. The day of sampling varied from day 5 to day 11. Four weeks after the dinner a second blood sample was obtained from all persons. Sera obtained from these specimens were stored frozen on the day of collection, until serological investigations could take place.

For antigen, preparation cells were harvested from thioglycollate-sheep blood-agar plates, and suspended in 10 ml formol 0.5% v/v. After 24 hours at 4 °C the cells were washed three times with formol 0.25% v/v and resuspended in the same solution at a density of 8 on McFarland's scale. With these suspensions a tube (H-)agglutination test was performed with serum dilutions to 1/1280. The titres were read after 24 hours in a water-bath at 37 °C.

Clinical data. Information was obtained from all 19 people at the dinner, with regard to the presence of diarrhoea, fever, colon spasms, incubation time and duration of the illness. In addition, data on consumption of the various fish and meat ingredients of the meal was obtained from each individual within 3 days after the meal.

Statistics. Fisher's test on two-by-two tables was used for correlating the consumption of each food item with disease or positive faecal cultures.

RESULTS

Faecal cultures of 15 of the 19 dinner guests yielded *C. jejuni* (Table 1). Only one of these was not ill while one of four people with negative cultures did have diarrhoea. However, the faecal sample of this patient was obtained for examination 13 days after the dinner.

In Table 1 the data on the consumption of two of the food items e.g. chicken liver and pork liver are also given. In Fisher's tests there was a statistically significant relationship (p. 0.04) between consumption of chicken liver and the occurrence of disease (Table 2). There was no significant correlation between

ANALYSIS OF OUTBREAK OF CAMPYLOBACTER INFECTIONS

Table 1 Data on disease, faecal culture and food items of the 19 dinner quests

Pat. No.	Clinical symptoms	Faecal culture	Consumption of food item Chicken liver	Pork liver
1	+	+	+	+
2	+	−	+	+
3	−	−	+	+
4	−	−	−	+
5	+	+	+	+
6	+	+	+	+
7	+	+	+	+
8	+	+	+	?
9	+	+	+	+
10	+	+	+	?
11	+	+	?	+
12	+	+	+	−
13	+	+	+	−
14	+	+	+	?
15	+	+	+	+
16	+	+	+	+
17	−	+	−*	−
18	+	+	?	+
19	−	−	?	?

* Positive for lettuce served with the chicken liver

positive faecal cultures and chicken liver consumption. Of the other food items only the data on pork liver and shrimp consumption are tabulated, but Fisher's tests on the remaining food items also showed lack of correlation with disease.

Of 14 persons who definitely ate chicken liver, only one (no. 3) did not experience symptoms. This person had travelled widely and had experienced travellers' diarrhoea many times, so that immunity may have resulted in the lack of symptoms. There is therefore a high infection/contamination ratio of 0.93. More specific clinical data are given in Table 3. Four weeks after the dinner another faecal specimen of each of 14 of the 15 victims of the outbreak was

Table 2 Correlation between consumption of food item and disease or faecal culture

		Disease +	−	p*	Faecal culture +	−	p
Chicken liver	+	13	1	0.04	12	2	NS
	− or ?	2	3		3	2	
Pork liver	+	10	2	NS	9	3	NS
	− or ?	5	2		6	1	
Red shrimps	+	14	4	NS	14	4	NS
	− or ?	1	0		1	0	

* Fisher's test on two by two tables

Table 3   Clinical data of 15 patients

Clinical data	No. (%)	Mean duration (No. of pat.)
Diarrhoea	11 (73)	
Fever	4 (27)	4.2 days (11)
Cramps	13 (87)	(range 2–14)
Incubation time		3.1 days (13)
		(range 2–5)

examined for *C. jejuni*. Five of these 14 control specimens were still positive (no's. 6, 7, 9, 10 and 16). No correlation with any of the symptoms, incubation time or duration of disease could be found.

The results of serotyping are given in Table 4; apparently identical strains are grouped together. At least seven different types could be identified. Absorption experiments are now being performed to exclude the presence of even more serotypes. We have refrained from assigning numbers (O-types) to the respective strains.

The serological investigations were performed without knowledge of bacteriological data. The results of these tests were disappointing; in many instances the method described did not lead to reproducible results. Therefore these will not be presented in full. In six patients no's. 5, 7, 9, 14, 16 and 17 a four-fold or greater titre rise was observed in repeated tests.

DISCUSSION

We had the rare opportunity to obtain precise data on the morbidity/ingestion ratio of this small outbreak, be it in only a small number of exposed people. This ratio will be dependent on the number of ingested bacteria, but even with a large dose an infection/contamination ratio of 0.93 is remarkably high. The ratio and the data of Table 2 indicate that consumption of chicken liver, served and prepared in the way described, seems to be an almost certain way to contract the disease. This is also in agreement with the findings of Simmons and Gibbs[8] and of Grant *et al.*[9] who found about 80% of chickens to be positive for *C. jejuni*.

Although the liver was undoubtedly cooked inadequately, we assume that bacteria on the surface were killed, so that bacteria within the liver may have been the cause. Alternatively, secondary contamination after cooking (on the plates of the consumer) may have taken place. Since many chickens must have been used to serve livers to 19 people we conclude that the majority of them must have been contaminated, probably via the bloodstream. The data on patient no. 17 suggests that the raw livers were highly contaminated, since this patient may only have been infected by lettuce served with the chicken liver. However as the patient was asymptomatic he may also have been a carrier.

The presence of seven or more serotypes strongly suggests that most, if not all, livers were contaminated from the start and that contamination of all the

Table 4 Titres of haemagglutination reactions with antisera against ten selected strains

AG → AS ↓	8	14	16	5	18	6	11	7	12	1	15	13	9	10	17
14	160	1280	80	320	—	—	—	—	—	—	—	—	—	—	—
6	320	1280	640	320	320	1280	320	—	—	—	—	—	—	—	—
11	160	1280	320	40	640	640	1280	320	320	640	—	—	—	—	—
12	320	≥1280	≥1280	≥1280	≥1280	≥1280	320	≥1280	≥1280	≥1280	—	—	—	—	—
7	≥1280	≥1280	≥1280	≥1280	640	≥1280	320	≥1280	640	≥1280	—	—	—	—	—
15	—	—	—	—	—	—	—	—	—	≥1280	≥1280	1280	—	—	—
13	—	—	—	—	—	—	—	—	—	320	≥1280	640	—	—	—
9	—	—	—	—	—	—	—	—	—	—	—	—	640	320	—
10	—	—	—	—	—	—	—	—	—	—	160	—	640	640	—
17	—	—	—	—	—	—	—	—	—	—	—	—	—	—	≥1280

livers was not due to one or two contaminated livers serving as a source for the others. In this outbreak of campylobacter infection, caused by contaminated chicken, the infection and the features of the outbreak are due rather to a lack of care in preparation than to the spread of a single strain contaminating the meat to be consumed.

References

1. Hayek, L. J. and Cruickshank, J. G. (1977). Campylobacter enteritis. *Br. Med. J.*, **2**, 1219
2. Robinson, D. A., Edgar, W. J., Gibson, G. L., Matchett, A. A. and Robertson, L. (1979). Campylobacter enteritis associated with consumption of unpasteurised milk. *Br. Med. J.*, **1**, 1171–1173
3. Porter, I. A. and Reid, T. M. S. (1980). A milk-borne outbreak of campylobacter infection. *J. Hyg. (Cambridge)*, **84**/3, 415–419
4. Oosterom, J., Becker, H. J., van Noorle Jansen, L. M. and van Schothorst, M. (1980). Een explosie van campylobacter-infectie in een kazerne, waarschijnlijk veroorzaakt door rauwe tartaar. **124**/39, 1631–1634
5. Severin, W. P. J. (1978). Campylobacter en Enteritis. *Nederlands Tydschrift voor Geneeskunde (Amsterdam)*, **122**/15, 499–504
6. Skirrow, M. B. (1977). Campylobacter enteritis: a 'new' disease. *Br. Med. J.*, **2**, 9–11
7. Butzler, J. P. and Skirrow, M. B. (1979). Campylobacter enteritis. Clinics in Gastroenterol, **8**/3, 737–765
8. Simmons, N. A. and Gibbs, F. J. (1979). *Campylobacter* spp. in oven-ready poultry. *J. Infect.*, **1**/2, 159–162
9. Grant, I. H., Richardson, N. J. and Bookenheuser, V. D. (1980). Broiler chickens as potential source of campylobacter infection in humans. *J. Clin. Microbiol.*, **11**/5, 508–510

DISCUSSION

Dr Taylor pointed out that in animal outbreaks of campylobacter enteritis, multiple serotypes are habitually found. Dr Watson asked if more than one serotype was isolated from each patient. In reply Dr Butzler said that this possibility had not been investigated and that *C. jejuni* was frequently isolated from healthy chickens.

47
The isolation of *C. jejuni* from babies with or without gastroenteritis

N. J. RICHARDSON*, H. J. KOORNHOF* and V. D. BOKKENHEUSER†
* South African Institute for Medical Research, Johannesburg.
† St. Luke's Hospital Center, New York, USA

Stools from 111 children up to the age of 2 years together with matched controls were investigated primarily for the presence of *Campylobacter jejuni*. The presence of other possible bacterial pathogens was noted. Of 70 children with diarrhoea, *C. jejuni* was isolated as the only bacterial pathogen from 20 (29%). The recovery rate was similar in two age groups (31% in those between 0–8 months and 26% in those 9–24 months old). In the non-diarrhoeal control group, however, the younger babies showed only a 10% isolation of *C. jejuni* as compared with 31% of those with diarrhoea of the same age ($p = <0.05$).

There was little difference in the isolation pattern of the older children in the two groups (diarrhoea 26% and control group 24%).

Identified strains of *C. jejuni* were recovered from the blood clot and stool of only one child.

All 20 children infected with *C. jejuni* only, had diarrhoea and nearly all vomited. Stools were soft to watery, some were mucoid but blood was rarely seen. All babies showed mild to moderate dehydration and their temperatures were slightly to moderately elevated.

On admission, dehydration was treated immediately. Antibiotic treatment was administered only if the case developed respiratory complications. By the seventh day in most cases, infected patients had made an uneventful recovery and were discharged from hospital.

Of the 34 children with diarrhoea from whom *C. jejuni* was isolated, either as the only pathogen or in association with other possible pathogens, 12 excreted *C. jejuni* 3 weeks later. These were examined weekly until a negative result was obtained from the faeces. One baby boy aged 11 months excreted *C. jejuni* weekly in the initial stages and then intermittently up to 40 weeks, when the last isolation was obtained.

48
Campylobacter fetus ssp. *fetus*

V. D. BOKKENHEUSER

St. Luke's – Roosevelt Hospital Center, New York, U.S.A.

Campylobacter fetus ssp. *fetus* in contrast to *Campylobacter jejuni*, is usually recovered from patients with disseminated infections. It is a comparatively rare condition. Most patients are immunologically compromised. Babies suffering from *C. fetus* ssp. *fetus* are usually premature or born with congenital defects. Virtually all cases of *C. fetus* ssp. *fetus* meningitis occur in this group. Mortality is 50%. Bacteraemia is the predominant feature in all other age groups. The only known predisposing factor in children is malnutrition. Predisposing factors in adults are cardiovascular diseases, malignancies, endocrinological disorders, and hepatorenal disorders. In general, the clinical picture is mild, and often overlooked. The prognosis is good although relapses are frequent. The underlying condition is often terminal. Erythromycin is the choice of drug. It should be given for 4 weeks to prevent bacteriological relapse. The patients form antibodies in high titres provided they are not on antimetabolites.

DISCUSSION

Dr Butzler stated that bacteraemias may occur in up to 50% of *C. jejuni* cases and that some blood isolates previously diagnosed as *C. fetus* ssp. *fetus* have recently found to be *C. jejuni*. Dr Bokkenheuser in reply said that his figure of 90% bacteraemia in *C. fetus* ssp. *fetus* was for infections without accompanying diarrhoea. Professor Mouton describing two cases of *C. fetus* ssp. *fetus* meningitis in newborns reminded the meeting of the presence of centrochromic cerebral spinal fluid as a diagnostical feature of the disease.

In reply to a question from Dr Payne, Dr Bokkenheuser said that the infection in neonatal cases may come from the mother's genital tract, but routine swabbing for campylobacter is unlikely to be rewarding. However, neither Dr Butzler nor Dr Bokkenheuser have been able to isolate campylobacters from the genital tract.

Dr Taylor commented that *C. fetus* ssp. *fetus* infection in cattle is similar to the disease caused by *C. jejuni* except that systemic infection is most frequent in the former.

49
Long-term infection with *Campylobacter jejuni*

V. D. BOKKENHEUSER* and N. J. RICHARDSON†

* *St Luke's-Roosevelt Hospital Center, New York, U.S.A.*
† *South African Institute for Medical Research, Johannesburg, South Africa*

It is generally accepted that patients suffering from acute *Campylobacter jejuni* enteritis cease to excrete the organisms in the faeces within 5–7 weeks. Nevertheless, from a 2-year-old child we recovered *Campylobacter jejuni* at weekly intervals over a 6 month period. The organisms disappeared following erythromycin treatment, but re-appeared again 10 weeks later.

Prompted by these findings, we examined 120 healthy rural school children at regular intervals over a period of 16 months. *Campylobacter jejuni* was isolated intermittently from five of the children for at least 9 months and from three for more than 1 year. Available microbiological techniques do not permit a clear-cut distinction between re-infections and carriers. Epidemiological evidence tends to support the contention that the long-term infected individuals were carriers.

50
Campylobacter enteritis: epidemiological and clinical data from recent isolations in the region of Freiburg, West Germany

M. KIST

Institute for General Hygiene and Bacteriology, Freiburg

The epidemiological features of the campylobacter enteritis are not well understood. Animals, such as cats and dogs, as well as food of animal origin, especially poultry or unpasteurized milk, have been incriminated as possible sources of infection. Little data is available about the role of patients or asymptomatic human carriers as sources of infection or the frequency of person-to-person spread.

We started to look routinely for *C. jejuni* in stools of patients with diarrhoea in 1979.

METHODS

Selection and processing of stool specimens

From December 1979, all soft or liquid stools were cultured for campylobacter using selective culture techniques. The material was directly inoculated onto a yeast-extract cystein blood agar, containing Skirrow-supplement (Oxoid) and growth-supplement (Oxoid). Three 30 µg cephalothin discs were placed in the inoculation area to provide additional selection for *C. jejuni*.

The plates were examined after 48 hours incubation at 37 °C and 42 °C in an atmosphere of 5% oxygen, 10% carbon dioxide and 85% nitrogen. Currently only 42 °C is used as the incubation temperature. Colonies with positive oxidase and catalase reactions were examined under phase-contrast microscopy for typical morphology and motility.

Organisms were considered as *C. jejuni* when they exhibited typical morphology, positive oxidase and catalase reactions, and growth at 42° and 37 °C but not at 25 °C. Further tests, such as growth in broth containing 1%

glycine, for sensitivity against nalidixic acid, growth inhibition by 3.5% NaCl and H_2S production were used as confirmation.

Evaluation of clinical and epidemiological data

Clinical and epidemiological data were obtained in a retrospective study using appropriate questionnaires. A random group of healthy people were interviewed by a local health officer and used as controls.

RESULTS

Frequency, age and sex distribution of campylobacter enteritis infections

From December 1979 to March 1981, 166 cases of campylobacter enteritis were diagnosed by isolation of *C. jejuni* from stool specimens, and in one case from a blood culture. In the same time period *C. fetus* ssp. *fetus* was recovered from blood cultures in only three cases and from a stool specimen in one case of septicaemia.

The average isolation frequency of *C. jejuni* was 4.9% of all diarrhoeal stool samples cultured for campylobacter. Within the first 10 days after onset of symptoms, 90.5% of all campylobacter isolations were made. Two patients had concomitant infections with salmonella and two with shigella.

In 22% of the patients more than one culture was positive for campylobacter. The average excretion lasted 18.4 days, though one patient excreted campylobacter over a period of 58 days. Ten (6%) of the campylobacter infections were probably contracted abroad, predominantly in India and North-Africa. Campylobacter isolations showed a summer peak, most isolations being made during July.

Fifty-three per cent of all patients investigated were male and significantly more males (63%) than females (37%) were infected with campylobacter. Forty-eight per cent of the patients examined came from urban areas and 52% came from rural areas, but the latter group provided 70% of all positive patients.

Table 1 shows the absolute and relative isolation frequencies within different age groups. The highest number of campylobacter isolates was obtained from 0–5-year-old infants, but the infection incidence was highest within 6–10-year-old patients (11.2%) followed by the 11–20-year-old patients (8%).

Clinical features

The evaluation of 114 patient questionnaires is shown in Table 2. The main clinical symptom was diarrhoea (92%). The stools were mostly of watery consistency (77%), mucoid (49%) or bloody (33%). Diarrhoea was usually not seen before the second day after onset of symptoms. Average duration of diarrhoea was 2–7 days. Fever was observed in 69% of the cases followed by

Table 1 Age distribution of campylobacter enteritis

Age groups (years)	Number of patients with campylobacter enteritis (n)	Campylobacter isolation rate (% of stools investigated)
0–5	40	5.3
6–10	21	11.2
11–20	25	8.0
21–30	31	5.1
31–40	16	4.6
41–50	15	4.9
51–60	11	3.6
61–70	2	0.6
71–80	3	1.1
81–90	2	3.4

abdominal pain, predominantly in the lower quadrants (66%). Vomiting was a less frequent symptom, pseudoappendicitis and extraintestinal symptoms such as arthritis or myalgia were only rarely observed. Half of the patients investigated showed a raised erythrocyte sedimentation rate and 31% had leukocytosis. The clinical symptoms showed some interesting age dependent variations (Table 3).

Table 2 Clinical symptoms of 114 patients with campylobacter enteritis

Symptom	Frequency	Symptom	Frequency
Diarrhoea	92	Headache	38
– watery	76	Vomiting	31
– mucoid	49	Myalgia	22
– bloody	33	Arthralgia	16
Fever	69	Appendicitic signs	6
Abdominal pain			
– lower	66	Leucocytosis	31
– upper	64	Raised ESR	60

Table 3 Frequency (%) of clinical symptoms in various age groups

Symptoms	0–5	6–10	11–20	21–60
Diarrhoea				
– watery	65	80	77	82
– mucoid	69	60	15	37
– bloody	42	33	15	37
Vomiting	42	33	38	22
Arthralgia	0	0	8	25
Pseudo-appendicitis	0	20	0	7

Bloody and mucoid stools and vomiting were more frequent in 0–5-year-old infants. Pseudoappendicitis was observed almost exclusively in 6–10-year-old children and extraintestinal symptoms occurred predominantly in adults.

Most infections were self-limiting and antibiotic treatment with erythromycin was only necessary in a few cases. This therapy was unsuccessful in only one case when the campylobacter strain isolated was also erythromycin resistant *in vitro*.

Epidemiological data

To investigate possible sources and routes of campylobacter enteritis transmission all patients were questioned as to the occurrence of enteric infections in their families and contacts, whether they possessed, or had contact with, pets or household animals and their consumption of potentially contaminated food, especially poultry.

The data obtained from the patients was compared with corresponding data from a healthy control group using the four-fold contingency table test (Table 4). Contacts of compylobacter patients had a higher, but statistically not significant, frequency (26%) of febrile enteritis. In six cases, contacts were shown to have positive-stool cultures. Statistically significant differences were seen in connection with the consumption of poultry, particularly broiler chickens, within 48 hours before the onset of illness. Two patients had most probably contracted their campylobacter infection by eating poultry as aircraft-passengers returning from abroad.

Table 4 Frequency (%) of epidemiological data of patients with campylobacter enteritis compared with a control group

Epidemiological data	Campylobacter patients (n = 114)	Control group (n = 90)	Statistical evaluation
Contact with dogs	38	33	n.s.*
Consumption of poultry	22	9	p 0.05†
Illness of contact persons	26	16	n.s.

* Statistically not significant
† Statistically significant (fourfold contingency table test)

Three members of a family fell ill 2 days after consumption of a roasted Christmas goose. There were no statistically significant differences concerning contact with pets, especially dogs.

The epidemiological data from various age groups are shown in Table 5. Enteric infections in contacts occurred most frequently (33%) in the 0–5-year-old patient group. Poultry as a possible source of infection seems to play a special role in 21–60-year-old patients.

Table 5 Frequency (%) of epidemiological data in various age groups (years) compared with a control group.

Epidemiological data	Campylobacter patients (n = 114) 0–5	6–20	21–60	Control group (n = 90)
Contact with dogs	48	57	33	33
Consumption of poultry	19	17	25	9
Illness of contact persons	33	23	25	16

CONCLUSIONS

The data shows that *C. jejuni* is a common enteric pathogen in West Germany, the micro-organism being isolated in about 5% of all cases of diarrhoeal diseases, which is an isolation frequency lower than found in England[6] or Sweden[10] but comparable with those found in Belgium[4] and the United States[2].

Male patients were more frequently infected than females and the 6–20-year-old patients showed the highest infection incidence. Campylobacter enteritis seems to be more common in rural areas than in urban areas.

Despite the previously published associations between infected animals, especially dogs, and campylobacter enteritis[1,7], we were unable to find any statistically significant difference between the patients and a control group with regard to the possession of, or contact with, animals.

Consumption of poultry seems to play a key role as a cause of foodborn campylobacter enteritis, which may reflect the high contamination rate for poultry[3,5,8].

Infants were found to be more involved with person-to-person spreading of infection than adults, which may indicate a higher susceptibility of the infant to enteric infections or that infants are a more frequent source of infection for the rest of the family.

References

1. Blaser, M. J., Powers, B. W., Cravens, J. and Wang, W. L. (1978). *Lancet*, **2**, 979–981
2. Blaser, M. J., Berkowitz, I. D., Laforce, F. M., Cravens, J., Reller, L. B. and Wang, W. L. (1979). **91**, 179–185
3. Grant, I. H., Richardson, N. J. and Bokkenheuser, V. D. (1980). *Microbiol.*, **11**, 508–510
4. Lauwers, S., De Boeck, M. and Butzler, J. P. (1978). *Lancet*, **I**, 604–605
5. Simmons, N. A., De Gibbs, F. J. (1979). *J. Infect.*, **1**, 159–162
6. Skirrow, M. B. (1977). *Br. Med. J.* **2**, 9–11
7. Skirrow, M. B., Turnbull, G. L., Walker, R. E. and Young, S. E. J. (1980). *Lancet*, **I**, 1188
8. Smith II, M. V. and Muldoon, P. J. (1974). *Appl. Microbiol.*, **27**, 995–996
9. Sticht-Groh, V. and Rohland, I. (1979). *Dtsch. med. Wschr.* **104**, 1375
10. Svedhem, A. and Kaijser, B. (1980). *J. Infect. Dis.*, **142** 353–358

DISCUSSION

The means whereby campylobacters were transmitted from cooked chickens to man were discussed. The most likely factors were undercooking particularly of frozen birds and the contamination of cooked foods on uncleaned work surfaces or with uncooked foods.

51
Susceptibility of *Campylobacter jejuni* to 19 antimicrobial agents

F. W. GOLDSTEIN, T. LAMBERT, L. DELORME and J. F. ACAR

Hôpital Saint-Joseph, Université Pierre et Marie Curie, Paris, France

---

Campylobacter jejuni is recognized as a common bacterial cause of gastroenteritis. In a 12-month period, 29 strains of *C. jejuni* have been isolated from stools (28 strains) and blood culture (1 strain) of patients with acute diarrhoea. The minimal inhibitory concentrations (M.I.C.'s) of 19 antimicrobial agents were evaluated on Mueller–Hinton agar after 48 hours incubation at 37 °C under microaerophilic conditions. Erythromycin, rosaramycin and gentamicin were active on all the strains. Nalidi ic acid, sulphonamides, pencillins and cephalosporins, including cefotaxime and moxalactam had a rather poor activity. Tetracycline was effective on all the strains but one (M.I.C. 64 µg/ml). Two strains were resistant to chloramphenicol (M.I.C. 32 µg/ml). All the strains were resistant to colistin, trimethoprim, vancomycin and rifampicin.

52
Colitis and campylobacter infection – a clinico-pathological study

B. K. MANDAL

Monsall Hospital, Manchester, U.K.

Colonic involvement in campylobacteriosis has now been demonstrated by several groups of workers. This paper describes the sigmoidoscopic-and rectal-biopsy appearances in 12 patients who had colitis and campylobacter infection. The classification of rectal biopsies into various diagnostic categories was according to the criteria previously described[1].

The patients could be separated into three clinico-pathological categories. In the primary campylobacter colitis group (Table 1), sigmoidoscopy revealed all grades of severity and contributed little in deciding whether a patient had infective colitis or inflammatory bowel disease. The histological changes varied from typical infective colitis to that of inflammatory bowel disease (IBD).

Table 1 Primary campylobacter colitis (9 patients)

Sigmoidoscopy:	Grade 1 (Oedema/erythema)	3 patients
	Grade 2 (Oedema/erythema/granularity)	3 patients
	Grade 3 (Oedema/granularity/friability)	3 patients
Rectal biopsy:	Infective Colitis	3 patients
	IBD	2 patients
	Non-specific	4 patients

In the second group, the patients had IBD as well as campylobacter infection (Table 2). Campylobacter infection was clearly responsible for causing flare-up of pre-existing inflammatory bowel disease in one patient and his rectal biopsy was characteristic of ulcerative colitis in spite of the superimposed infection. In the other however, the initial clinical presentation and rectal biopsy were suggestive of campylobacter colitis but the subsequent behaviour of her illness and serial rectal biopsies revealed the true nature of her illness.

The patient in the final category (recurrent colitis due to campylobacter infections) was a 14-year-old boy who had 2 days history of bloody diarrhoea

Table 2 IBD with concurrent campylobacter infection

Patient 1: 30-year-old man, diagnosed ulcerative colitis 3 years ago. Remission for 1 year. Presented with 24 hours history of bloody diarrhoea. Sigmoidoscopy – grade 2. Faeces – campylobacter. Settled on erythromycin. Rectal biopsy – ulcerative colitis.

Patient 2: 20 year old girl. Previous health — good.

		Sigmoidoscopy	Rectal biopsy
22.3.79	Bloody diarrhoea of 3 weeks Campylobacter in stool	grade 2	?Infective colitis
30.4.79	Well	grade 1	Infective colitis
16.4.80	Relapse. Stools negative	grade 3	Infective colitis
13.11.80	Relapse. Stools negative	grade 3	Ulcerative colitis

and abdominal pains. Active colitis was demonstrated by sigmoidoscopy, barium enema and rectal biopsy. Campylobacter was grown from his faeces. Intravenous fluids and erythromycin led to rapid recovery. Two years later, the boy suffered a relapse of colitis which initially raised the question of underlying inflammatory bowel disease but faeces again grew campylobacter. Rapid spontaneous recovery followed.

Problems facing the clinician in differentiating primary campylobacter colitis from inflammatory bowel disease with concurrent campylobacter infection is thus self-evident as sigmoidoscopic, barium enema and even histological changes can be identical in the two conditions. The existence of such patients highlights the need for additional studies of the relationship between infection and subsequent development of inflammatory bowel disease.

References

1. Day, D. W., Mandal, B. K. and Morson, B. C. (1978). The rectal biopsy appearances in salmonella colitis. *Histopathology*, **2**, 117–131

DISCUSSION

Asked how patients who were treated with steroids for inflammatory bowel disease, but who were subsequently shown to have concomitant campylobacter infection, fared clinically, Dr Mandel said that his experience with such cases was limited but that all were treated with erythromycin and recovered without incident. Experience however with I.B.D. cases with superimposed salmonella or shigella infections is that they come to no harm in spite of the steroids.

53
Campylobacter infections in patients presenting with diarrhoea, mesenteric adenitis and appendicitis

A. D. PEARSON*, D. P. DRAKE†, D. BROOKFIELD, S. O'CONNEL*, W. G. SUCKLING*, M. J. KNILL*, E. WARE* and J. R. KNOTT †

*Public Health Laboratory, Southampton. † Southampton University Medical School

The relative importance of campylobacter as compared to salmonella and shigella was assessed by a study of faecal specimens submitted to the Southampton Public Health Laboratory. A clinical and epidemiological study was undertaken on patients from whom *Campylobacter jejuni* was isolated. In a second study children presenting with abdominal pain were investigated for evidence of infection with *C. jejuni*.

MATERIALS AND METHODS

Study I

Faecal specimens from 5494 patients submitted to the Southampton Public Health Laboratory from patients with abdominal pain and/or diarrhoea were cultured between April 1977 and October 1978. Fifty-five of those patients from whom *C. jejuni* was isolated were interviewed by a clinical microbiologist or a nurse epidemiologist. Information gained from asking about events which might have significance led to the examination of avian and animal excreta and carcasses, effluents from fields sprayed with human sewage, and water from swimming pools, rivers and the sea.

Study II

Rectal swabs were taken from 251 children presenting to the paediatric surgical unit with acute abdominal pain. *C. jejuni* was found in six children and from these peritoneal swabs and appendix tissue were obtained at laparotomy.

CAMPYLOBACTER: CLINICAL ASPECTS

Histories were taken and recorded as in Study I. Agglutination tests were done with paired sera using the campylobacter strain isolated from the patient.

RESULTS

Study I

C. jejuni was isolated from 117 (2.1%) of the specimens as compared to 95 (1.7%) and 21 (0.4%) for salmonella and shigella respectively. The seasonal variation in isolation is given in Figure 1. This variation did not relate to the number of specimens examined. Peaks occurred in July and August in 1977 and in June, August and November in 1978. Table 1 gives the age distribution of patients from whom campylobacters were isolated in relation to the total number of faecal specimens examined in that age group. Fifty-two per cent of the isolates came from the two age groups 0–9 (27%) and 20–29 (25%).

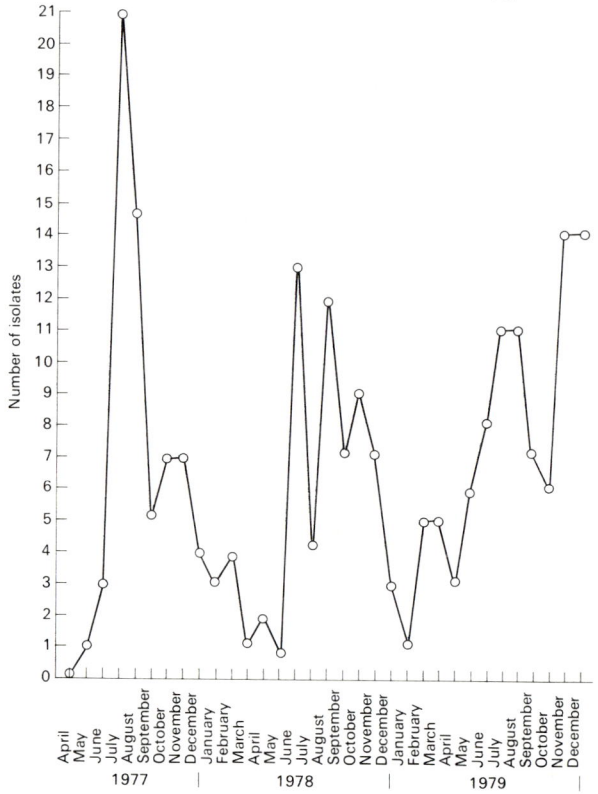

Figure 1 Faecal isolates of heat tolerant campylobacter April 1977–December 1979

During the June 1977 peak of cases, 66% of the cases were in the 0–39-year-old age group. The smaller autumn peak was particularly associated with people who gave a recent history of foreign travel, the majority of whom were in age groups between 10 and 39 (Table 2).

Environmental studies

Epidemiological histories were assessed in 35 patients (Table 3). The results of follow-up sampling from potentially relevant sources are given in Table 4.

Table 1 Age distribution of faecal specimens and campylobacter isolates (Study I, Southampton PHL, 17th April–31st October 1978)

Age group	Faecal specimens numbers	% Total	Campylobacter isolates	% Total	% Campylobacter/ total examined
0–10	1642	29.8	34	26.4	2.1
11–20	628	11.4	19	14.7	3.0
21–30	666	12.1	33	25.6	5.0
31–40	373	6.8	15	11.6	4.0
41–50	340	6.2	10	7.8	2.9
51–60	333	6.1	8	6.2	2.4
61+	734	13.4	10	7.8	1.4
Not known	778	14.2	—		
Totals	5494		129		2.3

Study II

C. jejuni was isolated from six out of 251 children: the findings are summarized in Table 5. Acute appendicitis was confirmed in three cases and mesenteric adenitis found in the others. In the four cases in which sera were available, antibody to the homologous strain was demonstrated.

Table 2 Seasonal occurrence of campylobacter presumed to be imported (Study I, Southampton PHL 1977)

Month in 1977	June	July	Aug	Sept	Oct	Nov	Dec
No. Campylobacter isolates	2	17	14	5	8	7	4
History recent foreign travel	0	2	2	1	3	5	1
% presumed acquired abroad Total	—	12%	14%	20%	38%	71%	25%

Table 3 Epidemiological findings in 55 patients with campylobacter information taken from patient questionnaire

No. of patients	
22	Swimming, paddling pool, fishing, drank raw milk, natural water, camping, trekking and occupation.
10	Sick animals or birds, multiple factors.
3	Sick animals with diarrhoea.

Table 4 Environmental and animal samples relating to the epidemiological histories of patients in Study I

Source	Campylobacter isolations/ total samples
Canary pen droppings	1/1
Pigeon	1/1
Fox	1/1
Horses	0/26
Cows	0/26
Human sewage effluent from fields	0/12
Swimming/Paddling pool water	0/19
Sewage contaminated seawater	6/13
Seawater	0/105
Mud	1/63
Freshwater	56/114

CONCLUSIONS

(1) *C. jejuni* was the commonest intestinal pathogen identified.
(2) Campylobacter enteritis occurs predominantly in the summer and autumn. Cases in summer are predominantly in the 0–39-year-old age group. Campylobacter enteritis in the autumn was associated with a history of foreign travel.
(3) *C. jejuni* infection in children may present with acute appendicitis or with mesenteric adenitis.
(4) Campylobacter infection in man is acquired from a variety of sources.
(5) It is suggested that *C. jejuni* infections in man occur at that time of year when people are on vacation and are involved in outside recreational activities.

It is tempting to try to explain seasonality on the basis of water temperature and its potential consequences, i.e. camping, swimming, drinking, washing etc., in polluted waters. There is however no evidence at the moment to support any

Table 5 Campylobacter from children with appendicitis and mesenteric adenitis (Study II)

Age	Clinical details	Source of campylobacter	Antibody response
10	Acute appendicitis	Rectal swab	320–80
11	Acute appendicitis	Rectal swab	160–20
10	Acute appendicitis and peritonitis	Peritoneal and rectal swabs	
8	Mesenteric lymphadenitis	Rectal swab appendix tissue	
4	Mesenteric lymphadenitis	Rectal swab	320–320–40
10	Mesenteric lymphadenitis Diarrhoea	Appendix tissue	320

of these factors. Blaser[1] found a marked relationship between water temperature and the isolation rate of campylobacters. Knill et al.[2], however, found no seasonal variation in isolation rates of campylobacter in polluted waters around Southampton.

References

1. Blaser, M. J., Hardesty, H. L., Powers, B. and Wang, W.- LL. (1980). Survival of *campylobacter fetus* subsp. *jejuni* in biological milieus. *J. Clin. Microbiol.*, **11**, 309–313
2. Knill, M., Suckling, W. G. and Pearson, A. D. (1978). Environmental isolation of heat-tolerant campylobacter in the Southampton area. *Lancet*, **ii**, 1002–1003

DISCUSSION

Dr Butzler noted that the 21–30-year-old age group included these people who travelled most but Dr Pearson said that in this group there was no significant history of recent travel. There was considerable discussion on the relevance of seasonality in campylobacter infections especially in relation to water, drinking and recreation, as a source of infection.

54
Incidence and clinical features of campylobacter infection in Alsace

Y. PIEMONT

Faculté de Médecine, Strasbourg, France

In 1972, Dekeyser and Butzler[1] isolated *C. jejuni* from stool specimens of two patients. Since then, many reports indicate that *C. jejuni* is one of the most common bacterial causes of gastroenteritis. As the incidence of this infection in France is not known, we examined 39 000 stool specimens for *C. jejuni* over a 2-year period. The majority of these specimens were obtained from hospital patients. During these investigations 231 strains of *C. jejuni* were isolated from 172 patients. In the same period, we isolated 897 salmonellas, 200 enteropathogenic *E. coli* in children, 89 shigellas, 35 *Yersinia enterocolitica* and one *Vibrio el tor*. *C. jejuni* is, therefore, one of the most frequently encountered enteropathogenic bacteria in our region. Eighty-one per cent of our patients were under 15 years old. In adults, men and women were equally infected, while 59% of the infected children were boys. In the children, *C. jejuni* was associated with other intestinal pathogenic agents (salmonella, enteropathogenic *E. coli*, shigella, lamblia) in 13% of the cases, while this was less frequently observed in adults (3% of the cases).

Rotaviruses were not found in any of the 16 stool specimens positive for *C. jejuni*.

Symptomatic patients infected by *C. jejuni* only, had, in decreasing frequency, diarrhoea (72%), abdominal pain (54%), fever (32%), nausea or vomiting (15%) and rectal pain (15%). Rectal pain was more frequent in children (18%) than in adults (6%). Most of these patients were otherwise healthy and their symptoms disappeared spontaneously within a few days with a symptomatic treatment alone. However, in a few cases, antibiotics (aminoglycoside, erythromycin and nalidixic acid) were needed. Three patients, who were not given antibiotics have had up to three relapses of the infection.

Healthy carriers represented 15% of the cases and were infected for a few days. These healthy carriers can infect the neighbouring population and represent a public health problem. Therefore, *C. jejuni* should be looked for in all stool samples.

References

1. Dekeyser, P, Gossuin-Detrain, M., Butzler, J. P. and Sternon, J. (1972). *J. Infectious Dis.*, **125**, 390

55
Clinical and laboratory aspects of acute campylobacter infections in children

M. ROGOL*, S. BRANSKI† and L. GRINBERG†

*Ministry of Health, Jerusalem, Israel. † Bikur-Cholim Hospital, Jerusalem, Israel

The fact that *Campylobacter jejuni* is one of the aetiological agents of diarrhoea in children, is now well established. In this report we present some clinical and bacteriological data concerning 17 cases of infants who have suffered from campylobacter infections.

All 17 cases had severe diarrhoea with liquid stools while six of them had mucus and blood in their stools. Besides diarrhoea, some of the infants suffered from additional illnesses such as pneumonia, otitis media and bronchitis.

Neither salmonella, shigella nor enteropathogenic *E. coli* could be isolated from any of the infants. A modified Skirrow medium (containing 25 iu polymyxin-B sulphate and 5 μg novobiocin per ml) was employed for the initial isolation of *C. jejuni* whose identity was confirmed by well established techniques. Fifteen out of the 17 cultures reacted with the polyvalent antisera prepared by the Central Laboratories, Ministry of Health. The serotyping of the cultures was based upon a provisional scheme of 14 sera: five cultures belonged to serogroup 8 and the others to serogroups 3, 9, 10, 11, 13 and 15.

The blood samples that were obtained from nine patients at 7–10 days after onset of their illness had antibody titres of 1/32–1/128 against the homologous culture.

All cultures were found to be susceptible to the same antibodies: chloramphenicol, colistin, erythromycin, tetracycline and gentamicin, and resistant to cephalothin, and penicillin.

All the infants were treated with erythromycin and the diarrhoea stopped within 5–7 days.

56
Resistance pattern of different antimicrobial agents in *Campylobacter jejuni* from man and animals

R. VANHOOF*, H. COIGNAU†, G. STAS† and J. P. BUTZLER†

Institute Pasteur, Brussels, Belgium. † Department of Microbiology, St Pieters Ziekenhuis, Brussels, Belgium

---

We have compared the *in vitro* bacteriostatic activity of different antimicrobial agents on *C. jejuni* from human origin with their activity on strains from animal origin. The following agents were tested on 426 human strains, 95 ape strains, 65 bovine strains, 107 chicken strains and 9 sheep strains; ampicillin, chloramphenicol, clindamycin, erythromycin, furazolidone, gentamicin and tetracycline. In general the distribution of sensitivities of the human strains was similar to those of the animal strains (total number of strains = 276); i.e. the difference of the geometric mean MIC values was less than one dilution except for ampicillin and clindamycin.

The animal strains had a bimodal distribution for ampicillin, clindamycin and tetracycline. The second peak for ampicillin was mainly due to the ampicillin-resistant ape strains and to a lesser extent to the ampicillin-resistant bovine strains. The tetracycline resistance in the animal population occurred exclusively in the chicken strains. The distribution patterns for tetracycline for the human and chicken strains were similar erythromycin-resistance was also found in chicken strains.

Although there is no substantial evidence from this study, it is possible that animal strains act as a potential epidemiological reservoir for resistant strains.

57
An epidemiological study of campylobacter enteritis in the Bath Health District

D. G. WHITE* and P. GILL†

*Public Health Laboratory, Bath, U.K. † Public Health Laboratory, Dorchester, U.K.

A study was undertaken of 175 consecutive sporadic cases of campylobacter enteritis diagnosed by the Public Health Laboratory, Bath, between January 1978 and July 1979. Clinical and epidemiological information was collected by means of a survey questionnaire, which was completed by an Environmental Health Officer at interviews with the patients (usually within 48 hours of diagnosis). Follow-up samples were collected from confirmed cases at approximately 7–10-day intervals and their household contacts were screened for carriage. Less detailed information from a further 199 patients, diagnosed between August 1979 and November 1980, was obtained from the routine Environmental Health Officer's report. The age/sex distribution of the second group was comparable with the first, and the data from both groups was combined for further analysis.

The laboratory serves a population of around 400 000. About 7000 specimens of faeces were examined annually of which 70% were submitted by general practitioners. Campylobacter cultures were performed using direct plating onto Skirrow's medium and incubation at 42 °C for 48 hours under microaerophilic conditions.

The following findings may be of epidemiological significance:

(1) Campylobacter was the commonest bacterial pathogen isolated.
(2) The peak prevalence was from June–September. The monthly isolation rate of *C. jejuni* varied from an average of 2–3%, to a maximum at the time of peak prevalence of 5–6% of samples tested. The peak prevalence for *Salmonella* sp. was different, extending from July–October. There were smaller peaks of campylobacter both in November and January/February (Figure 1).
(3) The male:female ratio was 1.5:1. The peak prevalence was seen in children aged 1–4 years and young adults aged 15–34 years. A slight excess in both these age groups remains when allowing for the age/sex distribution of the population. Eleven per cent of cases developed

EPIDEMIOLOGICAL STUDY OF CAMPYLOBACTER ENTERITIS

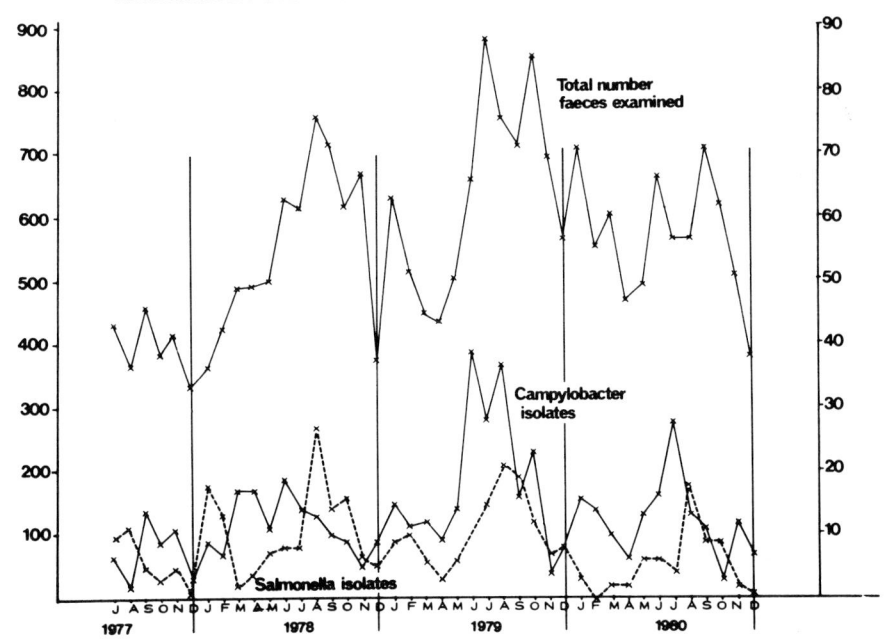

symptoms whilst abroad or within 1 week of returning to the U.K. These cases were evenly distributed throughout the year, and do not account for any of the peaks of prevalence.

(5) 12.5% of cases consumed unpasteurised milk regularly or within 1 week of onset of illness.

(6) 10% of cases drank untreated water prior to illness.

(7) 10.3% of adult cases were employed in the poultry-processing industry, and 8% in the meat industry. The food industry only employs 2.5% of the working population in this area (Population Census 1971–Wiltshire).

(8) Salmonella/campylobacter mixed infections were only seen in three cases – all acquired overseas.

(9) In 9.8% of cases, one or more household contacts were also infected (both cases and carriers). In only 30% of such households was a possible common source suspected (e.g. unpasteurised milk and farm animal contact).

DISCUSSION

Dr Feldman asked what proportion of people in the Bath area drank unpasteurised milk. Dr White could give no data on this but estimated that about 6% of farmers can retail pasteurised milk in that area.

58
General discussion

Dr Kusonen in the course of investigating 600 patients, from whom campylobacter was isolated, found 1–2% had an arthritis. These cases appeared to be reactive and were not septic. A possible relationship to histocompatibility type B27 was suggested, with 12 out of 17 arthritic patients being type B27. The arthritis cured spontaneously after several weeks or months. The 'arthritis' inducing strains were found to be quite different in preliminary serological typing schemes. Interest in common antigens which could produce such immunological responses was expressed.

Erythromycin therapy reduced the average duration of excretion from 10 days to a little over 2 days. Occasional resistant strains were found after treatment.

Dr Butzler referred again to the 24 published cases of meningitis due to campylobacter infections, the majority of which were due to *C. fetus* ssp. *fetus*. There was some discussion on the age distribution of this disease but the majority of cases appear to be in the newborn.

A discussion was initiated on the treatment of campylobacter enteritis with erythromycin. Dr Mandel described a hospital-based trial in which only 40 of 110 patients were included because the disease was so mild, even in hospitalized patients that recovery preceded the report of a positive culture. Dr Butzler commented that although the disease is generally mild erythromycin should be considered for treatment of abdominal pain especially in children. Additionally as erythromycin terminates excretion it should be considered in situations of potential person-to-person spread, i.e. in nurseries, to prevent transmission. However, the relevance of person-to-person transmission in campylobacter enteritis was questioned.

59
Editorial discussion

The clinical presentation of *C. jejuni* infections in humans has been well described in these presentations. Diarrhoea is the most prominent feature of the disease with liquid stools frequently containing mucus, blood and polymorphonuclear cells. The diarrhoea is usually preceded, for about 2 days, by prodromal fever and malaise. Severe abdominal pain is also a feature of the disease occasionally leading to hospitalization and appendicectomy. Although pseudo-appendicitis is the usual diagnosis in these cases campylobacter infections may be associated with mesenteric adenitis and appendicitis (Pearson *et al.*, Clinical Aspects, p. 147). Other clinical symptoms may occur including vomiting, rectal pain, reactive arthritis, hallucinations and convulsions. Disseminated infections rarely occur but bacteraemia may be more frequent than reported, as in animals it occurs within the first 2 days of infection (Taylor, Pathogenesis, p. 163).

Many of these clinical symptoms have been shown to be age related: for example bloody and mucoid stools predominantly occur in the 0–5-year age group, pseudo-appendicitis in the 6–10-year group and the extra intestinal symptoms, like arthritis, in adults (Kist, Clinical Aspects, p. 138). Rectal pain also occurs more frequently in adults (Piedmont, Clinical Aspects, p. 152) while meningitis probably only occurs in the newborn.

Insufficient histological data is available for identification of the disease process in humans. Original reports suggested involvement of the terminal ileum with haemorraghic necrosis but more recent investigations involving sigmoscopy and biopsy (Lambe and Ferguson, Serology, p. 113) indicate involvement of the colon with histological changes varying from typical infective colitis to inflammatory bowel disease (Mandal, Clinical Aspects, p. 145). The application of some of the recently developed immunoperoxidase techniques to the identification of antigens in paraffin-embedded tissue may provide considerable detail regarding association of campylobacter with these intestinal lesions.

Emphasis for further investigation must be placed on the occurrence of asymptomatic infections and the possibility of carriers with long-term, occasionally intermittent, excretion of campylobacters which may be related to immune status (Bokkenheuser and Richardson, Clinical Aspects, p. 137) and who may provide a source of infection and a public health problem.

Some epidemiological data suggests that the clinical symptoms experienced may be related to the pathogenicity of the strain involved (Itoh *et al.*, Geographical Epidemiology p. 5) although host response and dose may also affect the clinical presentation (Mounton *et al.*, Clinical Aspects, p. 129).

The majority of cases of campylobacter enteritis recover spontaneously (General discussion – Clinical Aspects, p. 158) within 2–7 days of the start of diarrhoea. The average excretion period in developed areas is about 18 days (Kist, Clinical Aspects, p. 138) but longer excretion periods are frequently found in underdeveloped countries (Bokkenheuser and Richardson, Clinical Aspects, p. 137). In only a few cases is antibiotic treatment required and the antibiotic recommended is erythromycin. Patients not given antibiotics are susceptible to multiple relapses of infection. Erythromycin resistant strains of *C. jejuni* have been reported (Vanhoof *et al.*, Clinical Aspects, p. 155 and Taylor *et al.*, Molecular Biology, p. 211) and the incidence of erythromycin resistance may be as high as 9%. The erythromycin treatment of patients in outbreaks, as suggested in the General discussion, should be reconsidered in the light of resistant strains.

Considerable epidemiological data is now available from both small point-source outbreaks and sporadic cases which allow definition of the disease process and the population groups at risk. It is apparent from Professor Mouton's fortuitous study and confirmed by Dr Robinson's human experimental study (Epidemiology, p. 274) that the incubation period is 2–3 days. There is obviously considerable controversy about the age peak of prevalence which may be accountable by the communities under study, i.e. their recreational activities, access to raw milk and water, tendency to travel and eating habits.

In summary we are still unaware of the reasons for the considerable variations observed in the clinical disease. However, studies centred on well-defined outbreaks and adequate knowledge of the pathogenic mechanisms and the immunological responses involved may provide some of the answers.

SECTION VI
PATHOGENESIS

Chairmen: Dr S. Dekeyser and Dr D. J. Taylor

60	Natural and experimental enteric infections with catalase-positive campylobacters in cattle and pigs D. J. Taylor	163
61	Experimental *Campylobacter jejuni* infections in calves and lambs B. D. Firehammer and L. L. Myers	168
62	Experimental pathogenesis of *Campylobacter jejuni* enteritis – Studies in gnotobiotic dogs, pigs and chickens J. F. Prescott, K. I. Manninen and I. K. Barker	170
63	Natural and experimental enteric infections with *Campylobacter jejuni* in dogs L. Macartney, I. A. P. McCandlish, R. R. Al-Mashat and D. J. Taylor	172
64	*Campylobacter sputorum* ssp. *mucosalis*, an atypical campylobacter infection G. H. K. Lawson	173
65	Campylobacter mastitis in the cow K. P. Lander	175
66	Fetopathogenicity of *Campylobacter jejuni* in sheep I. G. Shaw and M. Ansfield	177
67	Onset of resistance to pathogenic strains of *Campylobacter jejuni* in the chicken embryo J. A. Davidson and J. B. Solomon	178
68	Experimental *Campylobacter jejuni* infection in rhesus monkeys R. B. Fitzgeorge, A. Baskerville and K. P. Lander	180
69	Pathogenesis of campylobacter enteritis: animal model S. L. Welkos	182

CAMPYLOBACTER: PATHOGENESIS

70 Experimental morphology and colonization of the mouse intestine by *Campylobacter jejuni*
B. R. Merrell, R. I. Walker and J. C. Collbaugh 183

71 Intestinal colonization of neonatal animals by *Campylobacter jejuni*
L. H. Field, J. L. Underwood, L. M. Pope and L. J. Berry 184

72 Endotoxin-like activity associated with heat-killed organisms of the genus *Campylobacter*
D. Fumarola, G. Miragliotta and E. Jirillo 185

73 Enterotoxin activity of campylobacter species
M. Gubina, J. Zajc-Satler, A. Z. Dragas, Z. Zeleznik and J. Mehle 188

74 Pathogenicity of *Campylobacter jejuni* – An *in vitro* model of adhesion and invasion?
D. G. Newell and A. D. Pearson 196

75 General discussion 200

76 Editorial discussion 202

60
Natural and experimental enteric infections with catalase-positive campylobacters in cattle and pigs

D. J. TAYLOR

University of Glasgow, Veterinary School

Studies of the bacteria associated with enteric lesions in cattle and pigs have been carried out at Glasgow University Veterinary School. Catalase positive campylobacters were isolated from inflammatory lesions and, at times, from grossly normal mucosa[1]. Isolation was carried out using samples of mucosa obtained by shearing the lumenal surface and culturing on 7% horseblood-agar plates with or without Oxoid campylobacter supplement SR69 and incubation under microaerophilic conditions. Campylobacters were isolated most frequently from the ileal region of the intestine. All campylobacters isolated from the enteric lesions in cattle were catalase positive and were identified as *C. jejuni*, *C. fetus* ssp. *fetus* or *C. fecalis*, however some remained unclassified. The lesions from which the different species were isolated could not be differentiated and on some occasions more than one type of campylobacter was isolated from the same area of affected mucosa (*C. fecalis* and *C. jejuni*) or from different regions of the same alimentary tract (*C. fetus* ssp. *fetus* and *C. jejuni*).

Campylobacters isolated from the pig were found primarily in the ileum and were especially common in piglets with diarrhoea of 3 days to 3 weeks of age.

In both cattle and pigs the isolation of large numbers of campylobacters from the mucosa was often associated with gross changes, such as thickening and erythema of the mucosa particularly in the distal portion of the ileum, and enlargement of the mesenteric lymph nodes.

Histological changes such as stunting of the villi, the accumulation of plasma cells and polymorphonuclear leucocytes in the lamina propria, crypt abscesses and massive hypertrophy of the submucosal lymphoid tissue were commonly present in areas from which large numbers of campylobacters were isolated.

A number of other potential pathogens were also present on the lesions, including rotaviruses, coccidia, nematodes and clostridia in cattle and coccidia, cryptosporidia, rotaviruses, coronaviruses, clostridia and pathogenic spirochaetes in pigs.

Although *C. jejuni* (as '*Vibro jejuni*') was recognized as a cause of enteric disease in cattle[2], the isolation of the other campylobacters from lessions of the bovine intestinal tract suggested that they might also be potential pathogens. Therefore, cattle (both ruminating and milk-fed calves) were fed with pure cultures of *C. jejuni*, *C. fetus* ssp. *fetus* or *C. fecalis* in controlled experiments to assess the pathogenicity of bovine isolates of these organisms for that species and to determine the clinical and pathological features of the infection with these organisms.

C. jejuni was fed to three milk-fed calves and six ruminating calves in three experiments[3]. All infected animals developed clinical signs within 1–3 days of inoculation. Clinical signs included elevation of rectal temperature (to 41 °C) and the passage of dark-fluid faeces containing clear mucus and occasional spots of blood. No depression of appetite was noted and rumenal movements were apparently unaffected. *C. jejuni* was isolated from the faeces of all inoculated animals within 24 hours of inoculation and could still be isolated from the faeces of most infected animals 10–13 days post infection. At postmortem examination the changes seen were restricted to the gastrointestinal tract and associated lymph nodes. The small intestine was flaccid and, in its distal portion, thickened with a pale reticulated serosal surface. The mesenteric lymph nodes were enlarged and pale. The contents of the ileum, caecum and colon were generally dark in colour and contained varying quantities of blood-stained mucus. The wall of the jejunum and ileum was thickened and fleshy and there was patchy erythema of the mucosal surface. The mucosa of the large intestine was normal in appearance. Stunting of the small intestinal villi, the presence of inflammatory cells in crypts and in the lamina propria and enlargement of the lymphoid tissues in the submucosal tissues were seen in histological sections and resembled the findings in natural cases.

Curved gram-negative bacteria could be seen in smears of the ileal mucosal epithelium and *C. jejuni* was isolated from the gastrointestinal tract. Large numbers of campylobacters were isolated from the ileum and the organism was also isolated from the gall bladder in some cases. Antibody to the inoculated strain was demonstrated by agglutination tests[4]. Titres ranging from 1:320–1280 were found within 10–20 days of infection. No antibody was detected in the serum of controlled calves although *C. jejuni* was isolated from two of these controlled animals.

In an attempt to determine whether or not bacteraemia occurred, blood was cultured 3 days post-infection, when the clinical signs were most acute, and daily thereafter for 7 days. No organisms were isolated from blood.

Six calves known to be free from *C. jejuni* were infected and one was then killed at 24-hour intervals with appropriate controls. Gross lesions were first present in the calf killed at 48 hours after infection as well as the remaining calves in the study. *C. jejuni* was isolated from the gastrointestinal tract of all infected calves but isolation of campylobacters from lungs, gall bladders, mesenteric lymph nodes and spleens occurred only in the first two animals killed (i.e. 24- and 48-hours post-infection).

No histological changes were noted at 24-hours post-infection, but at 48-hours post-infection inflammation of the mucosa became evident beginning with crypt abscesses and polymorph accumulation until, at 4 and 5 days post-infection, all features of the natural lesion were present. In silver-stained sections spiral micro-organisms were seen adjacent to the mucosal epithelium and in the crypts of the jejunum and ileum (particularly in animals killed from 48 hours–96 hours post-infection). Invasion of the lamina propria was seen only in the animals killed 72 and 96 hours post-infection.

Isolates of *C. jejuni*, *C. fetus* subsp. *intestinalis* and *C. fecalis* were all found to adhere to isolated brush-border preparations.

These studies suggest that *C. jejuni* infections in cattle are mainly restricted to the gastrointestinal tract, in particular the ileum and jejunum and that extra-gastrointestinal infection only occurs within 48 hours of inoculation. The organism appears to adhere to the mucosal epithelium and invasion of the lamina propria appears to be transient and to occur after clinical signs have appeared.

Using pure cultures of *C. fetus* ssp. *fetus* to infect milk-fed and ruminant calves in controlled experiments the disease produced was clinically and pathologically indistinguishable from that associated with *C. jejuni* infections while cultures of *C. fecalis* caused a similar but milder disease in both milk-fed and ruminant calves[5]. Additionally the rise in body temperature seen in *C. jejuni* infections was less marked in *C. fecalis* infections.

C. coli was isolated from the ileum of unweaned piglets with diarrhoea and from weaned pigs with colitis following drug treatment[6]. An isolate of *C. coli* from an unweaned piglet was used to infect experimental animals in three controlled experiments. Three non-immune piglets produced by hysterectomy and deprived of colostrum were infected in the first experiment. Within 48 hours of post-infection, creamy mucoid diarrhoea containing occasional spots of blood was seen and a rise in rectal temperature occurred. These signs continued until the animals were killed 8 days later. Lesions were most obvious in the small intestine, particularly in the ileum, the contents of which were mucoid, the walls thickened and the mucosa inflamed. *C. coli* was isolated from the lesions which resembled those produced in cattle by oral infection with other catalase-positive campylobacters. No viruses or parasites were identified in either the inoculated pigs or in the controls.

Infection of conventional sucking piglets from a herd in which *C. coli* infection was endemic produced only mild clinical signs. The pathological findings resembled those in the 'non-immune' piglets but were less marked. *C. coli* was not isolated from the faeces of controls until 7 days of age but rotavirus infection was also identified in them.

In conventional weaned pigs no effect on the rate of daily live-weight gain or feed conversion ratio was seen although softening of the faeces was noted on two or three occasions following infection, and lesions resembling those seen in the younger pigs were present. Serum antibody to the inoculated strain could be demonstrated in all inoculated pigs.

The conclusions which can be drawn from these studies are as follows:
(1) Catalase-positive campylobacters can be isolated from lesions both in cattle and pigs.

(2) They are often accompanied in these lesions by other enteric pathogens.
(3) More than one subspecies may occur in the same lesions, e.g. *C. jejuni* and *C. fecalis*.
(4) All of the catalase-positive campylobacters used to infect 'non-immune' natural hosts were capable of initiating clinical and pathological changes.
(5) Following infection of cattle with *C. jejuni* the organism can only be demonstrated outside the gut during the 48 hours post-inoculation.
(6) The mechanism of disease production appears to be associated with adhesion but not to any great extent with invasion of the lamina propria.
(7) Clinical changes attributable to catalase-positive campylobacter infection include low fever, the presence of mucus and sometimes blood in diarrhoeal faeces and inflammatory changes and lymphoid hyperplasia in the small intestine especially in the distal ileum.

References

1. Al-Mashat, R. R. and Taylor, D. J. (1980). *Campylobacter spp.* in enteric lesions in cattle. *Vet. Rec.*, **107**, 31–34
2. Al-Mashat, R. R. and Taylor, D. J. (1980). Production of diarrhoea and dysentery in experimental calves by feeding pure cultures of *Campylobacter fetus* subsp. *jejuni*. *Vet. Rec.*, **107**, 459–464
3. Al-Mashat, R. R. and Taylor, D. J. (1981). Production of enteritis in calves by the oral inoculation of pure cultures of *Campylobacter fecalis*. *Vet. Rec.*, in press.
4. Butzler, J. P. and Skirrow, M. B. (1979). Campylobacter enteritis. *Clin. Gastroenterology*, **8**, 137
5. Jones, F. S., Orcutt, M. and Little, R. B. (1931). Vibrios (*Vibrio jejuni* NSp.) associated with intestinal disorders of cows and calves. *J. Exp. Med.*, **53**, 853
6. Taylor, D. J. and Olubunmi, P. A. (1981). A re-examination of the role of *C.f. subspecies coli* in enteric disease of the pig. *Vet. Rec.*, in press.

DISCUSSION

Dr Blaser enquired about the ages of the calves used in the experimental studies and the criteria used to identify the campylobacter isolates. Dr Taylor replied that the milk fed calves were 3–4 weeks of age when infected and the ruminating calves 3–6 months of age. The clinical signs of infection were indistinguishable in *C. jejuni* and *C. fetus* ssp. *fetus* infections but were less marked in *C. fecalis* infections. The isolates were identified on the basis of the characters described in Bergey's Manual.

Mr David asked Dr Taylor to speculate on the importance of campylobacters in diarrhoea in the field and asked whether he had carried out any epidemiological studies. Dr Taylor replied that in most field outbreaks of diarrhoea other agents such as nematodes, coccidia or viruses could also be isolated. The clinical signs, produced in the experimental calves, would not be significant to farmers observing calves on a high-roughage diet. It was likely that campylobacter infections could contribute faecal blood and mucus and a low fever to other syndromes and that primary, single infections would not be noticed. This probably also applied to campylobacter infection in the pig.

Mr David asked for details of screening of animals for campylobacter infection prior to experimental infection, and queried the effect of hydration of the culture plates used on the size of *C. fecalis* colonies. Dr Taylor replied that faecal samples from experimental animals had been monitored for 1 week prior to infection. No campylobacters had been found, which in his experience, was only a little guide as to the infected status of the animal. The inclusion of controls which were examined at post-mortem was of value in assessing the freedom from infection of the animals used.

Regarding colonial differences between *C. fecalis* and *C. jejuni* since the differences were seen on the same plates, hydration was presumably the same. *C. jejuni*-like colonies could be produced by *C. fecalis* at times. The colonial characters were of value in detecting *C. fecalis* in a mixed culture but individual colonies had to be picked and examined to detect *C. fetus* ssp. *fetus* in mixtures.

Professor Firehammer stated that agar concentration, the basal medium used, and oxygen tension could all drastically influence isolation of *C. fecalis*. He found that *C. fecalis* grew best at concentrations of oxygen of 1%. Dr Taylor used 4% which might explain the colonial differences found.

Dr Stowell asked whether cross-agglutinating antibodies between *C. fecalis* and *C. jejuni* had been found in experiments and for details of the preparation of the antigen used. Dr Taylor said that all sera were examined for agglutinating antibody to the isolate of *C. jejuni* used in the experiments. Antigens were whole-cell formolinized and standardized to Wellcome opacity tube 8. No cross-agglutinating antibody was detected between *C. jejuni* and the other organisms used, and in one study in which control animals were found to carry *C. jejuni*, no antibody to the inoculated strain was detected. In the *C. coli* studies, however, weaned carrier pigs did have low antibody levels of 1:10–1:40 pre-inoculation and in the control group. Infected animals seroconverted to a titre of 1:640. It was not clear whether this represented an anamnestic response or a primary response to infection with a new serotype.

Professor Glynn asked whether any recovered animals had been re-infected with the same strain of organism. Dr Taylor said that this had not been done; the nearest thing to this was the weaned pig experiment in which no, or slight, clinical signs had resulted from the infection of carrier animals but in which pathological changes had been found.

Dr Kosunen commented that he had found transient lung infections with *C. jejuni* in two patients and asked how soon the pneumonic changes seen in the calves had resolved. Dr Taylor said that the pneumonic lesions colonized were pre-existing and that *C. jejuni* had only been isolated from such lesions within 24 hours of infection. It was, however, of interest that the organism could persist even briefly in such a site.

61
Experimental *Campylobacter jejuni* infections in calves and lambs

B. D. FIREHAMMER and L. L. MYERS

Veterinary Research Laboratory, Montana State University, Bozeman, Montana, USA

Faecal samples from 127 diarrhoeic calves, representing 25 herds with enteric disease, were cultured for campylobacter. The samples were suspended in broth, centrifuged, and the supernatant fluid filtered through a prefilter over a 0.65 μm filter. The filtrate was cultured on blood-agar plates containing antibiotics[1]. The plates were incubated under reduced oxygen tension at 25 °C, and at either 37 °C or 43 °C. *Campylobacter jejuni* was isolated from 51 (40%) samples, representing 14 (56%) herds. All isolations were made from plates incubated at either 37 °C or 43 °C. No isolates of campylobacter were made from faecal samples taken from 36 diarrhoeic lambs (selected from 6 flocks with enteric disease) or from 20 healthy lambs (selected from two healthy flocks). *Campylobacter fetus* ssp. *fetus* was not isolated from either calves or lambs. However, retrospective experiments revealed that colony counts of *C. fetus* ssp. *fetus* were reduced by filtration to a greater degree than were counts of *C. jejuni*, which might explain the failure to make isolations of *C. fetus* ssp. *fetus*.

Three cultures of *C. jejuni* isolated from human faeces, one from an aborted lamb and 19 from the faeces of diarrhoeic calves were evaluated for enterotoxin production using the lamb intestinal-loop test. None of the 23 cultures produced distention of loops. Smears and tissue sections from loops containing nine cultures of *C. jejuni* from diarrhoeic calves were compared with control loops injected with sterile broth. Intraluminal leucocytes were markedly increased in six of the loops containing *C. jejuni*: four of these had increased numbers of free epithelial cells, and three contained relatively large amounts of mucus. Necrosis of villus tips and prominent hypercellularity of the lamina propria due to accumulation of neutrophiles were observed in inoculated segments.

Ten isolates of *C. jejuni* were evaluated for enterotoxigenicity with the infant-mouse gastric test[2] with negative results.

Twelve colostrum-fed calves, varying in age from 1–12 days, were fed broth cultures of *C. jejuni*. The dosage varied from 10^8–10^{11} colony-forming units per calf. All 12 calves became colonized with *C. jejuni*. Whilst two of the calves remained free of clinical signs the remainder had either frank blood in the faeces or a positive test for faecal occult blood. Two calves that developed severe diarrhoea were found to be compromised by other disorders at the time of inoculation; one had an umbilical infection and the other had just recovered from cryptosporidiosis, and a third calf developed mild diarrhoea.

Five lambs, between the ages of 12 hours and 3 days, were each given 5×10^9 colony-forming units of *C. jejuni* and returned to the ewes. The faecal samples from all the lambs were positive for *C. jejuni* the day after inoculation and remained positive for the 5–17 days the individual lambs were retained on experiment. None of the lambs developed diarrhoea but the faeces became mucoid and intermittently contained flecks of blood.

The evidence suggests that *C. jejuni* is well adapted to the intestinal tract of the calf, causes enteritis, and under certain conditions may cause diarrhoea.

References

1. Skirrow, M. B. (1977). *Brit. Med. J.*, **2**, 9
2. Moon, H. W., Fung, P. Y., Whipp, S. C., Isaacson, R. E. (1978). *Infect. Immun.* (*Washington*), **20**, 36

A published account of this work can be found in the following paper.

Firehammer, B. D. and Myers, L. L. (1981). *Am. J. Vet. Res.*, **42**, 918

DISCUSSION

Dr Blaser (CDC Atlanta, Georgia) asked Professor Firehammer the ages of the diarrhoeic lambs and whether *C. jejuni* could be detected in the faeces of healthy calves. Professor Firehammer replied that the diarrhoeic lambs sampled were all less than 4 weeks of age. He explained that the faecal samples from diarrhoeic calves had been collected on field trips to herds with diarrhoea problems and that there had been no intention to carry out a survey of the incidence of campylobacter infection. Examinations for the presence of campylobacters had merely been added to existing examinations for enteropathogenic *E. coli* and salmonellae. He was, however, aware that campylobacters could be isolated from clinically normal calves.

62
Experimental pathogenesis of *Campylobacter jejuni* enteritis – Studies in gnotobiotic dogs, pigs and chickens

J. F. PRESCOTT, K. I. MANNINEN and I. K. BARKER

Department of Veterinary Microbiology and Immunology, and Department of Pathology, Ontario Veterinary College, University of Guelph, Guelph, Ontario N1G 2W1, Canada

---

Campylobacter jejuni of human and canine origin were inoculated orally into six gnotobiotically-reared beagle puppies and reactions were compared with two controls. Inoculated dogs developed transient lassitude, inappetance, mild diarrhoea and tenesmus between 36 and 72 hours following inoculation. Pairs of dogs killed 43 hours, and 5 and 7 days after inoculation had lesions limited to typhlitis and colitis. Congestion of the colonic mucosa, associated loss of goblet cells, attenuation and exfoliation of surface epithelium with micro-erosions, hypertrophy of glands and neutrophil infiltration of lamina propria were seen during the acute phase. Less severe surface and inflammatory lesions were evident at 5 and 7 days than at 43 hours, with hyperplasia of the proliferative compartment in the mucosal glands. Campylobacter was recovered at over 10^{10} organisms per gram of colonic content but did not invade the mucosa.

It was concluded that *C. jejuni* caused a mild superficial colitis in the gnotobiotic puppies with associated mild diarrhoea, malaise and tenesmus and that these changes were similar to, but less severe than, those described in cases of campylobacter colitis in man. The organism was not invasive in this model.

Two experiments were carried out in 2–3-week-old gnotobiotic piglets to determine the effect of oral inoculation of pig or human isolates of *C. jejuni*. Isolates colonized the intestine (10^{8-9}/gram of colonic content) but no effect was observed on temperature, behaviour or appetite of inoculated piglets. Piglets were killed at serial intervals; the only gross pathological change was mild mesenteric oedema and a mild increase in fluidity of content throughout the intestine, which was more marked in the second experiment when freshly recovered human isolates were used. Histopathological changes of moderate inflammation were present in the colon of inoculated pigs and were similar to those described in the puppies but were in contrast more transient, being seen only 2–3 days after infection. The increased liquid nature of the intestinal content and associated diarrhoea was observed from the 5th–6th day after infection, in the absence of any histopathological changes.

Two experiments have been carried out to infect 5-day-old gnotobiotic chickens with two human isolates of *C. jejuni*. The organism became established in the intestine but the chickens remained unaffected by their presence. The presence of low-level antibodies to *C. jejuni* may be a significant factor in the failure to produce disease in chickens. Histologically the only feature of note was the increased number of neutrophils in the caecal lamina propria and submucosa. Further studies are planned.

References

Prescott, J. F., Barker, I. K., Manninen, K. I. and Miniats, O. P. (1981). *Campylobacter jejuni* colitis in gnotobiotic dogs. *Can. J. Comp. Med.*, **45**, 377–383

Prescott, J. F. and Bruin-Mosch, C. W. (1981). Carriage of *Campylobacter jejuni* in healthy and diarrhoeic animals. *Am. J. Vet. Res.*, **42**, 164–165

DISCUSSION

Dr Lawson asked whether any change in faecal counts of *C. coli* had occurred in the pig experiments in which delayed fluidity of the faeces had been noted. Dr Prescott replied that either no change, or possibly a slight increase, in numbers had occurred.

63
Natural and experimental enteric infections with *Campylobacter jejuni* in dogs

L. MACARTNEY, I. A. P. McCANDLISH,
R. R. AL-MASHAT and D. J. TAYLOR

Department of Veterinary Pathology, University of Glasgow Veterinary School

---

Campylobacter jejuni was isolated from dogs with naturally occurring enteric disease both alone and in combination with other potential pathogens such as canine parvovirus and coronavirus. The clinical syndrome observed was one of vomiting with diarrhoea and occasional dysentery. Gross lesions consisting of mild hyperaemia and thickening of the intestinal mucosa in the jejunum and ileum and enlarged mesenteric lymph nodes were seen. Histological changes noted included stunting of the small intestinal villi, infiltration of the lamina propria with polymorphonuclear leucocytes and mononuclear cells and enlarged Peyer's patches. These lesions were distinct from those found in animals with virus involvement. *C. jejuni* was isolated from the jejunum and ileum of all dogs examined and from the spleen, liver, gall bladder and mesenteric lymph nodes of some.

Pure cultures of *C. jejuni* of canine origin were fed to four experimental dogs. Watery mucoid diarrhoea occurred in two dogs and soft mucoid faeces were passed by the other two dogs within 7 days of inoculation. The organism was isolated from the faeces of all infected dogs but not from two controls.

At post-mortem examination, lesions resembling those described in the natural infections were seen in the experimentally infected dogs. *C. jejuni* was isolated from the duodenum, jejunum, ileum, caecum and colon in all infected dogs and from the kidneys in two. Campylobacters were not isolated from the controls however agglutinating antibody to *C. jejuni* (titres 1:320 and 1:640) was demonstrated in the sera of the controls. Experimental campylobacter infection in adult dogs therefore appears to be a relatively mild disease.

64
Campylobacter sputorum ssp. *mucosalis*, an atypical campylobacter infection

G. H. K. LAWSON

Royal (Dick) School of Veterinary Studies, Veterinary Field Station, Easter Bush, Roslin, Midlothian

Unlike many campylobacter infections in which the changes in either the genital or alimentary tract are primarily of an inflammatory or a degenerative character, infections associated with *C. sputorum* ssp. *mucosalis* do not have these features but are essentially proliferative in nature.

The organism is also unusual in that its 'normal' habitat appears to be the oral cavity, and infection at this site is distinct from the site at which it is associated with pathological change, the lower intestinal tract of the pig. Both experimental and natural exposure of pigs results in infection of the oral cavity for a similar period of time. Such infections may take place without detectable symptoms or alimentary tract lesions. Oral colonization does not appear to be commonly associated with extensive colonization of the remainder of the alimentary tract and it is exceptional to recover the organism from this latter site in healthy animals.

In intestinal adenomatosis, however, the organism can be recovered in large numbers from the diseased intestine and is often strictly confined to the site of the lesion. The cells involved carry intracellular vibrios and are unusually hyperplastic and immature but healthy. The organisms lie free in the cytoplasm and there is little inflammatory response in the tissues.

Some references to the condition

Rowland, A. C. and Rowntree, P. G. M. (1972). *Vet. Rec.*, **91**, 235
Rowland, A. C. and Lawson, G. (1975). *Vet. Rec.*, **97**, 178
Rowland, A. C. and Lawson, G. (1974). *Res. Vet. Sci.*, **17**, 323

DISCUSSION

Dr Newell asked whether organisms were in the cell, penetrating the cell surface or present in invaginations of the cell surface. Dr Lawson considered that by inference, the bacteria seen were within the cells. Dr Newell then asked whether thorium colloid-labelling of the cell surface glycoproteins had been carried out to establish the position of the organisms. Dr Lawson replied that it had not but that it might be possible to do it on fixed tissue.

65
Campylobacter mastitis in the cow

K. P. LANDER

Ministry of Agriculture, Fisheries and Food, Central Veterinary Laboratory, New Haw, Weybridge, Surrey KT15 3NB.

Mastitis in cows has been produced experimentally by inoculating a strain of *Campylobacter jejuni* originally isolated from the faeces of a child into the udder.

Seven cows were used, two Guernseys and five Jerseys, and ages ranging from 3–10 years. Most were in mid- to late-lactation but two were only about 3 months in lactation.

Thirteen quarters were infected, with doses of approximately 3–1000 organisms but two quarters of one cow were given doses of over 10^9 organisms.

The clinical effects varied from severe mastitis with systemic illness to mild inapparent disease. The appearance of the milk was grossly abnormal in the later stages of the severe cases with the secretion becoming straw-coloured with numerous large clots. In some of the milder cases no abnormalities were seen in the milk, whilst in others only a few small clots were noticed.

At its peak the excretion rate of campylobacters ranged from more than 10^6 organisms per ml of milk, in the severe cases, to as few as 200 per ml. Most of the milder cases had peak excretion rates of about 10^4 per ml.

In some cases, particularly the severe, organisms were excreted for only about a week but in milder cases low-level excretion continued for up to 75 days.

Reference
Lander, K. P. and Gill, K. P. W. (1980). Experimental infection of the bovine udder with *Campylobacter coli/jejuni. J. Hyg.*, **84**, 421–428

DISCUSSION

In his oral presentation Mr Lander added that until 3 months previously there had been no evidence that campylobacter mastitis occurred in the field however the Worcester Veterinary Investigation Centre had isolated large numbers of campylobacters and *Staphylococcus epidermidis* from a sample of mastitic milk. In a further incident, campylobacters had been isolated on two occasions, 12 hours apart, from raw bulk milk from a single farm but that 300 other samplers had been negative. He speculated that an infected cow was present in the herd on those occasions.

Dr Prescott raised the possibility that campylobacters in milk were of faecal origin. Mr Lander said that it was, in his opinion, unlikely that sufficient campylobacters to infect 2000 people could be present in milk without causing changes in keeping quality etc., if they were of faecal origin. He added that in most cases low concentrations of the organisms are normally present in bovine faeces.

66
Fetopathogenicity of *Campylobacter jejuni* in sheep

I. G. SHAW and M. ANSFIELD

Worcester Veterinary Investigation Centre

A strain of *C. jejuni* (11384), recovered from an outbreak of ovine abortion and from the farmer[1] who attended the flock, was used to investigate experimental fetopathogenicity in sheep.

Two groups of ten ewes were infected with 2×10^{10} CFU in a milk vehicle at 80 and 120 days post-conception. Sero-conversion occurred in both infected groups but the antibody response appeared higher in the '80-day' group.

In the '80-day' group, campylobacters were recovered only from day 3 to day 4 post-infection (4/10 ewes) whilst in the '120-day' group campylobacters were recovered from day 3 to 3 weeks post-infection (7/10 ewes). In this latter group, campylobacters were also recovered from 3 ewes at parturition and the jejunum, ileum, jenium and gall bladder of 1 ewe at slaughter. Although no abortions were observed two still-births occurred in the '120-day' group.

In the two still-born fetuses cholangitis lesions and lymphoreticular hyperplasia characteristic of campylobacter infections were observed. All other lambs survived the infection but some survivors, especially in the '120-day' group showed a neutrophil reaction in the liver together with lymphoreticular hyperplasia. Only a mononuclear response was observed in the livers of the '80-day' group. Nine out of ten lambs in the '80-day' group showed areas of pumonary collapse which were not artefactual or related to atalectasis. The significance of this lesion is not known.

Reference

1. Duffell, S. J. and Skirrow, M. B. (1978). Shepherd's scours and ovine campylobacter abortion – a 'new' zoonosis. *Vet. Rec.*, **103**, 144

67
Onset of resistance to pathogenic strains of *Campylobacter jejuni* in the chicken embryo

J. A. DAVIDSON and J. B. SOLOMON

Immunology Unit, Bacteriology Department, University of Aberdeen, Aberdeen AB9 2ZD, Scotland

---

Campylobacter jejuni has only recently been implicated as a cause of human enteritis and as yet little is known about the pathology and epidemiology of campylobacter infections.

The chicken embryo was used as a model to study the pathogenicity of two strains of *C. jejuni* which had been isolated from human faeces. The campylobacter were inoculated on the chorioallantoic membrane of the embryo and the recovery of colony-forming units from the heart and liver measured 24 and 48 hours after inoculation. The ontogenetic pattern of increasing resistance, on the part of the embryo, to invasion by the bacteria was studied by inoculation of embryos at different ages from 11–17 days of incubation.

There was a significant decrease in the numbers of campylobacter of both strains recovered from embryos inoculated at 17 days compared with those inoculated at 11 days. This pattern of acquired resistance to infection occurs at the same time as the emergence of lymphocytes and is similar to results previously obtained with certain viruses, bacteria and fungi.

The two strains of campylobacter displayed differences in their ability to invade the chorioallantoic membrane which were most apparent in embryos inoculated at 11 days of incubation. It is hoped to be able to study the pathogenicity of different strains of *C. jejuni* by the inoculation of 11-day chicken embryos.

Reference

Davidson, F. A. and Solomon, J. B. (1980). In *Aspects of Developmental and Comparative Immunology*, Vol. I. (Edited by J. B. Solomon.) pp. 289–294. Pergamon Press, Oxford

DISCUSSION

Dr Taylor asked whether maternal immunity would affect the results obtained in this study and whether the immune status of the eggs used was known. Dr Solomon said that maternal immunity might, indeed affect colonization of the egg and that antibody might be mobilized in the period under consideration. The immune status of the eggs used was not known.

68
Experimental *Campylobacter jejuni* infection of rhesus monkeys

R. B. FITZGEORGE and A. BASKERVILLE

Centre for Applied Microbiology and Research, Porton Down, Salisbury, Wilts

K. P. LANDER

MAFF, Central Veterinary Laboratory, New Haw, Weybridge, Surrey

---

This report describes the experimental infection of rhesus monkeys with a strain of *C. jejuni* originally isolated from an outbreak of diarrhoea and vomiting in children. The aims were to determine whether infection could be established, the persistence and duration of excretion of bacteria, the clinical effects, the sites at which the organisms localized and the lesions produced.

Experimental results show that oral infection of rhesus monkeys with a human strain of *C. jejuni* is possible, although the clinical disease induced was milder than that seen in human infection. However, the rhesus monkey did prove to be a suitable experimental animal for studying the excretion of the bacteria and their distribution in the body.

C. jejuni was isolated from faecal samples of the monkeys at varying times after oral infection but ceased by the 43rd day after infection.

Bacteraemia occurred in most monkeys for the period 1–3 days after infection, but despite the bacteraemia, there was only one isolation from organs not associated with the digestive system. *C. jejuni* colonized principally the duodenum, ileum, caecum, colon, liver and gall-bladder; though in numbers which decreased with time. The only organ colonized at 46 days post-infection was the gall-bladder.

Although lesions attributable to *C. jejuni* were not present in the intestine, small foci of infiltration by polymorphs and lymphocytes, associated with the presence of bacteria were found in livers and bile-duct walls.

The humoral immune response detected was poor but monkeys were resistant to re-infection.

Reference

Fitzgeorge, R. B., Baskerville, A. and Lander, K. P. (1981). Experimental infection of rhesus monkeys with a human strain of *Campylobacter jejuni*. *J. Hyg.* (*Cambridge*), (in press)

DISCUSSION

In reply to questions from Dr Blaser, the authors stated that the monkeys were 1–2 years of age, were culturally negative prior to infection and that the same strain was used to re-infect the two animals used in the re-infection study.

69
Pathogenesis of campylobacter enteritis – animal model

S. L. WELKOS

Eastern Virginia Medical School, Norfolk Virginia

An animal model for the acute enteritis caused by *C. jejuni* would provide a valuable tool for research on the pathogenesis of this disease. The purpose of our research is to develop a model of campylobacter diarrhoeal disease using small laboratory animals. In preliminary studies, outbred mice were inoculated orally with either a human clinical strain of *C. jejuni* or a strain isolated from chicken faeces. Although overt illness was not induced, the organisms colonized the entire intestinal tract and were excreted for at least 48 days after inoculation. Other experiments provided more evidence that *C. jejuni* can colonize mice and is potentially invasive. When *C. jejuni* was injected intraperitoneally, the organism was recovered several days later from the spleen, liver and intestinal tract. Since *C. jejuni* can persistently colonize the intestinal tract of mice, overt enteric disease might be elicited by modifying the parameters of infection or the charactristics of the host. Possible modifications of the murine model was discussed. We are currently examining some of these variables in an attempt to develop a small animal model of campylobacter enteritis.

DISCUSSION

Dr Kosunen queried whether antibody to *C. jejuni* had been present in her mice prior to inoculation as it had been found in mouse colonies in Finland. Dr Welkos said that it had not been detected in her studies.

70
Experimental morphology and colonization of the mouse intestine by *Campylobacter jejuni*

B. R. MERRELL, R. I. WALKER and J. C. COOLBAUGH

Naval Medical Research Institute, Bethesda, Maryland, U.S.A.

A human isolate of *Campylobacter jejuni* (strain 840-Smibert) was inoculated into the upper ileum of laparatomized mice. Mice were sacrificed at intervals, and their ilea and colons examined for *C. jejuni* by electron microscopy and culture. In the ileum at 24 hours, large numbers of bacteria were observed by electron microscopy, and *C. jejuni* was isolated from samples of ileum adjacent to those examined by electron microscopy. By 48 hours post-inoculation, *C. jejuni* was no longer detectable by electron microscopy in the ileum although *C. jejuni* was isolated on culture. After 48 hours no organisms were observed in, or cultured from, the ilea. As *C. jejuni* disappeared from the ileum, there was a corresponding appearance of the organism in the colons of the mice. After 48 hours post-inoculation, dense continuous sheets of organisms were observed on the surface of the colon. This colonization persisted until the termination of the experiment at 21 days with no overt signs of illness in the mice. The organisms appeared in the colon as thin long, slightly curved rods, often paired to give a gull-wing appearance. Controls inoculated with sterile media were uncolonized with organisms of this morphology. In contrast when *C. jejuni* was inoculated directly into the colons of mice, severe necrosis and mucosal degeneration were observed in association with the mats of bacteria at 24 hour post-inoculation.

Attachment of the organisms to the intestinal epithelial cells may be mediated by a capsule possessed by *C. jejuni*, and identified by electron microscopy using ruthenium red staining. The fibrous network observed in the colons of the mice may be remnants of this capsular material since no pili or other attachment appendages have been observed on *C. jejuni*.

These observations in this experimental animal system may resemble the persistence of *C. jejuni* in some described cases of human intestinal infection caused by this organism.

71
Intestinal colonization of neonatal animals by *Campylobacter jejuni*

L. H. FIELD, J. L. UNDERWOOD, L. M. POPE and L. J. BERRY

Department of Microbiology University of Texas Austin

Infant mice were inoculated intragastrically with strain BO216, a human isolate of *Campylobacter jejuni*. At various time intervals post-inoculation, mice were sacrificed, and dilution plate counts performed on segments of the gastrointestinal tract. Mice were uniformly colonized with strain BO216 up to 2 weeks post-inoculation and an appreciable number of mice were still colonized after 3 weeks. The greatest number of organisms (10^7) was recovered from the caecum and large intestine of all animals. The small intestine had from 10^2–10^5 CFU. Colonization of the stomach was not found consistently. Similar results were obtained with infant rats and infant rabbits, but neonatal hamsters were less successfully colonized. Two additional strains AC1 and AC127 were also tested and they behaved similarly in newborn mice. Retarded weight gain was observed in some litters of neonatal mice but this was not found consistently. The association of campylobacters with the epithelial cell surface of the gut of infant mice was studied by using scanning electron microscopy.

(*This poster was displayed in the absence of the authors and was not discussed.*)

72
Endotoxin-like activity associated with heat-killed organisms of the genus *Campylobacter*

D. FUMAROLA, G. MIRAGLIOTTA and E. JIRILLO

Institute of Medical Microbiology, University of Bari, Bari, Italy

INTRODUCTION

Much is still unknown regarding the pathogenetic mechanism(s) involved in campylobacteriosis[1]. There are suggestions that an endotoxin, a possible enterotoxin, and invasive properties may represent causative factors in the variable severity of the illness. Early reports[2,3] rightly pointed out the relevance of an endotoxin or endotoxin-like substance in these bacteria. With the aim of adding to knowledge of the ability of these organisms to produce endotoxin we have investigated various campylobacters for activity in the Limulus gelation assay and the skin reaction in rabbits.

MATERIALS AND METHODS

Micro-organisms examined.
(These were kindly provided by Dr A. D. Pearson, Southampton, U.K. and Dr H. G. D. Niekus, Amsterdam.)

C. sputorum sp. *bubulus* (strain 9977): from genital tract of cattle and sheep
C. jejuni 1 (77/55420): from human
C. jejuni 2 (77/53729): from human
C. coli (IP coli, Inst. Pasteur): from human
C. coli (C Worcester W33): from animal

These micro-organisms were heat-killed by autoclaving for 15 minutes at 121 °C and then suspended in sterile saline at an estimated concentration of 1 × 10^9 organisms/ml.

Limulus gelation assay

Equal aliquots (0.1 ml) of Lysate (LAL, Microbiological Associated) and of killed bacterial suspensions were incubated in screw-capped test tubes (10 × 75 mm) at 37 °C. After 60 minutes of incubation the presence or the absence of a firm gel was observed. A comparative control was obtained using *E. coli* (1028) also at approximately 1×10^9 organisms 1 ml instead of the test organisms. Pyrogen-free saline was used for the negative controls. In further experiments the endotoxin activity of positive samples was determined by multiplying the lysate sensitivity by the reciprocal of the highest positive titre obtained.

Dermal Schwartzman reaction

A sensitising injection of 0.1 ml of heat-killed micro-organisms given intradermally was followed 24 hours later by a challenge injection of 0.1 ml of the same suspension given intravenously. The diameters of the haemorrhagic lesions were measured 0, 2, 5, 6 and 24 hours after the second injection. The areas of necrosis measured at 6 hours were compared with a positive control (i.e. saline suspension of heat-killed *E. coli*) and saline controls were negative or less than 5 mm in diameter on every occasion.

RESULTS AND DISCUSSION

The suspensions of heat-killed strains of campylobacter were highly reactive (firm gel) in the Limulus clotting assay. The suspensions presented a Limulus activity equivalent to 16–32 µg/ml endotoxin compared with 128 µg/ml endotoxin in the *E. coli* suspension (Table 1).

Furthermore, the campylobacter suspensions caused a positive dermal Schwartzman reaction in rabbits: a significant haemorrhagic lesion was observed 6 hours after the second injection. However, the area of skin reaction appeared to be less extensive than that found with the *E. coli* suspension ($p < 0.001$) (Table 2).

Table 1 Limulus gelation assay and endotoxin concentration in suspensions of campylobacters and *E. Coli*

Organism	Bacteria per ml	Strain source	Limulus assay	Endotoxin (µg/ml)
C. sputorum	1×10^9	sheep	+	16
C. jejuni 1	1×10^9	human	+	32
C. jejuni 2	1×10^9	human	+	16
C. coli	1×10^9	human	+	32
C. coli	1×10^9	sheep	+	32
Escherichia coli	1×10^9	human	+	128

Table 2 Skin reaction in rabbits challenged with campylobacter and E. coli suspensions

Organism	Peak area of necrosis (mm) at 6 hours Means ± S.D. (industrial values in parenthesis)
C. sputorum	10 ± 2 (12, 8, 10)
C. jejuni 1	12 ± 2 (14, 10, 12)
C. jejuni 2	11.3 ± 1.2 (12, 10, 12)
C. coli	10.7 ± 3 (14, 10, 8)
C. coli	11.3 ± 2.3 (14, 10, 10)
E. coli	20 ± 2 (22, 20, 18)
Saline	1.3 ± 2.3 (4, 0, 0)

CONCLUSIONS

Since the Limulus gelation assay and the dermal Schwartzman reaction are measures of endotoxic potency, we can confirm previous studies[4,5] suggesting that members of the genus *Campylobacter* possess some of the *in vitro* and *in vivo* classical endotoxic properties associated with gram-negative bacteria. It is suggested that further investigations into the mechanism of the virulence of the campylobacter are required to determine whether endotoxin acts independently of or in conjunction with, other toxic invasive properties.

References

1. Butzler, J. P. and Skirrow, M. B. (1979). *Clin. Gastroenterol.*, **8**, 737
2. Osborne, J. D. and Smibert, R. M. (1962). *Nature*, **195**, 1106
3. Osborne, J. C. (1965). *Am. J. Vet. Res.*, **26**, 1056
4. Winter, A. J. (1966). *Am. J. Vet. Res.*, **27**, 653
5. Smibert, R. M. (1978). *Ann. Rev. Microbiol.*, **32**, 673

DISCUSSION

Professor Hofstadt said that in his paper about the isolation of lipopolysaccharides the previous day (Molecular Biology session) he had shown that lipid A was present. Dr Jirillo agreed that the heat-killed cultures he used also contained endotoxin and considered that good agreement between biological and chemical results had been obtained.

73
Enterotoxin activity of campylobacter species

M. GUBINA, J. ZAJC-SATLER, A. Z. DRAGAS

Institute of Microbiology, Medical Faculty, Ljubljana, Yugoslavia

Z. ZELEZNIK and J. MEHLE

Institute for Microbiology and Parasitology, Biotechnical Faculty, Veterinary Department, Ljubljana, Yugoslavia

---

INTRODUCTION

Enteropathogenic bacteria can be classified into different groups regarding the characteristics of pathogenicity mechanisms.

(1) Local invasiveness is typified by acute shigellosis. The problem is an intense inflammatory process with the production of necrotic plaques, predominantly in colonic mucosa. The invasive capacity is demonstrated experimentally by guinea-pig conjunctivitis[1].

(2) Penetration is a process of mucosal invasion, where the ingested organisms pass through the lamina propria, followed by bacteraemia and the establishment of discrete foci of infection. An example is infection with salmonella or *Yersinia enterocolitica*[2].

(3) Enterotoxicity is a cause of watery diarrhoea without inflammatory reaction of the intestinal wall usually associated with the small bowel. The classic example of this type of diarrhoeal syndrome is infection with *V. cholerae*. Certain strains of *E. Coli* produce heat-labile toxin (LT) which acts like cholera toxin, heat-stabile toxin (ST) or both ST and LT toxins[3]. Enterotoxic activity has been reported in association with other gram-negative enteric infections: klebsiella, enterobacter, proteus, citrobacter, serratia, yersinia sp., aeromonas and pseudomonas[4,5,6]. Heat-labile enterotoxins can be detected by tissue-culture assays or immunologically. Heat-stabile toxins are detected by the suckling-mouse assay, and by increasing skin capillary permeability (PF).

Diarrhoea is one of the most prominent features of the clinical picture of campylobacteriosis caused by *C. jejuni*. Stools can be liquid or mucous and mixed with fresh blood. The patients have pains in the stomach and frequently have an increased body temperature. Other clinical symptoms are less frequent: hallucinations[7], convulsions[8] and meningitis[9,10]. Infection with *C. fetus* ssp. *fetus* may be associated with an intermittent fever, diarrhoea or signs in the central nervous system[11]. Campylobacteriosis is therefore an acute diarrhoeal syndrome which may affect systems other than the GI tract.

Involvement of the gut wall varies from slight inflammation of the ileum and jejunum[12] to haemorrhagic necrosis of the colon[13,14,15].

Strains used

The experiments were conducted using 19 strains of campylobacter of which 13 were *C. jejuni* and six were *C. fetus* ssp. *fetus* types.

(1) *C. jejuni*: eight strains (660, 161, 130, 603, 620, 774, 817 and 533) were isolated from stool cultures of patients with enterocolitis[16,17] and five reference strains (204 and 205 of avian origin, and 4115, Van de Pitte and Edinburgh, of unknown origin).

(2) *C. fetus* ssp. *fetus*: two strains (812 and 052) isolated from blood cultures, one (481) from cerebrospinal fluid[11] and three strains (FII, 369/6 and 33a) of bovine origin.

(3) Control organisms were five strains of *E. coli* and *Shigella sonnei*.

METHODS AND RESULTS

1 Local invasiveness

The strains were tested for local invasiveness in the conjunctival sac of guinea pigs into which a bacterial agar culture was inoculated by loop (Sereny Test). Three to 6 days later, no changes were observed in inoculated animals. Ulceration of the cornea was observed in the control animal which received a culture of *Shigella sonnei*.

2 Enterotoxic activity

In order to detect the enterotoxic activity, tests were carried out with cell-free dialysates using all 19 strains of campylobacters which were grown in a succinate broth[18,19] (Peptone (Tryptone-BIO-KAR) 2%, yeast extract 0.3%, sodium chloride 0.3%, magnesium chloride 0.5% and sodium succinate 0.2%.) The medium was poured into 50 ml tubes, autoclaved for 15 min at 121 °C (final pH 6.8). Culture filtrates were prepared as follows: campylobacter strains were grown for 4 days in thioglycollate medium (fluid thioglycollate medium-Difco). Each strain was inoculated into 50 ml of succinate broth. The bottles were incubated aerobically (without CO_2) in a shaker waterbath at 37 °C for 3 days until the media became turbid. They were centrifuged for 1 hour at 15 000 rpm at 4 °C. The supernatant was filtered through membrane filters (Sartorius 0.22 μm) and the filtrates dialysed, in order to eliminate the sodium chloride and succinate, in dialysis tubes which were then placed under running tap water for 2 days. On the third day they were placed in distilled water at 4 °C. The filtrate was concentrated as follows: polyethyleneglycol (Carbovaks, Fluka AG–S. G. Buchs and P. Schweis,

56928) was diluted with water (1:10) and the dialysis tubes with filtrate were submerged in this for 2 days at 4 °C. In order to reconstitute the substrate (toxin), enough distilled water was added to obtain a tenth of the original volume of culture filtrate, i.e. the toxin was concentrated × 10 as compared to the original bacterial culture filtrate.

Permeability factor (PF)

0.1 ml of campylobacter filtrate was injected intradermally into the clipped skin of an albino rabbit. The results were recorded after 24 hours. The diameter of the reaction produced by *E. coli* filtrate was 10 mm but the sites injected with campylobacter filtrates did not show any reaction.

Heat-stable enterotoxin test

A suckling-mouse assay test[21] was used to demonstrate the heat-stabile enterotoxin. Three- to 5-day-old white mice were inoculated with 0.1 ml of the filtrates using an intragastric catheter. Four mice were used for each test. Four hours later their gut weight was measured and its relation to the weight of the carcasses of all four mice was established. Since a quotient higher than 0.08 was considered as evidence of the presence of heat-stabile enterotoxin, and our results were persistently lower than 0.06 for all campylobacter strains, no evidence of heat-stabile toxin activity was demonstrated.

Heat-labile enterotoxin test

Tissue culture of a clonal line of mouse adrenal cell (Y-1) was used to test for heat-labile enterotoxin[22]. The monolayer culture of adrenal cells was cultivated in Ham's F-10 medium supplemented with 15% horse serum and 2.5% fetal-calf serum on the surface of glass tubes. After 4 days the original culture medium was replaced by 2 ml of fresh medium which contained 0.2 ml of the campylobacter filtrates, for control purposes *E. coli* LT+ and *E. coli* LT− filtrates were tested in the same system.

The morphological changes in the monolayer culture of adrenal cells (Y-1) were observed after 2-, 4-, 6- and 24-hour exposure to the bacterial filtrates. The transformation of cells from flattened to spherical forms was taken as evidence of an LT effect. Strains of *C. fetus* ssp. *fetus* (FII, 481 and 369/6) and of *C. jejuni* (161 and 817) produced the morphological changes in the monolayer of adrenal cells (Y-1) as shown in Figures 1–4.

Tests with heated filtrates (10 min, 100 °C) were performed. The transformation of adrenal cells was minimal or non-existent. The toxic properties of strains 481 and 161 were shown to be heat-labile (Table 1).

CONCLUSION

Heat-labile enterotoxin causing morphological changes in cultures of mouse adrenal cells (Y-1), similar to that caused by *E. coli* LT+ was found in three

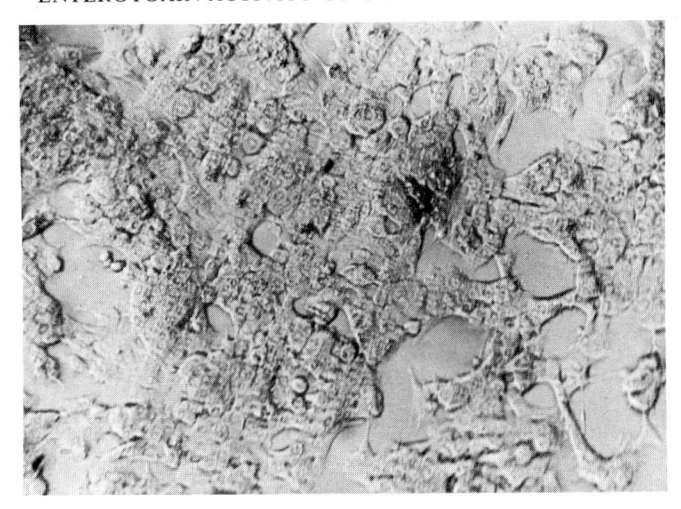

Figure 1 Monolayer culture of adrenal cells Y-1 (ATCC = CCL 79) 4 days old, unstained. Note the flattened epitheloid morphology of the cells. Magnification 500 ×

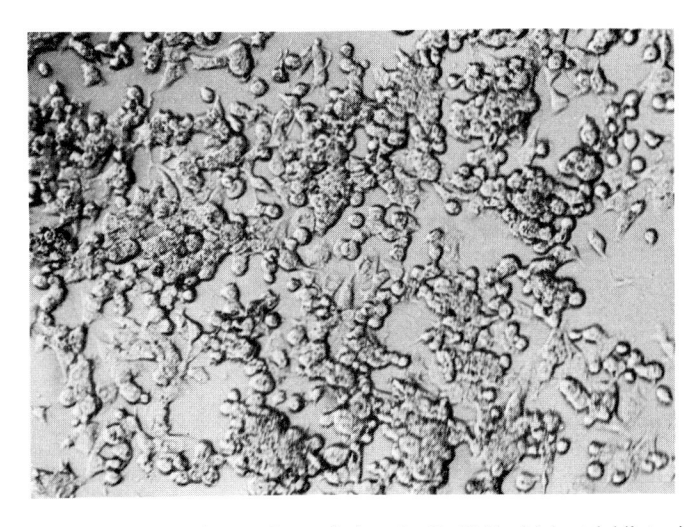

Figure 2 Four-day-old monolayer culture of adrenal cells (Y-1) with heat-labile toxin of *C. fetus* ssp. *fetus* (strain 481), unstained. Note the rounded morphology of the cells. Magnification 500 ×

strains of *C. fetus* ssp. *fetus* and in two strains of *C. jejuni*. Strain 481 was isolated from cerebrospinal fluid of a patient with meningitis. In the patient from whom the strain 161 was isolated, meningitis of unclear aetiology had been diagnosed 2 weeks earlier. The female patient from whom strain 817 was isolated had no neurological problems. However, it is not yet clear whether presence of heat-labile enterotoxin is connected with neurological abnormalities. Research is needed to confirm that these two species produce

CAMPYLOBACTER: PATHOGENESIS

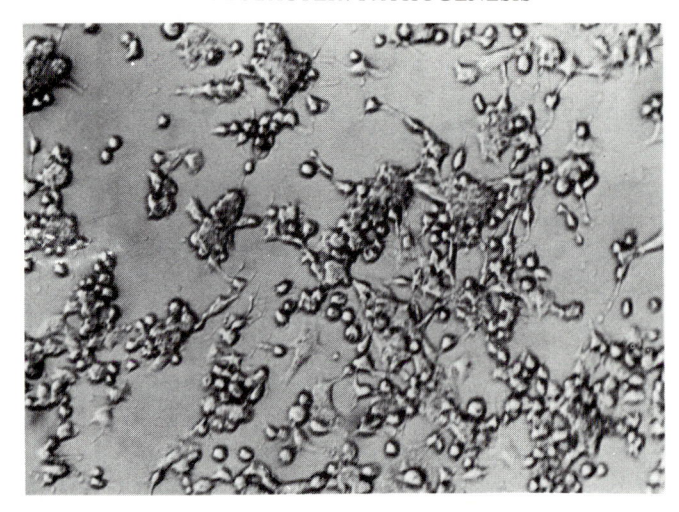

Figure 3 Four-day-old monolayer culture of adrenal cells (Y-1), with heat-labile toxin of *C. jejuni* (strain 161), unstained. Magnification 500 ×

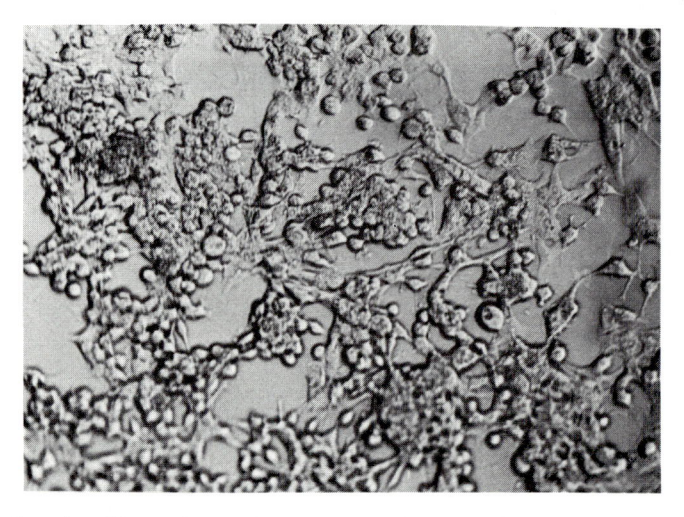

Figure 4 Four-day-old monolayer culture of adrenal cells (Y-1), with LT toxin of *E. coli* (serotype O149: K88, K91). Unstained. Magnification 500 ×

enterotoxin with the classical properties of *V. cholerae* and *E. coli* enterotoxins[6]. In addition the role of plasmids in the transmission of enterotoxic activity of campylobacters has yet to be established.

Acknowledgement

We are greatly indebted to Professor R. E. Weaver of the Center for Disease Control, Atlanta for confirming the identity of strains 812 and 481 *C. fetus* ssp.

Table 1 Enterotoxigenicity and invasiveness of campylobacter strains

Bacteria	ST (suckling mouse assay)	Enterotoxic assay		PF	Invasiveness (guinea-pig cornea cells)
		LT (% of spherical Y-1 cells)			
		Unheated filtrate	Heated filtrate*		
C. fetus ssp. *fetus*					
FII	0,0561	75	NT	—	—
369/6	0,0569	75	NT	—	—
481	0,0518	80	+?	—	—
C. jejuni					
161	0,0539	90	—	—	—
817	0,0450	50	NT	—	—
E. coli					
E-14	NT	NT	NT	+	NT
E-24	NT	50	NT	NT	NT
E-31	0,0604	NT	NT	NT	NT
E-33	NT	—	NT	NT	NT
E-42	0,1038	75	25	NT	NT
Shigella sonnei	NT	NT	NT	NT	+

NT = not tested, ST = thermo-stable enterotoxin, LT = thermo-labile enterotoxin, PF = permeability factor, Y-1 = tissue culture mouse adrenal tumour, − = negative, + = positive, +? = change not clear, * = heated 10 min at 100 °C

fetus and to Professor J. P. Butzler, Brussels for providing the reference strains of *C. jejuni* 4115, Van de Pitte and Edinburgh.

References

1. Sereny, B. (1957). Experimental keratoconjunctivitis shigellosa. *Acta Microb logica (Academiae Scientarium Hungaricae)*, **4**, 367–376
2. Carter, P. B. and Collins, F. M. (1974). The route of enteric infection in normal mice. *J. Exp. Med.*, **139**, 1189–1203
3. Klipstein, F. A., Rowe, B., Engert, R. F. and Short, H. B. (1978). Enterotoxigenicity of enteropathogenic serotypes of *Escherichia coli* isolated from infants with epidemic diarrhoea. *Infect. Immun.*, **21**, 171–178
4. Guerrant, R. L., Moore, R. A., Kirschenfeld, P. M. and Sande, M. A. (1975). Role of toxigenic and invasive bacteria in acute diarrhoea of childhood. *New England Journal of Medicine*, **293**, 567–573
5. Wadstrom, T., Aust-Kettis, A., Habte, D., Holmgren, J., Meeuwisse, G., Mollby, R. and Soderlind, O. (1976). Enterotoxin-producing bacteria and parasites in stools of Ethiopian children with diarrhoeal disease. *Arch. Dis. Child*, **51**, 865–871
6. Wadstrom, T. (1978). Advances in the purification of some bacterial protein toxins. In Jeljaszwicz, J. and Wadstrom, T. *Bacterial Toxins and Cell Membranes*. Academic Press, 9–57
7. Karmali, M. A. and Fleming, P. C. (1979). Campylobacter enteritis in children. *J. Pediat.*, **94**, 527–533
8. Havalad, S., Chapple, M. J., Kahakachchi, M. and Hargraves, D. B. (1980). Convulsions associated with campylobacter enteritis. *Br. Med. J.*, **280**, 984–985
9. Norrby, R., McCloskey, R. V., Zackrisson, G. and Falsen, E. (1980). Meningitis caused by *Campylobacter fetus* ssp. *jejuni*. *Br. Med. J.*, **280**, 1164
10. Thomas, K, Chan, K. N. and Ribeiro, C. D. (1980). *Campylobacter jejuni/coli* meningitis in a neonate. *Br. Med. J.*, **280**, 1301–1302
11. Gubina, M., Zajc-Satler, J., Mehle, J., Drinovec, B., Pikelj, F., Radsel-Medvescek, A. and Suhac, M. (1976). Septicaemia and meninigitis with *Campylobacter fetus* ssp. *intestinalis*. *Infection*, **4**, 115–118
12. Cadranel, S., Rodesch, P., Butzler, J. P. and Dekeyser, P. (1973). Enteritis due to 'related vibrio' in children. *Am. J. Dis. Child.*, **126**, 152–155
13. King, E. O. (1962). The laboratory recognition of *Vibrio fetus* and closely related vibrio isolated from cases of human vibriosis. *Ann. (New York) Acad. Sci.*, **98**, 700–711
14. Butzler, J. P., Dekeyser, P., Detrain, M. and Dehain, F. (1973). Related vibrio in stools. *J. Pediatr.*, **82**, 493–495
15. Lambert, M. E., Schofield, P. F., Ironside, A. G. and Mandal, B. K. (1979). Campylobacter colitis. *Br. Med. J.*, **1**, 857–859
16. Gubina, M. and Mehle, J. (1978). *Examples of human infection with Campylobacter fetus*. XII International Congress Microbiology, Munchen, *Abstracts* p. 179
17. Blatnik-Gubina, M. (1979). Disertacija: *Mikrobioloski vidiki kampilobakterioze pri cloveku*. Univerza V. Ljubljani, 1–127
18. Firehammer, B. D. (1978). Personal communication.
19. Berg, R. L. and Firehammer, B. D. (1978). Effect of interval between booster vaccination and time of breeding on protection against campylobacteriosis (vibriosis) in cattle. *J. Am. Vet. Med. Assoc.*, **173**, 467–471
20. Craig, J. P. (1965). A permeability factor (toxin) found in cholera stools and culture filtrates and its neutralization by convalescent cholera sera. *Nature*, **207**, 614–616
21. Dean, A. G., Yi-Chuan, Ching, Williams, R. G. and Harden, L. B. (1972). Test for *Escherichia coli* enterotoxin using infant mice: application in a study of diarrhoea in children in Honolulu. *J. Infect. Dis.*, **125**, 407–411
22. Donta, S. T., Monn, H. W. and Whipp, S. C. (1974). Detection of heat-labile *Escherichia coli* enterotoxin with the use of adrenal cells in tissue culture. *Science*, **183**, 334–336

DISCUSSION

Dr Lior stated that hundreds of isolates of *C. jejuni* had been tested for enterotoxin or cytotoxin in his laboratory over the preceding 2 years. None had been found. He inquired whether the results could be reproduced using Chinese Hamster Ovary or Vero cells using the casamino acid method of Evans. Dr Gubina said that she had not been able to use these methods and had, herself, been surprised that she had obtained positive results.

Dr Wells asked whether any attempt had been made to neutralize the activity found with cholera antitoxin or anti-heat labile toxin. Dr Gubina said that this had not been done and agreed that it would be of interest. Dr Wells then commented that this would establish whether the effect observed was cytotoxic or due specifically to heat-labile toxin. Dr Prescott said that a graduate student of his had used pig and calf gut-loops and had failed to demonstrate enterotoxin. He had not used Y-1 adrenal cells but doubted that Dr Gubina had detected enterotoxin and thought it more likely to be a cytotoxin. The invasion he had noted in Hela cells could not be detected using the guinea pig eye model. Dr Gubina replied that she had obtained similar results to those found with material prepared from enterotoxic *E. coli* strains and emphasized that the toxicity she had demonstrated was thermolabile.

Professor Butzler then said that when tests for ST and LT toxins were carried out in his laboratory on 700 strains of *C. jejuni* no LT or ST toxins could be demonstrated except on one occasion when ST activity was demonstrated. However, this result could not be repeated. All tests used – suckling mice, Y-1 adrenal cells and Sereny tests – were negative although Dr Newell (Poster 57) and now Dr Prescott had reported invasion in Hela cells and it had been observed in chicken embryo cells. In his laboratory Dr Gubina's strains had also been negative in the suckling mouse and Y-1 adrenal-cell tests. He therefore suggested that the effect observed was cytotoxic rather than enterotoxic.

Dr Gubina agreed that the observed effect was similar to the enterotoxic activity of *E. coli* and she found no changes in suckling mice as shown in Table 1. It is not clear how to reconcile the discrepancy between her and Professor Butzler's results. Possibly her strains had lost the cytotoxicity after several subcultures in the laboratory of Professor Butzler.

74
Pathogenicity of *Campylobacter jejuni* – an *in vitro* model of adhesion and invasion?

D. G. NEWELL and A. D. PEARSON

Public Health Laboratory, Southampton General Hospital, Tremona Road, Southampton SO9 4XY

The mechanism by which *Campylobacter jejuni* infection causes diarrhoea in man is, as yet, unknown but probably involves the production of an enterotoxin and/or destruction of intestinal epithelial cells by a cytotoxin or invasion. The clinical presentation of campylobacter enteritis suggests that the latter mechanism is the more likely as: (i) a high proportion of patients have blood, neutrophils and mucus in their faeces; (ii) fever and malaise generally precede diarrhoea; (iii) there is frequent dissemination to extra-gastrointestinal sites; and (iv) histological examination of fatal cases indicated the presence of haemorrhagic necrosis of the small intestine and numerous hyperplastic mesenteric lymph nodes. However, attempts to demonstrate invasion using the *in vivo* rabbit ileal-loop technique or the Sereny test have, so far, been unsuccessful[1] but invasion of chicken embryonic tissue has been claimed[2].

As the attachment of pathogenic organisms to epithelial cells is a necessary prerequisite to invasion of the intestinal mucosal surface, our preliminary studies have focussed on attempts to demonstrate the adhesion of campylobacter strains to epithelial cells. Two human epithelial cell lines have been used, HeLa 229 and INT 407 (derived from human fetal small intestine). Cells were cultured on 13 mm diameter glass coverslips in Costar 24-well trays with 1×10^5 cells/well, in Eagle's Minimum Essential Medium (MEM) containing 10% fetal calf serum (FCS). After incubation overnight at 37 °C in 5% CO_2 the medium was replaced with HEPES-buffered MEM with 5% FCS and a suspension of the campylobacter strain added (2.5×10^7 CFU/well). The trays were centrifuged at 1200 g for 1 hour at room temperature and incubated at 37 °C for a further 4–18 hours.

The attachment of campylobacters to tissue culture cells was detected by fluorescence microscopy using the Hoechst 33258 staining technique for specific staining of DNA[3]. Our preliminary studies indicate that all the strains tested so far, attach to HeLa 229 and INT 407 cells, after impaction by centrifugation, and that the degree of attachment varies between strains. However, little, if any, attachment was observed without centrifugation. The organisms appear to attach to the spread cytoplasmic areas of the cells and localize in small clumps or along the stress lines. Additional scanning electron microscopic (SEM) studies suggest that the flagella become closely associated with the cell surface during attachment such that they appear to penetrate the cell and are visible just beneath the cell surface (Figure 1). However, the possibility that this is an artefact of the preparation and means of observation cannot be ignored and further investigations are underway to establish the relationship between the flagella and the cell surface.

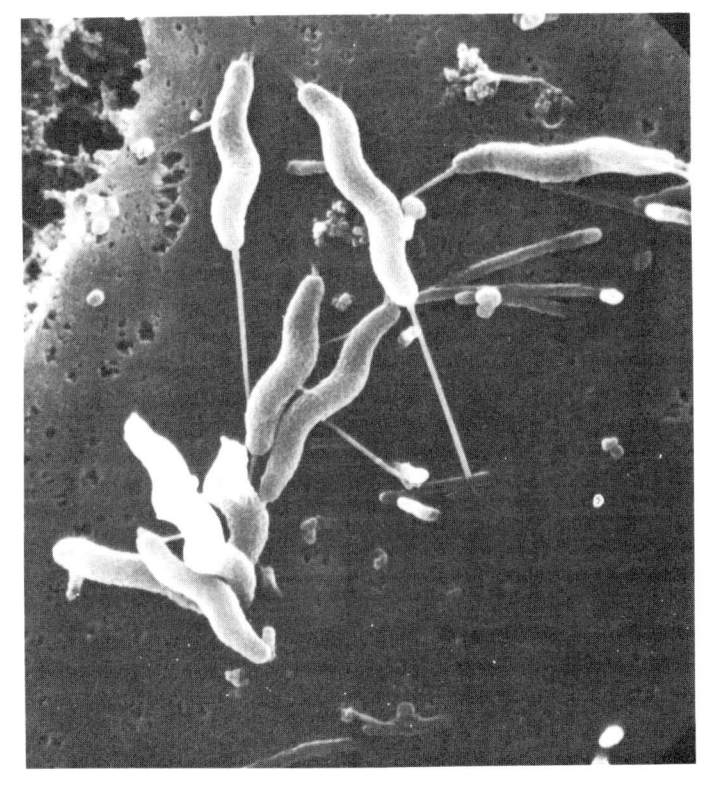

Figure 1 Campylobacter attached to HeLa cells after centrifugation. Note the apparent penetration of the cell surface by the flagella (× 34 000)

After 18 hours in culture, significant numbers of dead and dying cells were observed by SEM, as indicated by the presence of cell-surface blebs, pits and crevices. Cell-surface blebbing is an early indicator of acute cell injury and is usually associated with the presence of a toxic agent[4].

Additionally, by 18 hours, some strains produced elongated forms (10–15 µm) which were found associated with the tissue culture cells. These elongated forms frequently appeared to penetrate the cell surface (Figure 2). It is possible that penetration of, or entrapment in, the cell surface in some way inhibits cell division but it has previously been observed that some strains produce elongated forms, especially in broth cultures. It seems unlikely that invasive properties are restricted only to the elongated form.

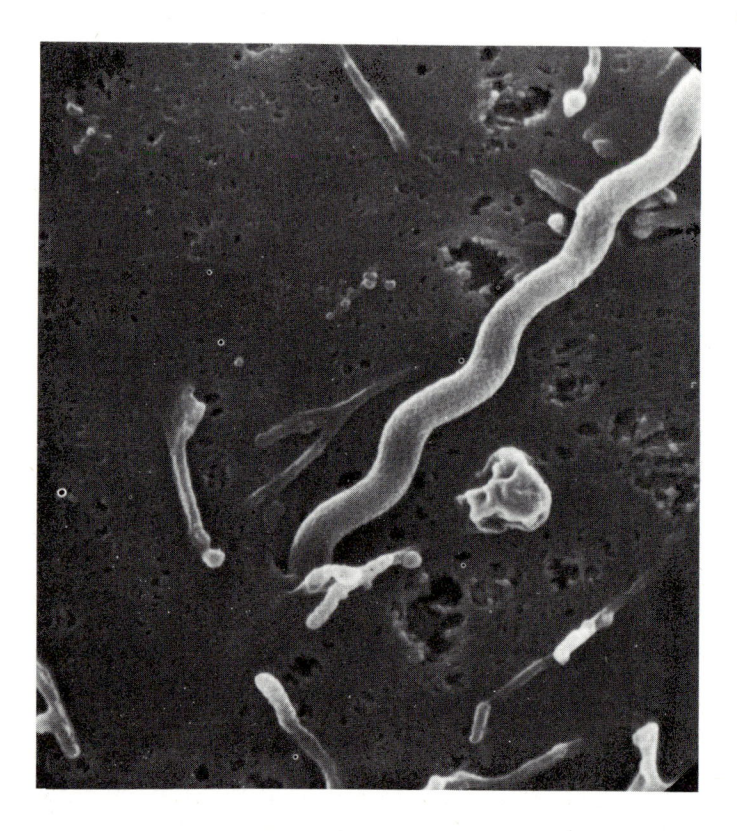

Figure 2 Elongated campylobacter apparently penetrating the cell surface (× 43 000)

Using transmission electron microscopy, campylobacter are observed in the vacuoles of both necrotic and intact cells after 18 hours incubation (Figure 3). Preliminary experiments using colloidal thorium to label the cell surface indicate that this is true internalization of organisms, and not just cell-surface attachment, which strongly supports the suggestion of invasion.

Although *in vitro* models using epithelial cell lines cannot be used to determine directional mobility or penetration of mucus gels by pathogens, provided the appropriate cell-surface receptors are expressed, they will be extremely useful for the quantitative evaluation of bacterial adherence and invasion.

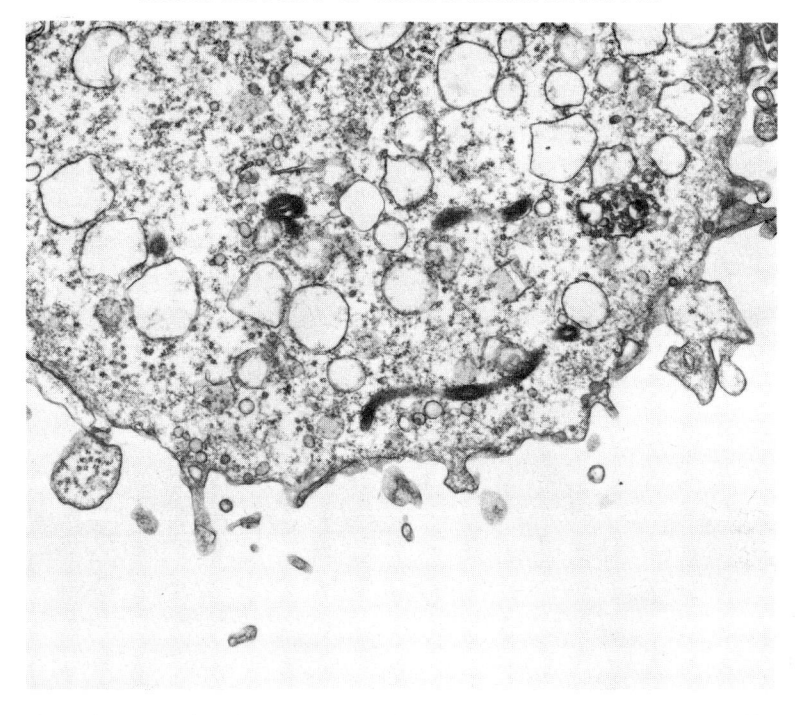

Figure 3 TEM of a relatively intact cell containing two campylobacter (× 22 000)

References

1. Guerrant, R. L., Lahita, R. G., Win, W. C. and Roberts, R. B. (1978). *Am. J. Med.*, **65**, 584–592
2. Butzler, J. P. and Skirrow, M. B. (1979). Clin. Gastroenterol., **8**, 737–765
3. Russell, W. C., Newman, C. and Williamson, D. H. (1975). *Nature*, **253**, 461
4. Trump, B. F., Penttila, A. and Berezesky, I. K. (1979). *Virchows. Arch. B. Cell. Pathol.*, **29**, 297

75
General discussion

Dr Park initiated a discussion on the environmental conditions prevailing in the gastrointestinal tract which allowed the production of large numbers of campylobacters in the faeces. Although some campylobacters, especially the *C. fetus* types, can grow in anaerobic conditions in the presence of substances like aspartate, most campylobacters are microaerophilic, and an adequate oxygen tension would be difficult to achieve in the gut. Small numbers of organisms could presumably grow on the intestinal epithelium and be shed in relatively small numbers but this could not account for the considerable numbers of campylobacters in the faeces. However, it was considered possible that during an increased flow of gut contents associated with diarrhoea the micro-environmental conditions would become less anaerobic providing a greater oxygen tension for campylobacter growth.

An hypothesis could therefore be developed whereby campylobacters attached to the intestinal epithelium could utilize the higher oxygen tension to divide and cause diarrhoea. The enhanced fluid flow through the gut would then cause a significant increase in campylobacter numbers. Such a situation may well account for the observation of systemic infections in humans and animals in the absence of, or preceding, diarrhoea. Additionally the concept implies a background campylobacter infection in man which has not yet been identified. This hypothesis was supported by investigations in pig infections where campylobacter colonization is easily detected in the early stages but is rarely associated with diarrhoea.

The relevance of oxygen tension to campylobacter infections was supported by Dr Telfer-Bruton who noted that fewer campylobacters were isolated from less diarrhoeic stools and that the redox potential was higher in diarrhoeic stools suggesting the presence of a higher concentration of oxygen.

Dr Telfer Bruton also considered the relationships between campylobacter infections and other diseases particularly relevant as 8–10 patients with severe campylobacter enteritis subsequently developed conditions such as Crohn's disease and ulcerative colitis. Some of these patients admitted to symptoms of mild gastroenteric disease prior to their illness and this may indicate some association previously unrecognized.

Returning to the comments about the growth conditions in the gut, Dr Prescott commented that in experimentally infected conventional animals campylobacters were always found in the intestinal crypts presumably because the lumen was anaerobic and the crypts were micro-aerophilic. He suggested that some of the difficulties experienced in establishing an infection in certain animals may have been due to the anaerobicity of the lumen. Following this

GENERAL DISCUSSION

point Dr Taylor said that the gnotobiotic pig gut was considerably less anaerobic than the conventional pig gut, and that *Clostridium perfringens*, an oxygen tolerant anaerobe could grow in the ileum in association with *C. coli*. This may account for the localization of campylobacters in the ileum in the conventional pigs whilst campylobacters occur in the colon in the gnotobiotic pig. Additionally the transient colonization of extragastrointestinal lesions, for example in the lung, may be associated with poor local-blood supply.

Dr Park reminded the meeting that the presence of large numbers of campylobacters in the gut with an essential requirement for oxygen by implication meant that small quantities of oxygen must be present in the gut.

Dr Taylor then suggested that iron might, perhaps, increase the availability of oxygen and that the feeding of blood-rich materials to animals or the leakage of blood into the gut lumen due to gastric ulcers, clostridial or coccidial infections might provide the required environmental conditions.

Finally, Dr Wilson observed that exudate from highly inflamed mucosa contains high concentrations of oxygen and that in such exudates large numbers of campylobacters were demonstrable.

76
Editorial discussion

This workshop primarily discussed investigations into the nature, development and mechanisms of campylobacter infections in animals and the relevance to the clinical situation. The contents of the workshop can be divided into three major, but overlapping areas of investigation: the natural infections, the experimental infections and the *in vitro* and *in vivo* models concerned with the elucidation of the pathogenic mechanisms.

Natural campylobacter infections in animals

The ubiquitous nature of campylobacter infections is a recurrent theme throughout this meeting with isolations from animals as diverse as reptiles and primates. The comparative aspects of these infections has yet to be investigated but in most animals campylobacter infection is associated with a relatively mild, generally enteric, disease usually unrecognized by the farmer and apparently of little economic importance, with the exception of ovine abortion. Despite the frequent observation of asymptomatic infections in domestic animals, little is known of the incidence of such infections or their significance in terms of immune status of the host or relative pathogenicity of the organism.

In man, however, campylobacter infections are usually associated with overt clinical disease, but asymptomatic infections and chronic excretion have been recorded, especially in underdeveloped countries, which may be closely related to the natural animal situation.

The significance of multiple infections in campylobacter enteritis generated considerable interest. The isolation of several campylobacter species from the intestinal lesions of cattle (Taylor, Pathogenesis, p. 163) and the association of *C. jejuni* with other potential enteric pathogens questions the role of *C. jejuni* in enteritis. However, the association of *C. jejuni* infections with other enteric pathogens in man is unusual, although epidemiological evidence suggests an association with salmonella and shigella infections in less developed countries (Richardson, Clinical Aspects, p. 135). Investigations using fresh biopsy material rather than faecal material may contribute to an understanding of the inter-relationships, if any, involved.

Experimental infections

A number of animal species have been infected with campylobacters with variable results. A clearly recognizable clinical syndrome is obtained in cattle infected with *C. jejuni, C. fetus* ssp. *fetus* and *C. faecalis* (Taylor, Pathogenesis, p. 163 and Firehammer and Myers, Pathogenesis, p. 168). Overt diarrhoea was also observed in experimental infections with *C. jejuni* in lambs (Firehammer and Myers, Pathogenesis, p. 168) and dogs (Macartney *et al.*, Pathogenesis, p. 172). However, milder clinical symptoms were observed by other investigators using rhesus monkeys (Fitzgeorge *et al.*, Pathogenesis, p. 180) and gnotobiotic dogs, pigs and chickens (Prescott *et al.*, Pathogenesis, p. 170). Other animals, such as adult and suckling mice or infant rabbits, rats and hamsters showed no obvious symptoms of infection with *C. jejuni* although recovery of the organism indicated that colonization had occurred (Welkos, Pathogenesis, p. 182; Merrell *et al.*, Pathogenesis, p. 183 and Field *et al.*, Pathogenesis, p. 184). Some of the observed differences in results may be due to a degree of species specificity in the pathogenicity of the organisms. In animal infections *C. coli, C. faecalis* and *C. fetus* ssp. *fetus* all appear capable of causing syndromes resembling those produced by *C. jejuni* in their natural host. Investigations on experimentally induced infections with *C. jejuni* which result in less common, but potentially more serious clinical manifestations, such as campylobacter mastitis in cows (Lander, Pathogenesis, p. 175) and ovine abortion (Shaw and Ansfield, Pathogenesis, p. 177) could have considerable veterinary importance in the future.

In vivo and *in vitro* studies of pathogenic mechanisms

Colonization of the intestine follows oral infection with *C. jejuni* on all species so far investigated. In the gnotobiote this colonization appears to occur predominantly in the colon (Prescott, Pathogenesis, p. 170) while in the conventional animal the site of infection is apparently in the terminal ileum (Taylor, Pathogenesis, p. 163). The role of available oxygen may be a relevant factor in the site of colonization as suggested by Dr Park (Pathogenesis – General discussion, p. 200). In those morphological studies of the earliest stages of infection, organisms have been observed attached to the intestinal epithelium using scanning electron microscopy (Welkos, Pathogenesis, p. 182 and Merell *et al.*, Pathogenesis, p. 183) and silver stains (Taylor, Pathogenesis, p. 163. Adhesion to isolated brush borders *in vitro* has been demonstrated by Taylor (Pathogenesis, p. 163) but not by Dijs and de Graaf (Molecular Biology, p. 243). Adhesion to, and penetration of, epithelial tissue culture cells by *C. jejuni* has been reported (Newell and Pearson, Pathogenesis, p. 196). Penetration was similarly observed in the intestinal epithelium of experimental infections of cattle (Taylor, Pathogenesis, p. 16?) and the chorioallantoic membranes of chick embryos (Davidson and Solomon, Pathogenesis, p. 178). The significance of these findings in relation to the failure of demonstrating invasion of the guinea pig cornea using the Sereny method has yet to be established.

The question of the production of an enterotoxin by *C. jejuni* was hotly debated. There appears to be little evidence for the presence of an enterotoxin using the ileal loop technique but biological (Fumarola *et al.*, Pathogenesis, p. 185) and chemical (Naess and Hofstad, Molecular Biology, p. 242) evidence of an endotoxin was presented. The morphological effect of a heat-labile toxin on

Y-1 cells described by Gubina *et al.* (Pathogenesis, p. 188) is unconfirmed by other workers and needs clarification. The cytotoxicity of *C. jejuni* to HeLa and other cells suggests that cell damage may be due to invasion and/or a cytotoxin. This is supported by changes in the gut of experimentally infected calves which suggest both invasion and endotoxin production as mechanisms. After the initial invasion the crypts apparently fill with polymorphonuclear leucocytes forming 'crypt abscesses' and leading to the lymphoid hyperplasia commonly observed in the later stages of disease.

Recovery from infection may occur in several stages. The demonstration of serum antibody to the inoculated strain is concomitant with the limitation of bacteraemia and colonization confined to the gastrointestinal tract. In rare cases, colonization of micro-aerophilic pre-existing lesions like in the lung (Taylor, Pathogenesis p. 163 and Kosunen, Taxonomy and Typing, p. 45) or the uterus or fetus in the sheep (Shaw and Ansfield, Pathogenesis, p. 177) can take place. Mastitis in the cow, however, appears to result from local invasion via the teat canal (Lander, Pathogenesis, p. 175). The level of serum antibody response varies considerably from 1:1280 in cattle (Taylor, Pathogenesis, p. 163) to barely demonstrable in the rhesus monkey (Fitzgeorge *et al.*, Pathogenesis, p. 180) although enteric infection may persist for periods of 30–40 days before the faecal shedding of campylobacters ceases. In a human-volunteer study antibody response, as indicated by raised complement fixation test and agglutination titres, occurred by 10 days after oral infection but there is considerable evidence for large variations in the serological response to *C. jejuni* infection in humans (Jones *et al.*, Epidemiology, p. 276; Mouton *et al.*, Clinical Aspects, p. 129 and Svedhem *et al.*, Serotyping, p. 118).

It is clear that considerably more effort must be put into the investigation of the mechanism(s) of pathogenesis. In particular, the relationship between attachment of the organism to the cell, invasion and cytotoxicity should be studied further in *in vitro* and *in vivo* models. The use of non-pathogenic strains and the development of laboratory animal models producing similar disease to the human will facilitate such studies. The sequence of events leading to recovery and antibody response are also worthy of further investigations especially in relationship to the limitation of systemic spread.

In most animal species oral infection was followed by a short period of 24–72 hours during which the organism could be recovered from sites outside the gut. This may reflect the bacteraemia observed in man during the prodromal phase of infection. Low fever and the presence of blood and mucus in the faeces occur in most animal infections with histological gastrointestinal changes indicative of mild inflammatory response in the ileum and/or colon (dependent on animal model) and lymphadenitis. These changes appear to resemble the situation observed in man at laparotomy though further investigations are necessary on the histological changes occurring in man during campylobacter enteritis. Preliminary studies indicate that the species in which the pattern of changes most closely resembles those in man are the rhesus monkey and dog. The manipulation of experimental animals, i.e. the use of non-immune animals, reduction of competitive gut flora or suppression of immunological responses, may provide more consistent, clinically significant and less expensive animal models.

SECTION VII
MOLECULAR BIOLOGY

Chairmen: A. A. Glynn and
V. Bokkkenheuser

77	Transmissible resistance in *Campylobacter jejuni* D. E. Taylor, S. A. De Grandis, M. A. Karmali and P. C. Fleming	207
78	Erythromycin resistance in *Campylobacter jejuni* D. E. Taylor, S. A. De Grandis, M. A. Karmali, P. C. Fleming, R. Van hoof and J. P. Butzler	211
79	The detection and frequency of beta-lactamase production in *Campylobacter jejuni* P. C. Fleming, A. D'Amico, S. De Grandis and M. A. Karmali	214
80	On the association between erythromycin resistance and the failure to hydrolyze hippurate in *Campylobacter jejuni* M. A. Karmali, S. A. De Grandis, D. E. Taylor and P. C. Fleming	218
81	Ultrastructure and antibiotic sensitivity of campylobacter A. J. Lastovica	221
82	Outer membrane protein composition of campylobacters R. A. Austen and T. J. Trust	225
83	The effect of growth conditions on total protein profiles of campylobacters H. M. McBride, D. G. Newell and A. D. Pearson	230
84	Total protein profiles — a method of identification and classification for campylobacters? B. Veal, D. G. Newell and A. D. Pearson	231
85	Fatty acid composition: a possible tool for typing different campylobacter species J. Johnsson, B. Kaijser and A. Svedhem	233
86	Cellular fatty-acid profiles of campylobacters M. A. Curtis	234

87 Immunochemistry of lipopolysaccharides isolated from *Campylobacter jejuni*
V. Naess and T. Hofstad — 242

88 In search of adhesive antigens on *Campylobacter jejuni*.
F. Dijs and F. K. de Graaf — 243

89 Auto-agglutination of *Campylobacter jejuni*: electron microscopic observations
A. E. Ritchie, J. H. Bryner and J. W. Foley — 244

90 Editorial discussion — 245

77
Transmissible resistance in *Campylobacter jejuni*

DIANE E. TAYLOR*, STEPHANIE A. DE GRANDIS,
M. A. KARMALI and P. C. FLEMING

*Department of Bacteriology, The Hospital for Sick Children,
555 University Avenue, Toronto, Canada M5G 1X8*

Erythromycin, tetracycline and furazolidone, a nitrofuran derivative, have been recommended for the treatment of severe cases of campylobacter enteritis[1,2]. Approximately 20% of *C. jejuni* strains isolated at The Hospital for Sick Children, Toronto, Canada, 1978–79 were resistant to 4 µg/ml of tetracycline and about 12% were resistant to high levels of tetracycline, with a minimal inhibitory concentration (MIC) from 6–256 µg/ml[3,4]. All strains of *C. jejuni* were susceptible to nitrofurantoin, and about 1% of strains were resistant to erythromycin. Resistance to ampicillin at 8 µg/ml was observed in approximately 24% and at 16 µg/ml in 16% of clinical isolates of *C. jejuni*[3].

Approximately 16% of strains produced β-lactamase (see Fleming *et al.*, Molecular Biology, p. 214).

Transmissible tetracycline resistance in *C. jejuni*

Resistance to tetracycline is plasmid-mediated in *C. jejuni* and intraspecies transfer, as well as interspecies transfer, to *C. fetus* was demonstrated[4,5]. Intraspecies transfer was compared at 42 °C by liquid- and filter-mating methods using strain MK22, a tetracycline-resistant isolate of *C. jejuni* (MIC of tetracycline = 128 µg/ml) as the donor strain of *C. jejuni* SD2, and a nalidixic acid-resistant mutant (MIC of nalidixic acid = 256 µg/ml) as the recipient strain. Transconjugants were selected on Diagnostic Sensitivity Testing agar (DST, Oxoid) containing 5% lysed horse blood, 50 µg/ml nalidixic acid and 16 µg/ml tetracycline. The filter-mating procedure gave approximately one-hundred-fold higher frequency of transfer than the liquid-mating method (5.0 × 10⁻⁴ transconjugants per recipient compared with 2.4 × 10⁻⁶ in a 48-hour mating period). The effect of temperature on transfer was tested by performing experiments at 37 °C and 42 °C, but there was no significant difference in the transfer frequency of tetracycline resistance when the temperature was reduced. Since the tetracycline resistance determinant appeared to transfer at a higher frequency on a solid surface, a plate-mating

---

* Present address: Department of Medical Bacteriology, University of Alberta, Edmonton, Canada

method was used for further studies of plasmid transfer in *C. jejuni*. Interspecies transfer was demonstrated from *C. jejuni* (MK 22) to *C. fetus* ssp. *fetus* (ATCC 27347). The frequency of plasmid transfer to *C. fetus* ssp. *fetus* was very similar to that observed in the intraspecies mating experiments (approximately 3×10^{-4} transconjugants per recipient in a 48-hour plate-mating experiment).

Demonstration of plasmid DNA in tetracycline resistant *C. jejuni*

Plasmid-enriched DNA fractions were prepared from four tetracycline-resistant strains of *C. jejuni* and from the tetracycline-susceptible strains *C. jejuni* (SD 2) and *C. fetus* ssp. *fetus* (ATCC 27374). Plasmid DNA was isolated initially by our modification[5] of the method of Meyers et al[6]. In subsequent experiments plasmid DNA yields were improved by using the isolation methods of Portnoy and White[7].

Tetracycline-resistant campylobacters harboured a plasmid with a molecular weight of 38 Mdal, whereas the susceptible strains were plasmid-free. Transconjugants of *C. jejuni* and *C. fetus* ssp. *fetus* also contained the 38 Mdal plasmid (Figure 1, Track A).

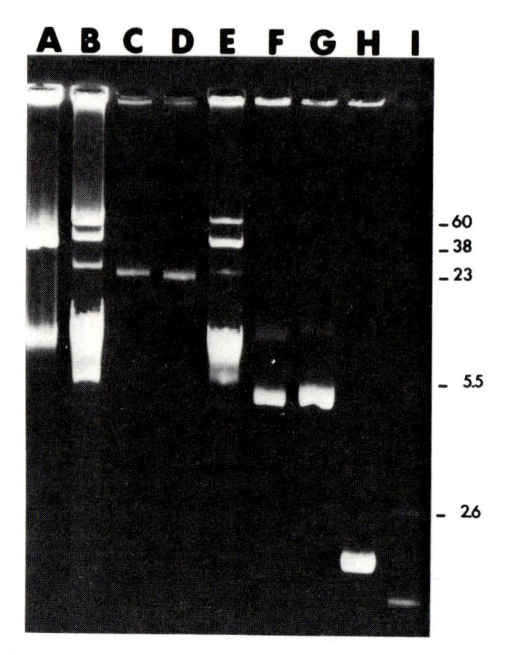

Figure 1 See page 212 for full description of this figure

Mechanism of tetracycline resistance transfer

Cell-free filtrates of tetracycline-resistant *C. jejuni* donor strains could not promote the transfer of tetracycline resistance determinants to plasmid-free recipient *C. jejuni* (SD 2) or *C. fetus* (ATCC 27374) ($<1 \times 10^{-8}$ transconjugants per recipient after a 48-hour mating period). This suggested that the transfer process was not bacteriophage-mediated. Moreover, the transfer frequency of the plasmids was not affected when DNAase (100 μg/ml) was added to the agar in the plate-mating experiments. It appears unlikely therefore that DNA transformation is involved in the transfer of tetracycline resistance between campylobacters. The process probably involves conjugation via cell-to-cell contact.

Attempts to transfer tetracycline resistance to *Escherichia coli*

Transfer of tetracycline resistance determinants from *C. jejuni* to *E. coli* was unsuccessful, even when strains of *E. coli*, which did not produce restriction enzymes, were used as recipients (*E. coli* C or strain NM 148, a restriction deficient mutant of *E. coli* K-12). Analogous host-range limitations are known in some other gram-negative organisms[5].

Ampicillin resistance in *C. jejuni*

Resistance to both ampicillin and tetracycline was exhibited by one clinical isolate of *C. jejuni* (MK 175). Although the tetracycline resistance determinant was transmissible in this strain, ampicillin resistance was never co-transferred from strain MK 175 to *C. jejuni* (SD 2) or *C. fetus* ssp. *fetus* (ATCC 27374). *C. jejuni* (MK 175) and tetracycline-resistant transconjugants, derived from this strain, contained a plasmid with a molecular weight of 38 Mdal. No other plasmid species was observed in *C. jejuni* (MK 175). Ampicillin resistance in this strain is associated with β-lactamase production, however, the B-lactamase enzyme was not detected in *C. jejuni* (SD 2) transconjugants which inherited the tetracycline resistance plasmid from MK 175. These results suggest that ampicillin resistance in *C. jejuni* (MK 175) is of chromosomal origin.

REFERENCES

1. Karmali, M. A. and Fleming, P. C. (1979). Campylobacter enteritis. *Can. Med. Assoc. J.*, **20**, 1525–1532
2. Vanhoof, R., Vanderlinden, M. P., Dierickx, R., Lauwers, S., Yourossowsky, E. and Butzler, J. P. (1978). Susceptibility of *Campylobacter fetus* subsp. *jejuni*. to twenty-nine antimicrobial agents. *Antimicrob. Agents Chemother.*, **14**, 553–566
3. Karmali, M. A., De Grandis, S. and Fleming, P. D. (1981). Antimicrobial susceptibility of *Campylobacter jejuni* with special reference to resistance patterns of Canadian isolates. *Antimicrob. Agents Chemother.* **19**, 593–97
4. Taylor, D. E., De Grandis, S. A., Karmali, M. A. and Fleming, P. C. (1980). Transmissible tetracycline resistance in *Campylobacter jejuni*. *Lancet*, **ii**: 797
5. Taylor, D. E., De Grandis, S. A., Karmali, M. A. and Fleming, P. C. (1981). Transmissible plasmids from *Campylobacter jejuni*. *Antimicrobial. Agents Chemother.* **19**, 831–35
6. Meyers, J. A., Sanchez, D., Elwell, L. P. and Falkow, S. (1976). Simple agarose gel electrophoretic method for the identification and characterisation of plasmid deoxyribonucleic acid. *I. Bacteriol.*, **127**, 1529–1537
7. Crosa, J. H. and Falkow, S. (1981). Plasmids. *In Manual of Methods for General Bacteriology. The American Society for Microbiology*, Washington, DC. P. Gehardt *et al.* eds. pp. 266 82

DISCUSSION

In answer to a question from Professor Trust, Dr Taylor said that they had not yet transferred a tetracycline resistance plasmid from campylobacter to *E. coli*.

78
Erythromycin resistance in *Campylobacter jejuni*

DIANE E. TAYLOR, STEPHANIE A. DE GRANDIS, M. A. KARMALI and F. C. FLEMING

Department of Bacteriology, the Hospital for Sick Children, 555 University Avenue, Toronto, Canada M5G 1X8

R. VANHOOF* and J. P. BUTZLER†

* Department of Medical Microbiology, Institute Pasteur, Stoomsleppersstraat 28, 1040 Brussels.
† Microbiology Laboratory, University Hospital of St Peter, 322 Rue Houte, 1000 Brussels, Belgium

---

Approximately 1% of *C. jejuni* strains isolated at the Hospital for Sick Children, Toronto were resistant to erythromycin (MIC > 1024 µg/ml). In the United Kingdom, about 0.5% of campylobacter isolates are resistant to erythromycin[1], whereas in Belgium[2] and Sweden[3] approximately 9% of *C. jejuni* strains are erythromycin-resistant.

We examined nine erythromycin-resistant isolates of *C. jejuni* for their plasmid DNA content (Figure 1). Four strains came from the Province of Ontario, two from animals (kindly supplied by Dr John Prescott) and two from humans. The other five strains originated in Belgium. No two strains belonged to the same serogroup, as determined by the system of Penner and Hennessey[4]. Most strains were also resistant to lincomycin (MIC > 100 µg/ml)[5]. Three erythromycin-resistant strains of *C. jejuni* harboured plasmids with molecular weights in the range of about 20–25 Mdal, including one human and one animal isolate from Ontario. Four other strains, including the other Ontario isolates, contained plasmids ranging from 1.5–5 Mdal, which are too small to encode their own conjugative transfer. The other two strains of *C. jejuni*, originating in Belgium, were found to be plasmid-free.

Transfer of erythromycin resistance from the three strains containing the larger plasmids was tested in plate-mating experiments with *C. jejuni* (SD 2) or *C. fetus* ssp. *fetus* (ATCC 27374) as the recipient strain. No transfer of the erythromycin resistance determinants was observed. Three other strains of *C. jejuni* resistant to both erythromycin and tetracycline were also tested for transfer of each of these resistance determinants. Although transfer of

CAMPYLOBACTER: MOLECULAR BIOLOGY

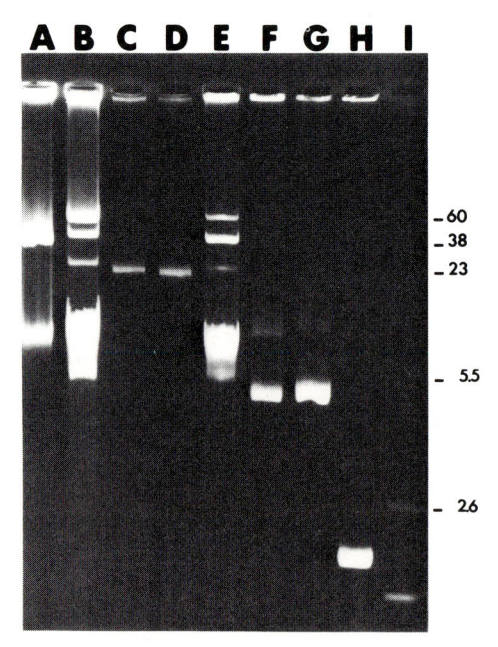

Figure 1 Agarose-gel electrophoresis of R plasmids from erythromycin-resistant *C. jejuni*. Plasmid-enriched DNA fractions from *C. jejuni* were isolated by the method of Portnoy and White (as described in reference 6). Some preparations were also extracted with acid-phenol as described by Zasloff *et al.*[7], to remove linear and open-circular (OC) DNA molecules. Samples were subjected to electrophoresis on agarose gels and the molecular weights calculated from the positions of the campylobacter plasmid relative to plasmids of known molecular weights[8].

Track A: *C. jejuni*, a tetracycline-resistant clinical isolate (MK 175), harbouring plasmid pMAK 175 (38 Mdal)

Track B: Reference plasmids RIP 69 (47 Mdal), RP 1 (38 Mdal), S-a (23 Mdal) and RSF 1030 (5.5 Mdal)

Track E: Reference plasmids RSF 1030, S-a and RP 1 as well as MP-10 (60 Mdal). Chromosomal DNA is present in Tracks A, B and E. The other six tracks contain DNA isolated from erythromycin-resistant *C. jejuni* strains after linear and OC forms were removed by acid-phenol extraction; note the absence of chromosomal DNA

Track C: 21 Mdal plasmid

Track D: 19.5 Mdal plasmid

Tracks F and G: 4.8 Mdal plasmid and a 9.5 Mdal plasmid, which may be the dimeric form of the smaller molecule

Track H: 2.0 Mdal plasmid and newly-formed open-circular derivative

Track I: 1.5 Mdal plasmid and OC DNA

tetracycline resistance was observed in these isolates, erythromycin resistance was not transferred either alone, or in association with, the tetracycline resistance determinant. The plasmid content of the erythromycin-tetracycline-resistant donor strains and the resulting tetracycline-resistant transconjugant strains remains to be determined.

Experiments are also in progress to determine if elimination of a particular plasmid is associated with loss of erythromycin resistance. The results of these experiments should clarify whether erythromycin resistance in *C. jejuni* results from a chromosomal mutation, whether it is plasmid-mediated, or whether erythromycin resistance determinants could reside in both locations.

References

1. Brunton, W. A. T., Wilson, A. M. M. and Macrae, R. M. (1978). Erythromycin resistant campylobacters. *Lancet*, **ii**, 1385
2. Vanhoof, R.,Vanderlinden, M. P., Dierickx, R., Lauwers, S., Yourossowsky, E. and Butzler, J. P. (1978). Susceptibility of *Campylobacter fetus* ssp. *jejuni* to twenty-nine antimicrobial agents. *Antimicrobial Agents and Chemotherapy*, **14**, 553–566
3. Walder, M. (1979). Susceptibility of *Campylobacter fetus* ssp. *jejuni* to twenty antimicrobial agents. *Antimicrobial Agents and Chemotherapy*, **16**, 37–39
4. Penner, J. L. and Hennessy, J. N. (1980). Passive haemaglutination technique for serotyping *Campylobacter fetus* ssp. *jejuni* on the basis of soluble heat-stable antigens. *J. Clin. Microbiol.*, **12**, 732–737
5. Karmali, M. A., De Grandis, S. and Fleming, P. D. (1981). Antimicrobial susceptibility of *Campylobacter jejuni* with special reference to resistance patterns of Canadian isolates. *Antimicrobial Agents and Chemotherapy*, in press
6. Crosa, J. H. and Falkow, S. Plasmid DNA purification and characterisation. In *Manual of Methods for General Bacteriology*, The American Society for Microbiology, Washington D.C. **19**, 593–97
7. Zasloff, M., Ginder, G. D. and Felsenfeld, G. (1978). A new method for the purification and identification of covalently closed circular DNA molecules. *Nucleic Acid Res.*, **5**, 1139–1152
8. Meyers, J. A., Sanchez, D., Elwell, L. P. and Falkow, S. (1976). Simple agarose gel electrophoretic method for the identification and characterization of plasmid deoxyribonucleic acid. *J. Bacteriol.*, **127**, 1529–1537

79
The detection and frequency of beta-lactamase production in *Campylobacter jejuni*

P. C. FLEMING, A. D'AMICO, S. DE GRANDIS and
M. A. KARMALI

Department of Bacteriology, The Hospital for Sick Children, Toronto

---

The iodometric, chromogenic cephalosporin (nitrocefin) and clover-leaf tests have been evaluated as methods for detecting beta-lactamase production in *C. jejuni*. Additionally, the incidence of beta-lactamase production in 120 strains of *C. jejuni* and its effect on the susceptibility of those strains to ampicillin and cephaloridine was determined.

Materials and Methods

One hundred and twenty clinical isolates of *C. jejuni* were studied. One-hundred of these strains were isolated in our laboratory from patients with diarrhoea. The remaining isolates were obtained from other laboratories. *C. jejuni* strains were cultured on blood agar (BA) consisting of Columbia blood-agar base (Gibco Ltd) with 7% horse blood and incubated at 37 °C under reduced oxygen tension.

Detection of beta-lactamases

Iodometrical method
The iodometric method used was a modification of the method of Perret[1]. Suspensions (turbidity approximately McFarland No. 6) of 48-hour BA cultures of each strain were made in 2 ml of a Penicillin-G solution (2.5 mg/ml in $KHPO_4$ buffer 0.1 M, pH 7.5). The suspensions were incubated for 1 hour at 37 °C before the addition of 150 µl of 0.4% soluble starch in distilled water. Then 0.025 M iodine in 0.125 M potassium iodide was added in 50-µl amounts until a blue-black colour persisted for at least 30 seconds with shaking. The volume of iodine required to reach this end-point was related to controls containing no organisms.

Chromogenic cephalosporin method
A technique based on the chromogenic cephalosporin substrate, nitrocefin, developed by O'Callaghan et al.[2] was used. Suspensions of 1 ml (turbidity approximately McFarland No. 6) from 48-hour BA cultures were made in $KHPO_4$ buffer (0.1 M, pH 7.5), five drops of nitrocefin solution (5 mg of nitrocefin dissolved in 0.5 ml of dimethyl sulphoxide then diluted in 9.5 ml of 0.1 M $KHPO_4$ buffer pH 7.5 and stored in the dark at 40 °C) was added to each suspension which were then incubated at 37 °C for 1 hour. The resulting colour reaction was interpreted as follows: a yellow colour = 0; weak orange-yellow = 1; strong orange = 2 and strong orange to red = 3.

Microbiologic method
The clover-leaf method of McGhie et al.[3] was used, with all 120 strains being tested against 10-μg ampicillin discs and 24 strains tested against 30-μg cephaloridine discs. The latter strains were selected on the basis of 12 that were positive and 12 that were negative for beta-lactamase activity by the iodometric method. The results were scored as: 0 = negative reaction; 1 = weak intermediate reaction; 2 = strong intermediate reaction and 3 = positive reaction.

Susceptibility and inoculum size effects

These tests were performed by the agar-dilution method using a Steer's replicator. The deposited organisms were cultured on DST agar (Oxoid) with 5% lysed horse-blood containing varying dilutions of ampicillin or cephaloridine.

RESULTS AND DISCUSSION

Table 1 shows the reactions, graded 1-3, of 120 strains of *C. jejuni* tested for beta-lactamase activity by the three different methods. In the iodometric test, results were recorded as either positive or negative, based on the volume of iodine required to reach an end-point compared with the controls. Twenty out of 120 (16.7%) strains were positive for beta-lactamase by the iodometric test.

In the chromogenic cephalosporin test, 21/120 (17.5%) strains gave a positive or strong intermediate reaction, whilst 52/120 (43.3%) strains gave a

Table 1 Reactions of 120 strains of *C. jejuni* according to three beta-lactamase testing methods

Reaction grade*	Iodometric	Nitrocefin	Microbiologic†
0	100	47 ⎫ 99	69 ⎫ 87
1		52 ⎭	18 ⎭
2		10 ⎫ 21	19 ⎫ 33
3	20	11 ⎭	14 ⎭

* 0 = negative; 1 = weak intermediate; 2 = strong intermediate; 3 = positive
† Using 10 μg ampicillin disc

weak intermediate reaction. A close correlation was seen between strains giving a positive iodometric reaction (20 strains) and strains giving a positive or strong intermediate reaction in the chromogenic cephalosporin test (21 strains).

In the clover-leaf microbiological method (using a 10 μg ampicillin disc), 33/120 (27.5%) strains gave a positive or strong intermediate reaction. Compared to the iodometric test, there were no false-negatives in the microbiological test, but 13/33 (39.4%) strains gave a false-positive reaction, being negative by the iodometric but positive by the microbiological test. A strong association was seen between beta-lactamase production and ampicillin resistance (Table 1), but no association was seen between beta-lactamase production and the susceptibility of strains to cephaloridine (Table 2). The susceptibility of beta-lactamase positive strains to ampicillin but not cephaloridine was markedly influenced by the inoculum size (Table 2). None of the 24 strains gave a positive reaction in the microbiological test when a 30 μg cephaloridine disc was used instead of ampicillin.

Table 2 Effect of beta-lactamase production and inoculum size on (geometric mean) MIC's to ampicillin and cephaloridine

Inoculum	Ampicillin (μg/ml) 10^6 10^4 10^2 cells	Cephaloridine (μg/ml) 10^6 10^4 10^2
Beta-lactamase positive (20 strains)	128 32 16	32 32 16
Beta-lactamase negative (100 strains)	16 8 4	32 32 32

The iodometric test was found to be the most satisfactory method for detecting beta-lactamase activity in *C. jejuni*. There was a close correlation between beta-lactamase production as determined iodometrically and ampicillin resistance. The susceptibility of beta-lactamase producing strains to ampicillin was markedly influenced by the inoculum size.

A positive iodometric reaction correlated closely with a positive or strong intermediate reaction in the chromogenic cephalosporin test, but did not correlate with a weak intermediate reaction. The difficulty of visually distinguishing a weak intermediate reaction from a strong intermediate reaction renders the chromogenic cephalosporin test less satisfactory than the iodometric test for routine use.

The clover-leaf microbiological test showed high sensitivity but poor specificity when compared to the iodometric test. About 40% of positive or strong intermediate reactions in the clover-leaf test were non-specific.

Beta-lactamase production did not correlate with resistance to cephaloridine. The susceptibilities of beta-lactamase producing strains to cephaloridine were not influenced by the inoculum size. There was no evidence of cephaloridine inactivation by beta-lactamase producing strains in the microbiological assay.

The frequency of beta-lactamase producing strains in our study was about 16%. This contrasts markedly with the observations of Severin[4] who found over 90% of his strains to be beta-lactamase producers. The characterization and classification of *C. jejuni* beta-lactamase(s) remains to be established. Whether the beta-lactamase activity is plasmid-mediated or chromosomally-mediated also remains to be elucidated. Our preliminary investigations[5] tend to support a chromosomal location for genes controlling beta-lactamase production in *C. jejuni*.

References

1. Perret, C. J. (1954). *Nature*, **174**, 1012–1013
2. O'Callaghan, C. H., Morris, A., Kirby, S. M. and Shingler, A. H. (1972). *Antimicrob. Agents. and Chemother.* **1**, 283–288
3. McGhie, D., Clarke, P. D., Johnson, T. and Huchison, J. G. P. (1977). *J. Clin. Path.*, **30**, 585–587
4. Severin, W. P. (1978). *Ned. Tijdschr. Geneesk.*, **122**, 499–504
5. Taylor, D. E., De Grandis, S. A., Karmali, M. A. and Fleming, P. C. (1980). *Lancet*, **2**, 797

DISCUSSION

Dr Skirrow commented that most hippurate-negative strains are *C. coli* and are isolated from pigs. It was therefore possible that the erythromycin resistance in these strains is related to the wide use of Tylocyn in pigs. His beta-lactamase results suggest that 80–90% of strains are positive by the nitrocefin test, which is in agreement with Dr Severin's results.

80
On the association between erythromycin resistance and the failure to hydrolyze hippurate in *Campylobacter jejuni* (*C. jejuni–C. coli*)

M. A. KARMALI, S. A. DE GRANDIS, D. E. TAYLOR and P. C. FLEMING

Department of Bacteriology, the Hospital for Sick Children, 555 University Avenue, Toronto, Canada M5G 1X8

Harvey[1] observed that some strains of *Campylobacter jejuni* (corresponding to the *C. jejuni–C. coli* group of Véron and Chatelain) were able to hydrolyze hippurate whereas other strains in the same group were hippurate-negative. We have examined 110 strains of *C. jejuni* for hippurate hydrolysis using the method of Hwang and Ederer[2]. There were 85 clinical isolates of *C. jejuni* (consisting of 73 isolates from our own Hospital, nine from J. P. Butzler and R. Vanhoof, and one each from R. M. Bannatyne, W. D. Leers and J. M. S. Dixon), and 25 animal isolates (supplied by J. F. Prescott and N. Luechtefeld). All strains were tested for susceptibility to erythromycin by the agar-dilution method[4]. Serotyping of strains was performed by J. L. Penner[3]. Seventy-eight strains (70 human and 8 animal strains) were hippurate-positive and 32 strains (15 human and 17 animal strains) were unable to hydrolyze hippurate (Table 1). Fourteen were highly resistant to erythromycin (minimal inhibitory concentration, 512 µg/ml). All erythromycin resistant strains were negative for hippurate hydrolysis, whereas erythromycin-sensitive strains (minimal inhibitory concentration, 2 µg/ml) were either hippurate-positive or hippurate-negative (Table 1). Table 2 shows the heterogeneous nature of the erythromycin-resistant strains with respect to geographical origin, source, and Penner serotype. In order to explore further the apparent association of erythromycin resistance in *C. jejuni* with the failure to hydrolyze hippurate, we examined the relationship between erythromycin susceptibility, hippurate reaction and serotype. Serotypes that contained at least three strains from our collection and included either erythromycin-resistant or hippurate-negative strains of *C. jejuni* were studied. An analysis of such serotypes showed that they

ERYTHROMYCIN RESISTANCE AND HIPPURATE HYDROLYSIS

Table 1 Erythromycin resistance (Ery^R) and the hippurate reaction (HIP) in C. jejuni (C. jejuni C. coli)

	Total	HIP^{+ve}	HIP^{-ve}
No. strains tested	110	78	32
No. strains Ery^S	96	78	18
No. strains Ery^R	14	0	14

Table 2 Sources and suppliers of erythromycin-resistant strains

Supplier	No. of strains	Source	Serotypes
R. M. Bannatyne (Toronto, Canada)	1	Human	26
W. D. Leers (Toronto, Canada)	1	Human	5
J. F. Prescott (Guelph, Canada)	3	Ovine (2) Porcine (1)	5; 25 24
J. P. Butzler and R. Vanhoof (Belgium)	9	Human	2; 5, 30; 6; 11; 14; 24; 28; 30;

could be divided into two groups. The first group (Table 3) contained serotypes (24, 26, 28 and 34) that were consistently negative for hippurate hydrolysis irrespective of erythromycin susceptibility. In the second group, (Table 4) the majority of strains in each serotype (2, 5 and 11) were hippurate-positive. Only a minority of strains in the latter group were hippurate-negative, and all of these were erythromycin-resistant. The remaining five erythromycin-resistant strains, not included in Tables 3 and 4, were all hippurate-negative and belonged to one of the serotypes 5, 30; 6, 14; 25 or 30. They were not suitable for analysis because the serotypes they belonged to contained less than three strains from our collection.

In conclusion, in serotypes 2, 5 and 11, there was a clear association between erythromycin resistance and the inability of strains to hydrolyze hippurate; in serotypes 24, 26, 28 and 34, all strains were hippurate-negative irrespective of erythromycin susceptibility although the frequency of erythromycin resistance

Table 3 Relationship between serotype, hippurate hydrolysis (HIP) and erythromycin resistance (Ery^R) in C. jejuni (C. jejuni C. coli)

1. Serotypes consistently negative for hippurate hydrolysis

Serotype (Penner and Hennessy)	No. of strains Total	HIP^{+ve}	HIP^{-ve}	No. of strains Ery^R
24	5	0	5	2
26	3	0	3	1
28	3	0	3	1
34	8	0	8	0

Table 4 Relationship between serotype, hippurate hydrolysis (HIP) and erythromycin resistance (Ery^R) in *C. jejuni* (*C. jejuni C. coli*)

2. Serotypes usually positive for hippurate hydrolysis

Serotype (Penner and Hennessy)	Total	No. of strains Hip^{+ve}	Hip^{-ve}	No. of strains Ery^R
2	20	18	2	2 (HIP^{-ve})
5	12	10	2	2 (HIP^{-ve})
11	8	7	1	1 (HIP^{-ve})

was higher than might be expected. The nature and significance of the association between erythromycin resistance and the inability of *C. jejuni* to hydrolyze hippurate, requires further study.

References

1. Harvey, S. M. (1980). Hippurate hydrolysis by *Campylobacter fetus*. *J. Clin. Microbiol.*, **11**, 435–437
2. Hwang, M. N. and Ederer, G. M. (1975). Rapid hippurate hydrolysis method for presumptive identification of Group B streptococci. *J. Clin. Microbiol.*, **1**, 114–115
3. Penner, J. L. and Hennessy, J. N. (1980). Passive haemagglutination technique for serotyping *Campylobacter fetus* subsp. *jejuni* on the basis of soluble heat-stable antigens. *J. Clin. Microbiol.*, **12**, 732–737
4. Karmali, M. A., De Grandis, S. A. and Fleming, P. C. (1981). Antimicrobial susceptibility of *Campylobacter jejuni* with special reference to resistance patterns of Canadian isolates. *Antimicrobiol. Agents and Chemotherapy*, (in press, April 1981).

81
Ultrastructure and antibiotic sensitivity of campylobacter

A. J. LASTOVICA

Department of Microbiology, Red Cross Children's Hospital, Rondebosch 7700, Cape Town, South Africa

Over an 18-month period 26 strains of campylobacter were selected from those campylobacters isolated from patients with acute diarrhoea. On the basis of temperature tolerance at 25 °C and 42 °C and susceptibility to a 30 µg nalidixic-acid disc, these strains were differentiated into four strains of *C. fetus* ssp. *fetus* and 22 strains of *C. jejuni*. Four of the strains were obtained from blood cultures, the rest from stools. The organisms were maintained at 37 °C under micro-aerophilic conditions on tryptose blood-agar plates or in liquid-culture medium. The antibiotic sensitivity of these strains was determined by an antibiotic disc-diffusion technique. All the strains tested were found to be resistant to novobiocin (5 µg), bacitracin (0.1 U), sulfadiazine (200 µg) and sulfamethoxazole/trimethoprim (25 µg). All but two of the strains were resistant to fusidic acid (10 µg). All of the strains tested were sensitive to clindamycin (2 µg), chloramphenicol (30 µg), erythromycin (15 µg), framycetin (100 µg), gentamicin (10 µg), neomycin (30 µg), nitrofurantoin (300 µg), nicene (30 µg) and tetracycline (30 µg). All of the strains were sensitive to a degree to amikacin (10 µg), kanamycin (30 µg) and tobramycin (10 µg). All but three strains were sensitive to ampicillin (10 µg) and amoxycillin (25 µg). Fourteen of the strains were sensitive to metromidazole (5 µg) and rifampicin (30 µg). All but six of the strains were sensitive to carbenicillin (100 µg). The 22 *C. jejuni* strains were resistant to cephalothin (30 µg) and sensitive to nalidixic acid (30 µg). With the four *C. fetus* ssp. *fetus* strains, the converse was true. Two strains each of *C. fetus* ssp. *fetus* and *C. jejuni* were chosen for further investigation. Replicate experiments were done by standard doubling-dilution techniques to determine the median minimal inhibitory concentration (MIC) of amoxycillin and gentamicin which were found to be, respectively, 0.93 µg/ml and 0.45 µg/ml.

Log-phase cultures of bacteria were incubated for various periods of time with various concentrations of amoxycillin or gentamicin or without these antibiotics. Samples were prepared for electron microscopy by established methods[1,2]. Under the transmission and scanning electron microscopes, control log-phase cultures of the campylobacter strains were found to consist of curved to spiral rods 1.4–3.1 μm in length by 0.25 μm–0.48 μm in width at the polar ends (Figure 1). Usually, a single flagellum 2.5–5.3 μm in length by 20 nm in width emerged from a conical pit at one or both ends of the cell. Membrane-bound osmiophilic granules or laminated structures 50–75 nm in diameter were noted in the cytoplasm of some of the cells in thin-section.

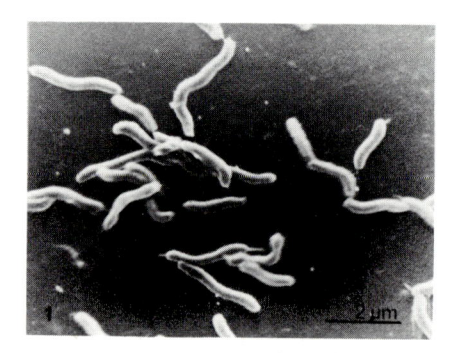

Figure 1 A control log-phase culture of *Campylobacter jejuni*

Campylobacter treated for 30 min at 37 °C with twice the MIC of amoxycillin were long and undulating, and were composed of interconnected chains of individual cells. These chains were 40 μm or more in length (Figure 2). Organisms treated for 90 min at 37 °C with five times the MIC of amoxycillin readily formed spheroplasts, usually from the centre of the cell (Figures 3 and 4). Campylobacter exposed to twice the MIC of amoxycillin for six or more hours degenerated into an amorphous mass.

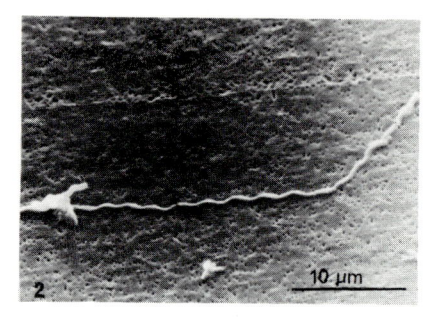

Figure 2 Filament formation; twice MIC amoxycillin for 30 min

Amoxycillin, like penicillin, probably acts at the final stages of wall synthesis as a structural analogue of the terminal portion of the peptide molecule attached to the *N*-acetyl-muramic acid. The Beta-lactam ring in the antibiotic successfully competes with the CO–N bond of the D-alanyl-D-alanine for the active site of the transpeptidase enzyme. Normal transpeptidation is inhibited,

ULTRASTRUCTURE AND ANTIBIOTIC SENSITIVITY OF CAMPYLOBACTER

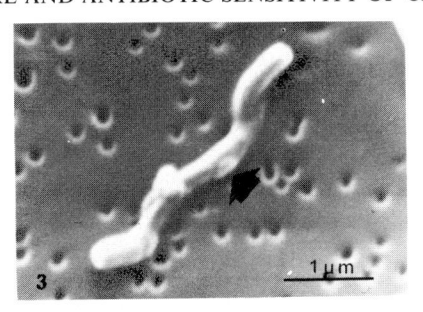

Figure 3 Beginning of spheroplast (arrow) formation with five times MIC amoxycillin for 30 min

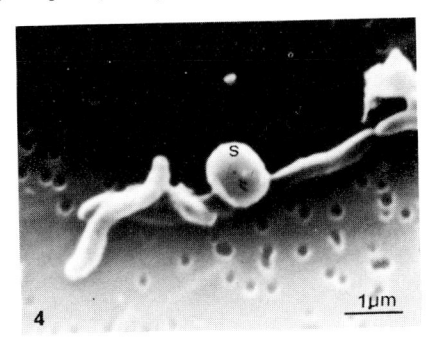

Figure 4 Spheroplast (S) formed after exposure to five times MIC amoxycillin for 90 min

consequently the cell-wall peptidoglycan lacks adequate cross-linkages[3]. In general, relatively low concentrations of amoxycillin for short periods of time convert susceptible campylobacter into elongated filaments, due to inhibition of cross-wall formation only, while higher concentrations of amoxycillin for longer periods of time produce spheroplasts. These observations are similar to those reported for another gram-negative bacterium, *E. coli*[4].

Campylobacter exposed for 30 minutes at 37 °C, with twice the MIC of gentamicin, did not readily divide and the cells lost their characteristic morphology, becoming much shorter and thicker (Figure 5). Bacteria exposed to four times the MIC for five or more hours lysed, degenerating into an amorphous mass (Figure 6).

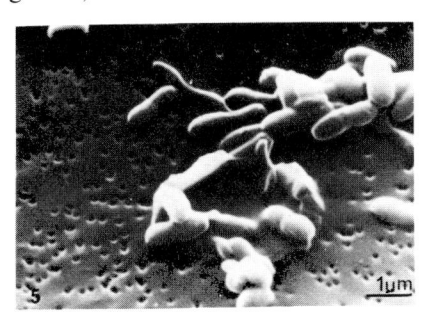

Figure 5 Twice MIC gentamicin for 30 min. Most cells are much shorter and thicker than normal

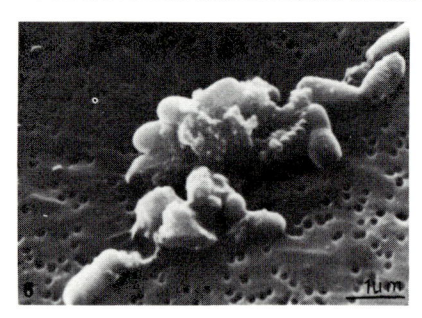

Figure 6 Gentamicin at four times MIC for 5 hours. Most of the campylobacter have lysed

Gentamicin is thought to affect the initiation step in protein synthesis by binding to the 30s ribosome, consequently the synthesis of protein chains on ribosomes cannot occur[5]. It therefore seems likely that in campylobacter those proteins involved with normal transverse and longitudinal cell-wall formation have been interfered with by gentamicin. Gentamicin may have also interfered with the biosynthesis of membrane lipoproteins in campylobacter, as has been demonstrated for *Pseudomonas*[6].

References

1. Lastovica, A. J. (1974). *Int. J. Parasit.*, **7,** 139
2. Lastovica, A. J. (1976). *Z. Parasit. Kde.*, **50,** 275
3. Selwyn, S. (1980). *Penicillins and cephalosporins in perspective.* Hodder & Stoughton, London, 363 pp.
4. Comber, K. R., Boon, R. J. and Sutherland, R. (1977). *Antimicrobiol Agents and Chemotherapy,* **12,** 736
5. Council for Interdisciplinary Communication in Medicine, Ltd. (1974). *Gentamicin: Review and commentary on selected world literature.* New York City, 209 pp
6. Dimitrou, L. I., Pitsin, D. G. and Gigova, N. D. (1979). Compes rendus de l'Academic bulgare des Sciences, **32**(7), p. 529

Acknowledgement

The author gratefully acknowledges the financial support of the South African Medical Research Council.

DISCUSSION

In reply to questions from Dr Hofstadt and Professor Bokkenheuser, Dr Lastovica said that he had seen no evidence of capsules in campylobacters and all his strains were chloramphenicol sensitive. Dr Wang noted that the morphology of these treated cells was similar to old cells but Dr Lastovica pointed out that he only used early log-phase cells.

82
Outer membrane protein composition of campylobacters

R. A. AUSTEN and T. J. TRUST

Department of Biochemistry and Microbiology, University of Victoria, Canada

---

The outer membrane of a gram-negative bacterial pathogen serves as an interface between the host and the pathogen. It therefore plays a critical role in the outcome of the host-parasite relationship. Studies with a number of pathogenic bacteria have shown that components of the outer membrane can participate in the adherence of the pathogen to host-epithelial cells, the invasion of host cells, resistance to the bactericidal activity of serum, resistance to phagocytosis and to intraphagocytic killing, and in the sequestering of iron[1,2].

The outer membrane is believed to be a highly asymmetric lipid bilayer containing lipopolysaccharide, which is located in the outer leaflet, and phospholipid, much of which is located in the inner leaflet[3,4]. Interspersed in this bilayer is a set of outer membrane proteins. Like the polysaccharide portion of the lipopolysaccharide, some of the outer membrane proteins can be exposed on the surface of the cell and both the polysaccharide and the protein can serve as antigens. This means that outer-membrane composition is important in host immunity, and is an important determinant in serotyping and bacteriophage typing schemes.

Little is known concerning the outer membrane composition of species of campylobacter. Although there have been reports of an antiphagocytic surface protein in the case of *Campylobacter fetus*[5,6], there have been no descriptions of the protein composition of the *Campylobacter jejuni* group. Here we report on the outer-membrane composition of these organisms.

The 'thermophilic' campylobacters examined included human faecal and blood isolates, canine, bovine and porcine isolates, and environmental isolates and were from Australia, Belgium, Canada, England and the U.S.A. Strain UVC 23 was a canine isolate (M. Blaser, 79–159). All stock cultures were maintained at $-80\,°C$ in 20% (v/v) glycerol-trypticase soy broth (BBL). Unless specified otherwise, cells for whole-cell protein profiles and for the preparation of outer-membrane proteins were grown for 36 hours at 37 °C on Meuller–Hinton agar (Difco). Reduced oxygen atmosphere was produced using anaerobic jars without catalysts and BBL H_2 and CO_2 generator envelopes.

Cell envelopes were prepared by passage of bacterial cells through a French pressure cell, removal of any remaining whole cells, and centrifugation at 40 000 g for 30 min at 4 °C. Outer membranes were prepared by differential solubilization of the bacterial envelopes using the detergent sodium lauryl sarcosinate (American Chemical and Solvent Co.) as described by Filip et al.[7]. An envelope protein:detergent ratio of 1:6 mg/mg was maintained,. The outer membrane 'bleb' or fragment fraction was prepared by differential centrifugation as previously described. Cell-free culture supernatants were centrifuged at 100 000 g for 1 hour at 4 °C. The supernatant was then centrifuged at 300 000 g for 8 hours at 4 °C. The resultant pellet was re-suspended in a small volume of 20 mM Tris-HCl, pH 7.4.

Intact bacteria were surface labelled with ^{125}I using the solid-phase lactoperoxidase-glucose oxidase system as described by the manufacturer (Biorad Laboratories).

Samples were prepared for sodium dodecyl sulphate polyacrylamide gel electrophoresis (SDS-PAGE) and separated on 14% acrylamide gels according to the methods described by Hancock and Carey[8] in their modification of Neville's method[9]. Gels were stained using Coomassie blue for protein and the periodic acid-Schiff procedure of Fairbanks et al.[10] for carbohydrate. The protein content of the membrane fractions was determined by the modified Lowry procedure developed by Markwell et al.[11] using bovine serum albumin (Sigma) as standard.

For electron microscopy, unfixed specimens were negatively stained on Formvar coated grids using 2% (w/v) phosphotungstic acid. They were examined in a Philips EM 300 electron microscope.

When whole-cell SDS-PAGE protein profiles of these various 'thermophilic' campylobacters were examined, a large number of bands were apparent. The major protein component of all isolates varied in the region of 40 000–45 000 molecular weight. Outer-membrane preparations revealed that this protein was also the major protein component of the outer membrane. In addition to this major band, a number of other minor bands were present. A typical outer-membrane protein profile, that of UVC 23, is shown in Figure 1. Examination of the outer membrane prepared from cells grown for 26 hours shows the presence of nine distinct protein bands. The approximate molecular weights of the upper doublet (a) are 75 000 and 73 000, and of the lower doublet (g) are 35 500 and 34 500. In between these two doublets are proteins of molecular weight 70 000 (b), 66 500 (c), 57 500 (d), 52 500 (e) and 44 000 (f). At the bottom of the profile is a 'wavy' band in the 18 600 region. This band, which is evident in profiles of cultures older than 18 hours, stained positively with periodate-Schiff reagent and likely corresponds to the location of LPS. In contrast, the 57 500 protein was much more pronounced in the early period of growth, i.e. in 18- and 26-hour profiles.

A survey of other campylobacters showed similar numbers of outer-membrane proteins, however some variations in molecular weights were apparent, as were variations in amounts of the various proteins. Initial radio-labelling experiments with several isolates revealed that the major protein was exposed on the surface of whole cells. Several of the minor outer-membrane proteins also radio-labelled suggesting that these were also surface exposed.

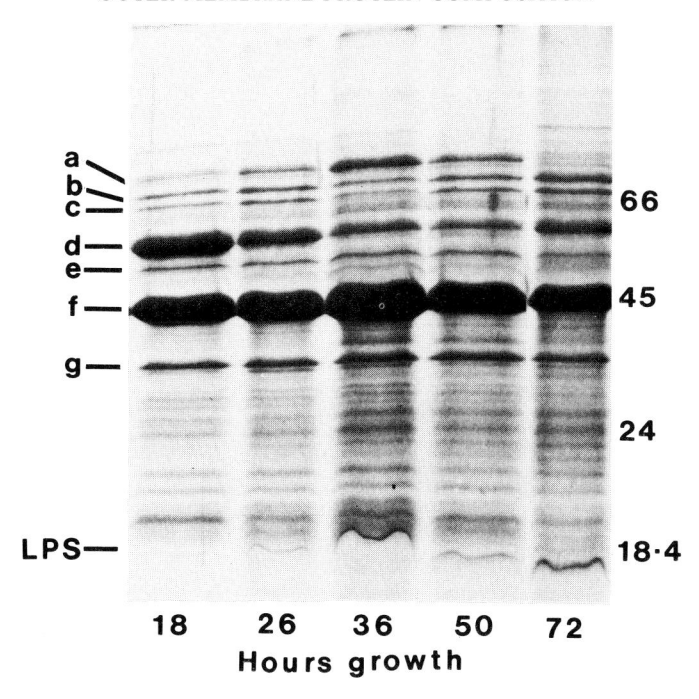

Figure 1 Outer-membrane protein profile of thermophilic campylobacter strain UVC 23 grown on Meuller–Hinton agar at 37 °C for varying times. The location of the major outer-membrane proteins is indicated (a–g) as is the lipopolysaccharide. Molecular weights ($\times 10^3$) are given on the right.

We also investigated the presence of heat-modifiable proteins. This was done by comparing the SDS-PAGE profiles of outer-membrane preparations treated for 1 hour at 37 °C with those treated for 3 min at 100 °C. Heat modifiable proteins are those whose mobility varies according to the heat treatment during SDS solubilization. The results obtained demonstrated the presence of one or more heat-modifiable proteins in the campylobacter outer membrane. The modification patterns obtained were quite complex, and varied from strain to strain. The mobility of the major outer-membrane protein was clearly altered in this procedure. These findings are of considerable interest since those proteins which constitute the diffusion pores through the outer membrane of other gram-negatives are heat modifiable[3]. Moreover, heat-modifiable outer-membrane proteins have been shown to have important roles in the virulence of *Neisseria gonorrhoeae*[2].

In some other gram-negative species, the outer membrane can be released during growth in the form of 'blebs' or vesicles[12,13]. These outer-membrane blebs can have more or less endotoxic activity depending on the LPS composition of the organism in question. Electron microscopic examination of several campylobacter strains at various stages of growth also revealed distinct outer-membrane blebbing. In the case of UVC 23, bleb formation was most pronounced at 36 hours. This outer-membrane bleb fraction was isolated by differential centrifugation. Electron microscopy revealed that this outer-membrane bleb fraction contained fragments of flagella. Preliminary examination of the protein profile of the blebs showed them to be similar but not identical to the outer membrane. The major outer-membrane protein was however present in the blebs. The toxicity of the bleb fraction is currently under investigation.

In summary, the outer membrane protein profiles of 'thermophilic' campylobacter species are variable. The predominant protein of most strains has an apparent molecular weight of 40–45 000. This protein is exposed on the surface and is heat modifiable. The protein profiles of the outer membrane differ from strain to strain, and the profile is altered with time of growth. Other heat-modifiable proteins are present. Some strains also release outer-membrane fragments which may contribute to virulence.

Acknowledgement

This investigation was supported (in part) by a grant from the British Columbia Health Care Research Foundation.

References

1. Buchanan, T. M. and Pearce, W. A. (1979). Pathogenic aspects of outer membrane components of Gram-negative bacteria. In *Bacterial Outer Membranes* (M. Inouye, ed.), pp. 475–514. John Wiley & Sons, New York
2. Lambden, P. R., Heckels, J. E., James, L. T. and Watt, P. J. (1979). Variation in surface protein composition associated with virulence properties in opacity types of *Neisseria gonorrhoeae*. *J. Gen. Microbiol.*, **114**, 305–312
3. Di Rienzo, J. M., Nakamura, K. and Inouye, M. (1978). The outer membrane proteins of gram-negative bacteria: biosynthesis, assembly, and functions. *Ann. Rev. Biochem.*, **47**, 481–532
4. Inouye, M. (1979). What is the outer membrane? In *Bacterial Outer Membranes* (M. Inouye, ed.), pp. 1–12. John Wiley and Sons, New York
5. McCoy, E. C., Doyle, D., Burda, K., Corbief, L. B. and Winter, A. J. (1975). Superficial antigens of *Campylobacter (Vibrio) fetus*: characterization of the antiphagocytic component. *Infect. Immun.*, **11**, 517–525
6. Winter, A. J., McCoy, E. C., Fullmer, C. S., Burde, K. and Bier, P. J. (1978). Microcapsule of *Campylobacter fetus*: chemical and physical characterization. *Infect. Immun.*, **22**, 963–971
7. Filip, C., Fletcher, G., Wulff, J. L. and Earhart, C. F. (1973). Solubilization of the cytoplasmic membrane of *Escherichia coli* by the ionic detergent sodium-laurylsarcosinate. *J. Bacteriol.*, **115**, 717–722
8. Hancock, R. E. W. and Carey, A. M. (1979). Outer membrane of *Pseudomonas aeruginosa*: heat- and 2-mercaptoethanol-modifiable proteins. *J. Bacteriol.*, **140**, 902–910
9. Neville, D. M. (1971). Molecular weight determination of protein-dodecyl sulfate complexes by gel electrophoresis in a discontinuous buffer system. *J. Biol. Chem.*, **246**, 6328–6334
10. Fairbanks, G., Steck, T. L. and Wallach, D. F. H. (1971). Electrophoretic analysis of the major polypeptides of the human erythrocyte membrane. *Biochemistry*, **10**, 2606–2617
11. Markwell, M. A. K., Naas, S. M., Biaber, L. L. and Tolbert, N. E. (1978). A modification of the Lowry procedure to simplify protein determination in membrane and lipoprotein samples. *Anal. Biochem.*, **87**, 206–210
12. Russell, R. R. B. (1976). Free endotoxin – a review. *Microbios Lett.*, **2**, 125–128
13. MacIntyre, S., Trust, T. J. and Buckley, J. T. (1980). Identification and characterization of outer membrane fragments released by *Aeromonas* sp. *Can. J. Biochem.*, **10**, 1018–1025

DISCUSSION

Outer-membrane blebs were prepared by differential centrifugation. In reply to questions about serum resistance, Professor Trust said that all 20 strains tested were resistant against normal rabbit serum but that specific immune serum had not been tried. Dr Taylor asked if the heat-modified protein had any relation to adhesion. Professor Trust said that they had not looked for adhesion but studies on one of the protein-2 family of gonococci outer membrane have been shown by Dr Heckles, Dr Lambden and Professor Watt (Southampton) to be related to adhesion.

83
The effect of growth conditions on total protein profiles of campylobacter

H. M. McBRIDE, D. G. NEWELL and A. D. PEARSON

Public Health Laboratory, Southampton

The classification of campylobacter species and the identification of associated virulence factors are areas of major interest in the epidemiology and pathogenesis of campylobacter enteritis. Protein profiles, using the high resolution of gradient sodium dodecyl sulphate-polyacrylamide gel electrophoresis, may contribute significantly to these investigations. However, the isolation and identification of surface proteins could be complicated by any changes in the proteins expressed, induced by growth conditions. Therefore five human campylobacter strains were cultured under various conditions including changes in temperature, time, atmospheric conditions and growth media.

In general, slight variations were found between all growth conditions, but the majority of these differences were seen in the minor bands only. However, a temperature-dependent protein with an approximate molecular weight of 68 000 daltons was quantitatively increased when the incubation temperature was altered from 37 °C to 43 °C. Few differences were observed between organisms grown micro-aerophilically on blood agar and broth or aerobically in broth containing sodium metabisulphate. However, organisms grown on G.C. base produced a number of extra bands, at least three of which were common to all five isolates (molecular weights 63 500, 39 000 and 18 500). A number of other extra bands were common to two or more of the isolates. As the organisms grew poorly on G.C. base these extra proteins probably reflected a response to an inadequate nutritional supply.

Although there were few qualitative differences in the major protein bands of organisms harvested as spiral or coccal forms there were quantitative differences and/or total loss of some minor proteins together with the production of two additional low-molecular weight bands associated with coccal development. These changes could reflect either loss of viability or a reduction in cell function associated with a 'resting state'.

Further investigations are in progress to identify and isolate the outer-membrane proteins and relate the expression of these proteins to pathogenicity.

84
Total protein profiles – a method of identification and classification for campylobacters

B. VEAL, D. G. NEWELL and A. D. PEARSON

PHLS, Southampton General Hospital, Southampton, U.K.

Despite the recent introduction of a simplified biotyping scheme based on hippurate hydrolysis and H_2S production in iron medium[1], the classification and identification of the thermophilic campylobacters is confused and inadequate for pathogenic and epidemiological studies.

We have, therefore, attempted to classify campylobacter strains, using total protein profiles of whole organisms, by gradient SDS-polyacrylamide gel electrophoresis. Campylobacter strains were isolated from human faecal material and compared with various campylobacter NCTC reference strains. All strains were tested for hippurate hydrolysis, H_2S production, nalidixic acid (30 µg disks) sensitivity and 2,3,5-triphenyl tetrazolium chloride (40 g/l) tolerance.

Sixty-five human isolates have been investigated for total protein profiles. Each isolate has a single major protein band in the 40 000–44 000 dalton range. Manipulation of the electrophoretic conditions indicates that although there are four proteins, identifiable in this region of the gel, only one is predominantly expressed in each isolate.

Comparison with the NCTC reference strains demonstrates that the *C. coli/jejuni* group can be readily distinguished from *C. fetus* ssp. *fetus*, *C. fetus* ssp. *venerealis* and *C. sputorum bubulus* on the basis of the 40 000–44 000 dalton protein bands.

Comparison of the three classes (*C. coli*, *C. jejuni* (biotype I) and *C. jejuni* (biotype II)) obtained by the biotyping technique of Skirrow and Benjamin (1980) indicates some, but not complete, correlation with the mobility of the major protein band. Considerable difficulties experienced with the reproducibility of the biotyping tests may account for the inconsistencies in correlation.

Preliminary studies on isolates of *C. coli* and *C. jejuni* from river and sea water show a similar protein profile to the human strains.

These investigations suggest that the technique of gradient SDS-polyacrylamide gel electrophoresis may be useful in the classification and identification of campylobacter isolates from a variety of sources and could be particularly relevant in future epidemiological studies.

Reference

1. Skirrow, M. B. and Benjamin, J. (1980). '1001' Campylobacters: cultural characteristics of intestinal campylobacters from man and animals. *J. Hyg.* (*Cambridge*), **85,** 427–442

85
Fatty acid composition: a possible tool for typing different campylobacter species

J. JOHNSSON, B. KAIJSER and A. SVEDHEM

Department of Clinical Bacteriology, Institute of Medical Microbiology, University of Gotenborg, Gotenborg, Sweden

---

The typing of campylobacter strains is important in epidemiological studies of campylobacter infections and several biotyping or serological schemes have been suggested. In the present investigation gas–liquid chromatography (GLC) has been used to type 150 different strains from chickens, pigs and humans including patients involved in an epidemic outbreak in Sweden. The results indicate that GLC could be a most valuable technique for distinguishing *Campylobacter jejuni* from other campylobacter species.

DISCUSSION

Dr Johnsson detailed his extraction method which included heating at 100 °C for 2 hours in 14% BF_3 in methanol.

Several questions were asked regarding the results obtained. All fatty acids are stable in the extraction procedure and although whole-cell extraction produces complicated pictures it was easier to examine whole cells and partially purified extracts might result in the loss of some components. He considered that any differences in fatty acids in relation to growth phase were probably quantitative rather than qualitative, and they had found no differences on incubation at 35 °C or 40 °C for 24 or 48 hours.

86
Cellular fatty acid profiles of campylobacters*

M. A. CURTIS

Public Health Laboratory, County Hospital, Hereford

MATERIALS AND METHODS

Methylated whole-cell extracts from 77 campylobacters were analyzed by gas–liquid chromatography (GLC).

The organisms represented three groups: 'thermophilic' campylobacters (*C. coli*, *C. jejuni*, nalidixic acid-resistant thermophilic campylobacters (NARTC)); *C. fetus* group (ssp. *fetus*, *venerealis*, 'atypical *C. fetus*'); *C. sputorum* group (ssp. *sputorum*, *bubulus*, *mucosalis*). Reference cultures of *Vibrio*, *Plesiomonas* and *Spirillum* were included for comparison.

Campylobacters were grown on Oxoid blood-agar base No. 2 and were incubated at 37 °C for 48 hours in an atmosphere containing approximately 10% oxygen. Freeze-dried cells were subjected to alkaline hydrolysis, methylation with boron triflouride-methanol followed by extraction with chloroform in hexane. Fatty acid methyl esters (FAMEs) were separated in a Pye Unicam 204 GLC fitted with a packed glass column (2.7 m × 2 mm internal diameter) containing 3% SP 2100 DOH on 100/120 Supelcoport (Supelco) and with a flame-ionisation detector. The carrier gas (N_2) flow rate was 20 ml/min and the column temperature was programmed to rise from 150–225 °C at 6 °C/min. Detected FAMEs were recorded as a series of peaks and their retention times, relative to 16:0 (RRt), and peak areas were calculated with the aid of a computing integrator. Peak identification was achieved by comparison of RRts with those of a standard mixture of FAMEs.

RESULTS

Six fatty acids were common to all campylobacters: 14:0, 3-OH–14:0, 16:1, 16:0, 18:1 and 18:0 (Table 1). In addition the 12:0 FAME occurred in members of the *C. sputorum* group and 'atypical *C. fetus*', whilst the cyclopropane-19:0 was found only among *C. coli* and *C. jejuni*. Profiles from reference strains of vibrios, *Plesiomonas* and *Spirillum* differed in general from campylobacters in producing 3-OH-12:0, several C_{17} acids and a low proportion of 18:1.

* This work formed part of a thesis submitted for Fellowship of the Institute of Medical Laboratory Sciences.

Table 1 Mean FAME peak areas of groups of campylobacters

Group	No. of strains	12:0	14:0	3-OH–14:0	16:1	16:0	18:1	18:0	cyc-19:0
C. coli	5	—	6.6	2.5	4.2	39.4	38.8	1.0	7.2
C. jejuni	12	—	7.8	2.2	3.9	35.9	37.1	1.1	11.4
NARTC	2	—	3.4	1.4	5.5	36.2	52.6	1.0	—
C. fetus ssp. fetus	29	—	8.7	2.1	18.6	33.4	35.0	0.5	—
C. fetus ssp. venerealis	6	—	11.6	1.9	21.0	37.6	27.4	0.4	—
C. fetus ssp. venerealis (intermediate)	5	—	8.1	1.4	14.0	31.1	40.6	0.4	—
C. fetus ssp. intestinalis	2	—	7.4	2.2	16.0	29.7	42.9	0.75	—
'atypical C. fetus'	6	3.2	3.8	3.6	26.8	32.0	22.0	1.2	—
C. sputorum	1	6.6	8.8	2.2	24.3	25.4	31.5	0.7	—
C. sputorum ssp. bubulus	3	0.4	24.5	4.2	7.2	26.1	36.3	0.5	—
C. sputorum ssp. mucosalis	3	8.2	9.9	3.0	25.5	27.3	23.8	0.5	—

The reproducibility of the GLC performance was assessed by repetitive injection of a single FAME preparation from a strain of C. jejuni (NCTC 11322) and the measurement of 'artificial peaks' by the computing integrator. Variation in peak areas from six repetitive injections of the extract ranged from 0–2.8%. An integrator variation of 0.2% was obtained during the study. The variation between profiles of ten extracts of the control strain (NCTC 11322) and seven extracts of C. fetus ssp. fetus (NCTC 10842) was found to be less than 1%. Individual peak area variation from these strains however ranged from 2–40%.

Forty campylobacter profiles were selected for numerical analysis, and their relationships were displayed in the form of a correlation matrix and dendrogram based on single linkage clustering (Figure 1). In this analysis, the rounded-up integer values for the peak areas of the eight predominant FAMEs were used. The highest threshold clustering level (0.99) was chosen as the one whose clusters most closely resembled the taxa under study. The six clusters (Figure 1) were brought together in a small correlation matrix in which clusters 1 and 2 were called Profile Groups 1 and 2 (PG 1 and PG 2), clusters 3, 4 and 5 were coalesced to form PG 3, and cluster 6 became PG 4. The validity of these groups was supported by studies of within-group and between-group correlation. The characteristic features of the four Profile Groups are illustrated in Figure 2 and Table 2. PG 1 contains C. sputorum and ssp. mucosalis with a characteristic 12:0 peak and approximately equal amounts of

CAMPYLOBACTER: MOLECULAR BIOLOGY

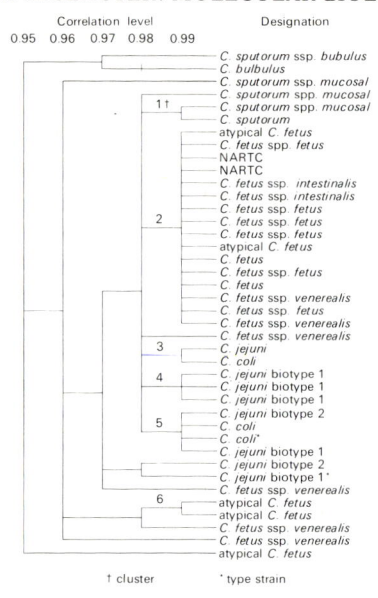

Figure 1 Dendrogram of FAME profiles of 40 campylobacters

Table 2 Differential characters of Profile Groups

Profile group	12:0	FAME cyc-19:0	16:1 to 16:0 ratio	Group
1	+	−	1:1	sputorum
2	−	−	1:2	fetus 1:6 NARTC
3	−	+	1:9	coli, jejuni
4	+	−	1:1	atypical fetus

the two C_{16} acids. PG 2 is typical of the *C. fetus* subspecies, two strains of 'atypical *C. fetus*' which conform to descriptions of *C. faecalis* (Skirrow, personal communication) and two representatives of the NARTC group. Members of this group lack 12:0 and have approximately twice as much 16:0 as 16:1, except for the NARTC group which produces six times as much 16:0 as 16:1. Profiles of *C. coli* and *C. jejuni* (PG 3) are characterized by the presence of cyc-19:0 and the large amount of 16:0 compared with 16:1. The fourth PG resembles PG 1 in the relative proportion of the two C_{16} acids and the presence of 12:0 but differs in the presence of a significant amount of an unidentified peak ('U', Figure 2d), the small amount of 14:0 and the presence of C_{15} and C_{17} acids. Correlation between the campylobacter profiles and the hypothetical mean profiles of the Profile Groups (Table 3) indicated that the majority (35/37) of the profiles not included in the matrix were correctly 'identified'.

Table 3 Profile Groups: hypothetical mean profiles

Profile group	No. of strains	\multicolumn{8}{c}{Mean FAME peak area (%)}
		12:0	14:0	3-OH-14:0	16:1	16:0	18:1	18:0	cyc-19:0
PG 1	2	7.0	9.5	3.0	24.5	25.0	30.0	0.5	—
PG 2	16	—	8.3	2.0	16.3	32.6	39.0	0.8	—
PG 3	9	—	7.0	2.1	4.2	38.0	39.3	1.0	7.8
PG 4	2	4.0	2.5	4.0	31.0	29.0	18.5	1.0	—

DISCUSSION

The predominant fatty acids common to all campylobacters were 14:0, 3-OH-14:0, 16:1, 16:0, 18:1 and 18:0. In certain profiles, 12:0 or cyc-19:0 also occurred. The findings of this study agree with those of Blaser et al.[3] in the identity of major acids of C. jejuni, and that these acids, except cyc-19:0, were present in members of C. fetus ssp. fetus and ssp. intestinalis. They did not, however, investigate the catalase-negative members of the genus and omitted 18:0 from their report.

Tornabene and Ogg[4] reported small (<1%) amounts of 18:0 from two strains of Vibrio fetus, of which one (3–17) was re-designated C. jejuni[1]. They also reported the identification of the major acids 14:0, 16:1, 16:0 and 18:1 with cyc-19:0 from 1–17 but did not observe 3-OH-14:0.

Smibert[5] has reported the major fatty acids for C. fetus ssp. fetus (14:0, 16:1, 16:0 and 18:1) for C. jejuni (10:0, 12:0 and 14:0 with larger amounts of 16:1, 16:0 and 18:1) and ssp. intestinalis, which in general, had the same acids as C. jejuni.

In this study a comparison of the mean peak areas of the eight predominant acids, according to strain designation, shows that there were three differential characters (Table 1). These were the presence or absence of 12:0 and cyc-19:0, and the ratio of the areas of 16:1 and 16:0. The C. coli and C. jejuni groups had cyc-19:0 but no 12:0 and with high ratios of the C_{16} acids (1:9.8 and 1:9 respectively). Blaser et al.[3] noted that C. jejuni contained less 16:1 (13%) than C. fetus ssp. fetus (26%) and C. fetus ssp. intestinalis, although the ratio of their peak areas for the C_{16} acids for C. jejuni was somewhat lower (1:2.2) than that found in the present study.

The C. fetus subspecies are characterized by the absence of both 12:0 and cyc-19:0 with a low ratio of the C_{16} acids (1:1.7–1:2.2). Members of the C. sputorum groups and 'atypical C. fetus' contained significant amounts of 12:0 no cyc-19:0 and low ratios (1:1–1:3.7) of C_{16} acids. Small amounts of 12:0 have been reported for C. fetus[3] and C. jejuni[3,5] but this was not confirmed in the present study. The suggestion that the NARTC group could be classified as a species[1] may be supported by their fatty-acid profiles. The profiles of two NARTC strains had a high correlation (0.998): both 12:0 and cyc-19:0 were absent and the ratio of C_{16} acids was moderately high (1:6). These profiles clustered in PG 2 which contains C. fetus subspecies and 'atypical C. fetus'. In the profile 'identification' study however they shared a high similarity with both the 'fetus' PG 2 and the 'coli/jejuni' PG 3.

PROFILE GROUP 1

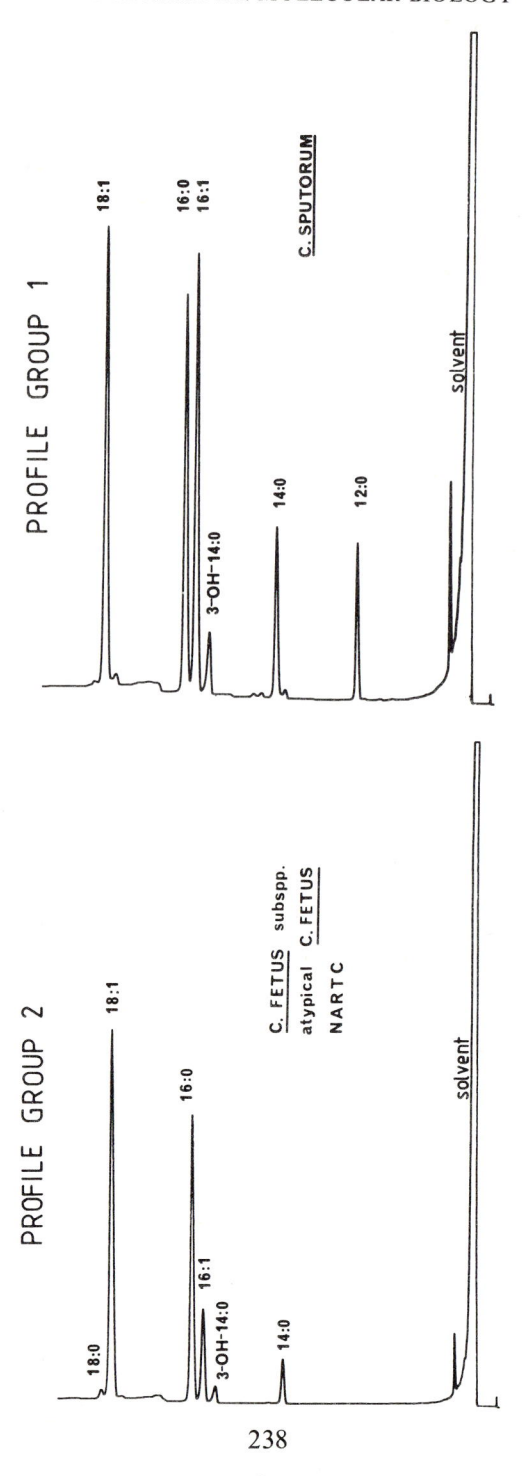

C. SPUTORUM

PROFILE GROUP 2

C. FETUS subspp. atypical
C. FETUS NARTC

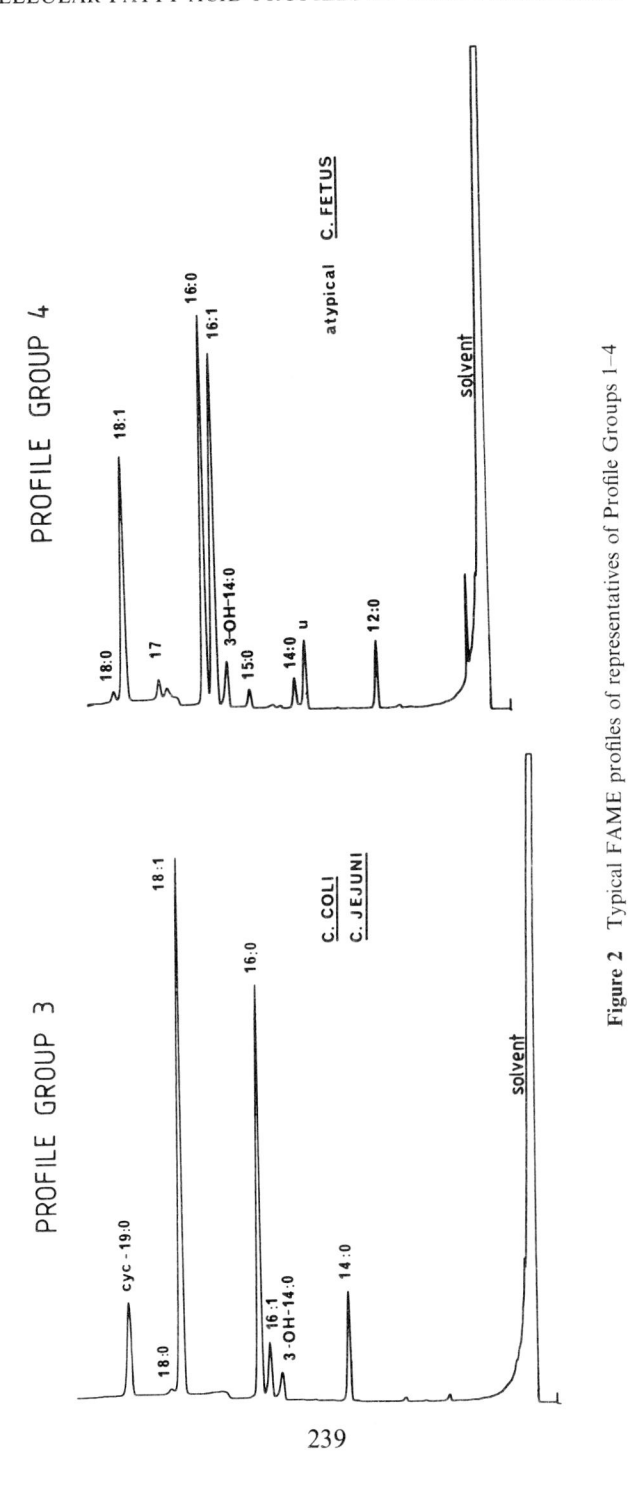

CELLULAR FATTY ACID PROFILES OF CAMPYLOBACTERS

Figure 2 Typical FAME profiles of representatives of Profile Groups 1–4

The peak area variation produced by repetitive injections of a single FAME preparation from C. jejuni (NCTC 11322) indicated that a systematic error is to be expected in the order of 3%. Integrator variation of 0.2% compares favourably with the manufacturer's limit of 2%. Repetitive extraction from subcultures of one strain produced considerable variation in individual peak area and there was a tendency for the smaller peaks to be the most variable. The profile reproducibility (<1% variation) compared favourably with a calculated figure of 1.7% based on Bøe and Gjerde's results[6].

A numerical analysis was undertaken to see whether the groups, formed from the profiles, would reflect the classification of the genus. The basis of similarity between profiles was the percentage peak areas, relative to the total FAME peak area, of the eight predominant fatty acids. The correlation coefficients between a pair of profiles could then be calculated using an equation similar to the one employed by Miyagawa et al.[7]. The 40 FAME profiles were displayed as a dendrogram. This 'tree' shows only the similarity between profiles and cannot therefore be a complete classification of the organisms. There were, however, relationships between the profiles clustering at the highest level of correlation (0.99) and the designation (or classification) of the corresponding organisms. The validity of the Profile Groups distinguishable at this level was confirmed by showing that the within-group correlations were higher than those between the groups, and that the difference between the lowest within-group value (0.96 for PG 2) and the highest value between groups (0.92 between PG 1 and PG 2) was approximately four times the expected level of profile variation.

In conclusion it was demonstrated that members of the genus *Campylobacter* produce eight predominant cellular fatty acids. Three groups of organisms corresponding to *C. coli/C. jejuni*, *C. fetus* ssp. and *C. sputorum* ssp. could be differentiated. In addition, there was evidence to support the view that the NARTC group may occupy an intermediate position between *C. coli/C. jejuni* and the *C. fetus* group. It was not possible, however, to separate *C. coli* and *C. jejuni*, or the subspecies of *C. fetus* or *C. sputorum*. There was some evidence that profiles of strains conforming to descriptions to *C. fecalis* were indistinguishable from those to *C. fetus* subspecies. The FAME profiles of the campylobacter were distinguishable from those of selected members of related genera.

The application of numerical analysis to the FAME profiles was useful in determining relationships. Four discrete Profile Groups were postulated based on profile clustering at the highest level of correlation. These groups corresponded to *C. sputorum* (PG 1), *C. fetus* ssp., 'atypical *C. fetus*' and NARTC (PG 2), *C. coli* and *C. jejuni* (PG 3) and 'atypical *C. fetus*' (PG 4). Correlation between all the campylobacter profiles and the Profile Groups indicated that the majority could be correctly 'identified' on fatty acid profile alone.

Addendum

The identities of the FAMEs reported have been verified by GLC–mass spectrometry and the unknown peak ('U', Figure 2d) is identified as the methyl ester of 14:1.

Acknowledgement

I am most grateful to Mr R. Wait of the Bacterial Metabolism Research Laboratory, Colindale for the determination and interpretation of mass spectra.

References

1. Skirrow, M. B. and Benjamin, J. (1980). '1001' Campylobacters: cultural characteristics of intestinal campylobacters from man and animals. *J. Hyg. (Camb.)*, **85**, 427–442
2. Skirrow, M. B. and Benjamin, J. (1980). Differentiation of enteropathogenic campylobacters. *J. Clin. Pathol.*, **33**, 1122
3. Blaser, M. J., Moss, C. W. and Weaver, R. E. (1980). Cellular fatty acid composition of *Campylobacter fetus*. *J. Clin. Microbiol.*, **11**, 448–451
4. Tornabene, T. G. and Ogg, J. E. (1971). Chromatographic studies of the lipid components of *Vibrio fetus*. *Biochim. Biophys. Acta*, **239**, 133–141
5. Smibert, R. M. (1978). The genus *Campylobacter*. *Ann. Rev. Microbiol.*, **32**, 673–709
6. Bøe, B. and Gjerde, J. (1980). Fatty acid patterns in the classification of some representatives of the families *Enterobacteriaceae* and *Vibrionaceae*. *J. Gen. Microbiol.*, **116**, 41–49
7. Miyagawa, E., Azuma, R. and Suto, T. (1979). Cellular fatty acid composition in gram-negative obligatory anaerobic rods. *J. Gen. Appl. Microbiol.*, **25**, 41–51

87
Immunochemistry of lipopolysaccharides isolated from *Campylobacter jejuni*

VIGFRID NAESS and TOR HOFSTAD

Department of Microbiology and Immunology, The Gade Institute, University of Bergen, Norway

---

Lipopolysaccharides (LPS) have been isolated from three strains of *Campylobacter jejuni* by extraction with 45% aqueous phenol, and purified by ultracentrifugation of the water phase and treatment of the pellet with ribonuclease.

The purified LPS are macromolecular compounds composed of a heteropolysaccharide and a lipid-A moiety. The heteropolysaccharide can be split off from the lipid-A part by mild-acid degradation. The following components have been identified in all three LPS preparations: glucosamine, L-glycero-C manno-heptose, 3-deoxy-C-manno-octulosonic acid, glucose, galactose, 3-hydroxy-tetradecanoic acid, hexadecanoic acid and phosphorus. Galactosamine was present in one LPS preparation. Untreated and alkali-treated LPS were able to sensitize sheep erythrocytes to agglutination in homologous antisera. The LPS from the three strains of *C. jejuni* did not cross-react, but antibodies to two strains were present in a few (but not the same) antisera made against other strains of *C. jejuni*. O-antigenic specificities are therefore present.

The preliminary results of this study indicate that indirect haemagglutination and inhibition of haemagglutination, using known LPS as inhibitors, may form a sound basis for a future typing of clinical isolates of *C. jejuni*.

DISCUSSION

Dr Jirillo asked if the strains with no polysaccharide chains were rough. Dr Hofstad said that they were not. Professor Trust commented that other organisms such as aeromonas have no O-side chains but may not look rough. Therefore, the rough/smooth concept derived from salmonella should not be applied to other genera.

88
In search of adhesive antigens on *Campylobacter jejuni*

F. DIJS and F. K. DE GRAAF

Biological Laboratory, Department of Microbiology, Free University, Amsterdam

Ten strains of *Campylobacter jejuni*, isolated from patients in two Dutch hospitals, were examined for the presence of adhesive antigens. Cultures of these strains, harvested during different phases of the growth cycle, both from liquid and solid media, were submitted to negative staining with phosphotungstic acid as well as platinum shadowing and studied under the electron microscope. So-called fimbriae or pili were not observed in any of these cases. Cell suspensions of the same strains, harvested in late log-phase and stationary-phase, showed agglutination of erythrocytes of man, guinea pig, chicken, horse, mouse and cow. This agglutination was mannose resistant and active at 0 °C, 20 °C and 37 °C. Shearing, extraction in glycine-hydrochloride buffer, extraction with 1% Triton X-100, or boiling of these suspensions did neither affect their haemagglutinating ability nor release an haemagglutinating agent. These results suggest the presence of a non-specific agglutinating agent in the cell wall of *C. jejuni*. By phase-contrast microscopy the same suspensions did not show adhesion of *C. jejuni* to epithelial cells or brushborders, isolated from the jejunum of piglets.

89
Auto-agglutination of *Campylobacter jejuni*: electron microscopic observations

A. E. RITCHIE, J. H. BRYNER and J. W. FOLEY

National Animal Disease Center, Ames, Iowa, U.S.A.

Serotyping of some *Campylobacter jejuni* isolants is aggravated by auto-agglutination. We have examined *C. jejuni* antigen cultures in phosphotungstic acid negative contrast to gain insight into any morphological basis for the auto-agglutination. Two observations appear to relate directly to the settling phenomenon. Most stationary growth-phase cells stained internally with phosphotungstic acid indicating a loss of permeability control. Many of these cells were 'leaky' with the extruded DNA closely adherent to the cell surface. Fused anastomosing networks of DNA also entrapped *C. jejuni* cells, possibly augmenting the precipitation. The second observation was that flagella were generally aggregated by protein-like materials, presumably phage gene product(s) released from ruptured cells. This conclusion was based on the observed specific affinity of contracted phage tails for flagella. We conclude that minimal auto-agglutination of *C. jejuni* antigen cultures can most practically be achieved by using young, log-phase cells (<27 hours) and cultures carrying a low phage multiplicity.

90
Editorial discussion

It is evident from the papers presented at this workshop that considerable advances are being made in knowledge of the biochemical characteristics of campylobacters. However, such work is still in the preliminary stages and more effort should be applied to understanding the growth characteristics, immunogenicity and antibiotic sensitivity at the biochemical level. Many of the participants have used techniques which may become applicable to taxonomy, for example the fatty acid and protein profiles. Such techniques will need to be related to established serotyping schemes in the future.

The relationship between surface components and pathogenicity markers, such as adhesion and invasion, is potentially a very interesting area of investigation which has provided considerable advances in the study of other infectious diseases. These investigations are dependent on detailed analysis of the outer-membrane proteins, flagella and lipopolysaccharides and await the development of adequate laboratory techniques for the quantitative determination of adhesion, invasion and/or toxin production *in vivo* and *in vitro*.

Preliminary investigations indicate that both plasmid-mediated and chromosomal antibiotic resistance may occur in campylobacters, and that the plasmid resistance may be transferable. Further studies are needed to demonstrate the significance of such findings in epidemiological and clinical terms.

SECTION VIII
EPIDEMIOLOGY AND ENVIRONMENTAL ASPECTS

Chairmen: M. J. Blaser and J. G. Cruickshank

91	Animal reservoirs of *Campylobacter jejuni* Nancy W. Luechtefeld and W-L. L. Wang	249
92	Campylobacters in cats and dogs D. Bruce	252
93	An epidemiological study of a campylobacter enteritis outbreak involving dogs and man M. S. Khan	256
94	Campylobacters in pig faeces V. Stich-Groh	259
95	Birds as a source of campylobacter infections D. R. Fenlon, T. M. S. Reid and I. A. Porter	261
96	Campylobacters and the broiler chicken J. G. Cruickshank, S. I. Egglestone, A. H. L Gawler and D. Lanning	263
97	Contamination of chicken meat with *Campylobacter jejuni* during the process of industrial slaughter J. Mehle, M. Gubina and B. Gliha	267
98	*Campylobacter jejuni* in poultry products from retail outlets and in poultry slaughterhouses B. J. Hartog and E. De Boer	270
99	*Campylobacter jejuni* in raw red meats. A Public Health Laboratory Service survey P. C. B. Turnbull and P. Rose	271
100	The occurrence of campylobacter on commercial red-meat carcasses from one abattoir W. R. Hudson and T. A. Roberts	273

CAMPYLOBACTER: EPIDEMIOLOGY AND ENVIRONMENTAL ASPECTS

101 Campylobacter infection in milking herds
D. A. Robinson — 274

102 Aspects of *Campylobacter jejuni* in relation to milk
S. Waterman and R. W. A. Park — 275

103 A large milk-borne outbreak of campylobacter enteritis in Luton
P. H. Jones and A. T. Willis — 276

104 A water-borne outbreak of campylobacter in central Sweden
L. O. Mentzing — 278

105 Campylobacters from water
M. J. Knill, W. G. Suckling and A. D. Pearson — 281

106 Epidemiology of campylobacter infection
W. P. J. Severin — 285

107 Campylobacter outbreak in a military camp: investigations, results and further epidemiological studies
J. Oosterom and H. J. Beckers — 288

108 Sero-epidemiological studies of *C. jejuni* infection
D. M. Jones, D. A. Robinson and J. Eldridge — 290

109 Serological epidemiology of campylobacter infection
T. M. S. Reid and I. A. Porter — 293

110 Duration of excretion period of *Campylobacter jejuni* in human subjects
E. P. Wright — 294

111 Comparison of the epidemiological characteristics of human illness from salmonella and campylobacter
R. A. Feldman and M. J. Blaser — 299

112 Editorial discussion — 301

91
Animal reservoirs of *Campylobacter jejuni*

NANCY W. LUECHTEFELD and WEN-LAN LOU WANG

Microbiology Laboratory, University of Colorado School of Medicine, U.S.A.

A number of animal species have been implicated as sources of human infection with *C. jejuni*. To determine the prevalence of this zoonosis we surveyed 3068 wild, domestic and zoo animal specimens for caecal or faecal carriage of the organism.

Specimens were collected from September, 1978 through December, 1980. Type of specimen (faecal, caecal, intestinal or rectal swab) and source of specimens are shown in Table 1. Approximately 100 of the zoo specimens were collected in sterile containers without transport media and then refrigerated; all other specimens were placed into transport media (either Campy-thio[1] or Cary Blair with decreased agar[2] immediately after collection and then refrigerated. Specimens were plated onto Campy-BAP selective medium then incubated for 48 hours at 42 °C in an atmosphere of 5% oxygen and 8% carbon dioxide. *C. jejuni* was identified by methods described previously[1].

Table 1 shows the rates of isolation of campylobacter from the various types of animals tested. Turkeys showed the highest rate of isolation and were 100% positive for the organism. The overall isolation rate from 1497 specimens from all mammals was 15%. Most of the birds and mammals were apparently healthy and showed no signs of enteritis or other illness, although some of the zoo animals, as well as some of the dogs, tested had diarrhoea or other illness. Rates of isolation of campylobacter from zoo mammals were higher from diarrhoeic specimens (31.8%) than from non-diarrhoeic specimens (5.6%) ($p < 0.001$). Although these statistics are not age-adjusted, the rates of isolation from zoo mammals were not significantly different between juveniles (less than 1-year-old) and adults, whether from diarrhoeal or normal stools.

At a local kennel where lost and unwanted pets are housed, 9% dogs and 27% puppies were positive for campylobacter. In contrast, only 2.2% of dogs ($p < 0.02$) and no puppies ($p < 0.01$) were positive at a nearby private veterinary clinic. At this clinic, 18% of the puppies and 4% of the dogs cultured had diarrhoea but campylobacter was not isolated from any of these diarrhoeic specimens. At the kennel, an estimated 6–15% of puppies and less

Table 1 Survey of animals harbouring *Campylobacter jejuni*

Type of animal	No. specimens tested	% positive for Cj	Source of specimens	Animals state of health*	Age of animal†	Type of specimen‡
Turkeys	650	100	Eight farms	H	18–24 wk	C
Ducks	445	35	Collected by hunters	H	M	C
Pigeons	153	17	Trapped at zoo	H	M	C
Various birds	62	10	Denver Zoo	H, D, O	M	C, F
Doves	80	0	Collected by hunters	H	M	C
Hogs	71	66	Two farms	H	A, J	F
Cattle	130	43	Slaughterhouse	H	A	C
Sheep	35	23	Stock show	H	A, J	F
Horses	50	0	Stable	H	A	F
Dogs	642	13	Kennel, vet. clinic	H, D, O	A, J	R
Hooved animals	203	6	Denver Zoo	H, D, O	A, J	R, F, C
Felines	89	2	Denver Zoo	H, D, O	A, J	R, F
Primates	277	5	Zoo and primate colony	H, D, O	A, J	R, F, C
Reptiles	26	4	Denver Zoo	H	A, J	F
Toads	55	0	Wild, captured	H	J	I
Snails	50	0	Freshwater stream	?	?	I
Trout	50	0	Fish Hatchery	H	A	I

* H = apparently healthy, D = diarrheic, O = other illness
† M = mature, A = adult, J = juvenile (<1-year old)
‡ C = caecal, F = faecal, R = rectal swab, I = intestinal

than 10% of dogs had diarrhoea, but we did not obtain data as to which specimens were from diarrhoeal animals.

Campylobacter was isolated from 6.6% of healthy celebes macaque monkeys at the Colorado Psychiatric Hospital's primate colony for behavioural studies. This rate is similar to that noted in healthy zoo primates (5.1%).

The only campylobacter isolate from 181 cold-blooded animals was from the faeces of a dwarf crocodile. Although salmonella and arizona are commonly isolated from reptiles[3], campylobacter was not common among the few reptiles we cultured. It is possible that since *C. jejuni* has a high optimum temperature of growth (42 °C), the organism may be quite uncommon among cold-blooded animals.

Serotyping (Table 2) of 39 isolates was performed by Dr John L. Penner by use of a passive haemagglutination technique[4].

Table 2 Serotypes of 39 Isolates of *Campylobacter jejuni* from Animal sources*

Animal	Serotype	Animal	Serotype
Dama gazelle	1	Dog	19
Dog	1	Bighorn sheep	21
Macaque monkey	2	Tapir	23
Red panda	2	Dwarf crocodile	23
Steer	2	Saki monkey	28
Saki monkey	3	Chimpanzee	34
Saki monkey	3	Colobus monkey	34
Saki monkey	3	Colobus monkey	34
Patas monkey	3	Turkey	39
Magellan goose	4	Turkey	39
Llama	5	Dama gazelle	41
Llama	5	Black lemur	5; 24
Dama gazelle	5	Roan antelope	13; 16
Dama gazelle	5	Steer	13; 16
Reindeer	5	American flamingo	Not typable
Black lemur	5	Dama gazelle	Not typable
Mallard duck	5	Mallard duck	Not typable
American widgeon duck	5	Dog	Not typable
Macaque monkey	8		
Turkey	8		
Turkey	8		

* Serotyping by passive hemagglutination technique, kindly performed by Dr John Penner, Toronto, Canada

Over the last 63 years, *C. jejuni* has been considered (at various times and by various authors) as being the pathological agent involved in bluecomb disease of turkeys, swine dysentery, abortion in sheep, winter scours in cattle, avian vibrionic hepatitis in chickens, and enteritis in dogs, cats, primates and horses. Of all these disease entities, only a sheep abortion has campylobacter been convincingly shown to be the aetiological agent. Conflicting reports exist regarding attempts at experimental infection and rates of campylobacter isolation in sick and well animals. Our studies show that *C. jejuni* can be frequently isolated from a wide variety of apparently healthy animals. In zoo animals, carriage rates of campylobacter were higher in diarrhoeic than in non-diarrhoeic animals, but individual case histories of these animals diminish the reliability of these statistics (Luechtefeld *et al.*, manuscript in preparation). A heterogeneous group of serotypes was found among the 39 isolates tested; since over half of these isolates belong to serotypes 1, 2, 3, 5, 8, or 13; 16, all of which are common serotypes of isolates from cases of human enteritis, animals may well represent a reservoir for campylobacter enteritis in humans. Further studies are required to settle the question of the pathogenicity of *C. jejuni* for various species of animals.

Acknowledgements

We thank Richard C. Cambre, DVM (Denver Zoological Gardens), Robert Taylor, DVM (Alameda East Veterinary Clinic) and Martin Reite, MD (CPH Primate Laboratory) for providing specimens for this study.

References

1. Blaser, M. J., Berkowitz, I. D., LaForce, F. M., Cravens, J., Reller, L. B. and Wang, W.-L. L. (1979). Campylobacter enteritis: clinical and epidemiological features. *Ann. Intern. Med.*, **91**, 179–185
2. Luechtefeld, N. W., Wang, W.-L. L., Blaser, M. J. and Reller, L. B. (1981). Evaluation of transport and storage techniques for isolation of *Campylobacter fetus* subsp. *jejuni* from turkey caecal specimens. *J. Clin. Microbiol.*, **13**, 438–443
3. Cambre, R. C., Green, E., Smith, E. E. and Montali, R. J. (1980). Salmonellosis and Arizonosis in the reptile collection at the National Zoological Park. *J. Am. Vet. Assoc.*, **177**, 800–803
4. Penner, J. L. and Hennessey, J. N. (1980). Passive haemagglutination technique for serotyping *Campylobacter fetus* subsp. *jejuni* on the basis of soluble heat-stable antigens. *J. Clin. Microbiol.*, **12**, 732–737

92
Campylobacters in cats and dogs

D. BRUCE

Public Health Laboratory, Hereford, U.K.

Dogs, especially puppies, have been shown to be responsible for the transfer of campylobacters to human contacts.

Four surveys were undertaken:

(1) An 18-month study[1] to determine the frequency of isolation of thermophilic campylobacters from the faeces of cats and dogs at the local RSPCA premises and of puppies seen in kennels and veterinary practice (Tables 1 and 2).
(2) A study of faecal samples from puppies taken during an outbreak of acute haemorrhagic enteritis at a kennel (Table 3).
(3) A study of asymptomatic dogs seen in private veterinary practice (Table 4).

Specimens were examined by direct culture and following enrichment in the following medium.

Liquid enrichment media (L.E.M.)

Oxoid nutrient broth No. 2	1 litre
7% horse blood	70 ml
Vancomycin	10 mg
Polymyxin B. sulphate	2500 iu
Trimethoprim lactate	25 mg

Comparative results are presented in Table 5.

Table 1 Isolation of *C. jejuni* from faeces of cats and dogs at R.S.P.C.A. premises

	Number of animals	Campylobacter isolated	Isolation rate
Cats	56	25	45%
Dogs	144	70	49%
Total	200	95	48%

Table 2 Isolation of *C. jejuni* from faeces of puppies from a veterinary practice and kennels

	Number of animals	Campylobacter isolated	Isolation rate
Asymptomatic puppies	38	15	39%
Diarrhoeic puppies	42	16	38%
Total	80	31	39%

Table 3 Isolation of *C. jejuni* from samples taken from puppies during an outbreak of acute haemorrhagic enteritis at a kennel

	Number of animals	Campylobacter isolated	Isolation rate
Puppies with diarrhoea clinically recovered	13	7	54%
Puppies dead from haemorrhagic enteritis	29	9	31%
Total	42	16	38%

Table 4 Faecal carriage of campylobacters in asymptomatic dogs

Number of animals	Campylobacter isolated	Isolation rate
36	8	22%

Table 5 Comparison of media
No. of specimens of cats and dogs examined = 305

	No. of campylobacters isolated	Isolation rate
Direct culture only	7	2%
Enrichment culture only	34	11%
Direct culture + enrichment	93	31%
Total no. of isolations	134	44%

References

1. Bruce, D., Zochowski, W. and Fleming, G. A. (1980). Campylobacter species in cats and dogs. *Vet. Rec.*, **107**, 200–201
2. Skirrow, M. B. (1981). Campylobacter enteritis in dogs and cats: a new Zoonosis. *Vet. Res. Commun.*, **5**, 13–19

DISCUSSION

Dr Skirrow has recently reviewed the literature concerning isolations of *C. jejuni* from dogs and cats[2]. In general, two points can be made. There is a much higher prevalence in kennel dogs than amongst household dogs, and human cases have almost exclusively been due to contact with diarrhoeal puppies.

93
An epidemiological study of a campylobacter enteritis outbreak involving dogs and man

M. S. KHAN

Pathology Laboratory, Warwick, U.K.

In the summer of 1979 there was an outbreak of campylobacter enteritis in a number of dogs and people from one street, the residents of which use a riverside meadow to exercise their dogs. This meadow is often flooded and wild ducks and various waterfowl feed there and breed nearby.

From January 1980, a 12-month survey of samples from the river and meadow area was carried out to establish base-line data on seasonal variation of biotype and the prevalence of 'thermophilic' campylobacters (Figure 1).

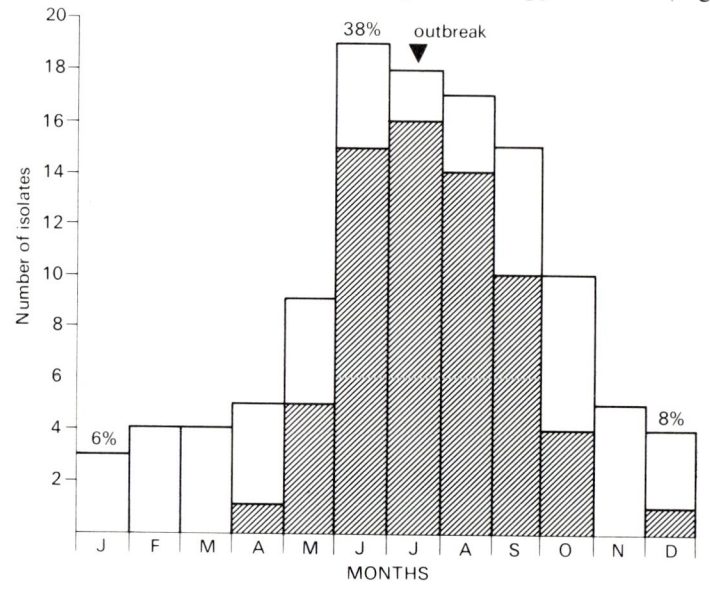

Figure 1 Seasonal variation of campylobacter isolates and biotype.

Every fortnight, 25 samples were taken for culture, three of river-bank mud, two of river water, ten of dog excreta and ten of fowl droppings from the nesting area and the river bank.

Biotyping was done using the method described by Skirrow[1]. In the first quarter of 1980, the average positive isolation rate was 8%. *C. jejuni* biotype 1, biotype 2, *C. coli* and a few untypable strains were found to be evenly distributed (Table 1). From May–August, there was a sharp rise of positive isolations reaching a peak of 38% in June. This increase was confined to *C. jejuni* biotype 1. The positive isolation rate gradually fell to 12% during the last quarter of 1980 (Table 2).

Table 1 Rate of isolation of thermophilic campylobacters from 50 environmental sites sampled each month in 1980 in Warwickshire

Month	J	F	M	A	M	J	J	A	S	O	N	D
Rate	6	8	8	10	18	38	36	34	30	20	10	8

Table 2 Number of 'thermophilic' campylobacter isolated from environmental samples during 1980

	C. jejuni 1	C. jejuni 2	C. coli	NRTC/NT
River mud	13	4	5	1
River water	12	1	3	0
Dog excreta	19	10	7	2
Fowl droppings	22	9	4	2

In the second week of July 1980, there was an outbreak of *C. jejuni* biotype 1 enteritis involving seven people and their five dogs. Four households from the same neighbourhood near the meadow area were involved. All human cases occurred within a period of 10–12 days and needed medical attention. The dogs developed diarrhoea on average 6 days before the first human contact became ill. All isolates were indistinguishable from each other by the biotyping method and designated as *C. jejuni* type 1. These 'epidemic' strains were serotyped at Manchester P.H.L. by the method described by Abbott et al.[2] and all were found to be serotype 3.

Except for the regular use of the meadow area, no other common factor was found. The exact starting point of the outbreak is still unclear. The increase in one biotype in the meadow and in fowl droppings 1 month before the first case was diagnosed in dogs and man suggest that the reservoir could be the environment.

References

1. Skirrow, M. B. and Benjamin, J. (1980). Differentiations of enteropathogenic campylobacter. *J. Clin. Pathol.*, **33**, 1122
2. Abbott, J. D., Dale, B., Eldridge, J., Jones, D. M. and Sutcliffe, E. M. (1980). Serotyping of Campylobacter jejuni/coli. *J. Clin. Pathol.*, **33**, 762–766

DISCUSSION

Dr Blaser pointed out that sampling from the same points throughout a year showed an increase in isolations in the warm months, which suggests a basis for the increase in isolations from humans during those times.

94
Campylobacters in pig faeces

V. STICH-GROH

Institute for Hygiene and Microbiology, The University, Wuerzburg, W. Germany

Since the first reports from Belgium[1] and Great Britain[2] it is now accepted that *C. jejuni* is a major cause of diarrhoeal disease in man. The mode of transmission is still uncertain, as the evidence is largely circumstantial. We postulate an additional means of spread from animal to man.

In Wuerzburg (Federal Republic of Germany, Bavaria) we have recovered campylobacter in great numbers from the faeces of healthy pigs at the time of slaughter. From one-hundred faecal samples (plates incubated at 42 °C in micro-aerophilic condition, using Skirrow's medium), 72 campylobacter strains were cultured.

In Germany, pig intestine is still used in sausage production therefore we followed the processing of sausage skins from the slaughterhouse to the butcher's shop. In the butcher's shop, after overnight salting, the intestines were washed before sausage making. From the samples obtained campylobacters were recovered from 30% of the specimens tested (Table 1). As a proportion of the pig campylobacters (*C. coli*) were probably really *C. jejuni* (one strain has been identified by Dr Skirrow, Worcester), it is likely that infection may spread from pig to man. In countries where a large amount of pork sausage and related products are consumed, this process may be an additional way of transmitting gastrointestinal infection to man.

References

1. Butzler, J. P., DeKeyser, P., Detrain, M. and Dehaen, F. (1973). Related vibrios in stools. *J. Paediatr.*, **82**, 493–495
2. Skirrow, M. B. (1977). Campylobacter enteritis, A 'new' disease. *Br. Med. J.*, **2**, 9–11

DISCUSSION

Dr Jorgenson found similar isolation rates in Germany. Dr Luechtefeld found that pig isolates in Denver, USA were hippurate negative. Dr Skirrow pointed out that hippurate-negative strains are isolated more commonly from humans in Belgium than in the UK.

CAMPYLOBACTER: EPIDEMIOLOGY AND ENVIRONMENTAL ASPECTS

Table 1 Isolation of campylobacters in a slaughterhouse for pigs

Source	No. tested	No. + for: C. jejuni	No. + for: C. coli
Faeces (slaughterhouse)	116	18	59
Water bowels washed in (slaughterhouse)	4	2	1
Washed pig bowels (slaughter house)	22	2	8
Water, salted bowels kept in overnight (butcher shop)	8	2	1
Washed pig bowels before treatment (butcher shop)	10	1	4
Washed pig bowels after salt treatment (butcher shop)	7	0	3
Floors, pots, pans, tables (butcher shop)	6	0	2
Sausage	6	0	0
Total no. of pig campylobacters isolated/No. specimens	103/173	25	78

95
Birds as a source of campylobacter infections

D. R. FENLON, T. M. S. REID and I. A. PORTER

North of Scotland College of Agriculture and City Hospital, Aberdeen

Interest has been shown in the possibility of wild birds carrying and transmitting pathogenic bacteria to domesticated livestock and man. A survey has therefore been undertaken into the incidence of pathogens, including the thermophilic campylobacters, in the faeces of wild birds. Attention was concentrated on those species (gulls, rooks, geese and pigeons) which feed and roost in large numbers on grazed pastures and so were a potential source of infection.

Only fresh faecal samples were taken, either beneath rookeries or by disturbing flocks of resting birds. Isolations and counts were made on Skirrow's medium supplemented with 4 mg/l actidione to suppress fungal growth, and incubated micro-aerophilically at 42 °C.

The carrier rates, numbers of organisms per gram of faeces and nalidixic acid resistance of the isolates from various species of birds are shown in Table 1.

Table 1 Numbers and frequency of campylobacter in the faeces of wild birds

Bird species	No. of samples	% positive	No. of isolates Nalidixic acid Res	Sens	Range of counts of campylobacter per gm. of faeces
Herring and great black-backed gulls	167	55	30	57	$1.8 \times 10^2 - 4.9 \times 10^6$
Black-headed gull	58	22	1	12	$7.4 \times 10^2 - 1.7 \times 10^5$
Pigeons (urban)	29	41	1	11	$1.4 \times 10^3 - 1.2 \times 10^6$
Rooks	45	40	0	18	$6.7 \times 10^3 - 2.9 \times 10^6$
Wild geese	24	33	0	8	$6.4 \times 10^4 - 3.0 \times 10^5$

Table 2 shows those isolates from wild birds which have so far been biotyped[1]. Nalidixic acid resistance is mainly confined to those isolates from the large gulls, but falls into two categories, biotype NARTC, and a larger H_2S negative campylobacter of unknown biotype.

Table 2 Biotypes of thermophilic campylobacters isolated from wild birds

Bird species	No. of samples	Nalidixic acid resistant/sensitive	H_2S	Hippurate hydrolysis	Biotype
Herring and black-backed gulls	5	R	−	−	untypable
Gull	1	S	+	+	*jejuni* II
Gull	2	R	+	−	NARTC
Gull	3 }	S	−	−	*coli*
Crow	1 }				
Wild goose	1 }	S	−	+	*jejuni* I
Crow	1 }				

The remaining isolates are scattered over the *C. jejuni* biotypes. Only two isolates fall into the *C. jejuni* I biotype which is responsible for most human infections and none of these were isolated from gulls.

This survey has also shown that whereas carriage of *Salmonella* ssp. and drug-resistant coliforms tend to be concentrated in gulls which scavenge near sources of sewage, and are absent or found only in low numbers in gulls and other bird species feeding on agricultural sources, this is not the case with carriage of *Campylobacter* ssp. Campylobacters are found frequently in all the bird species examined, suggesting that they are endemic in the general bird population, and some may be specific biotypes associated with birds.

The low incidence of the important human pathogen *C. jejuni* I in the isolates, especially its absence from gulls might suggest that the role of birds, scavenging or otherwise, in the spread of this organism must be open to question.

References

1. Skirrow, M. B. and Benjamin, J. (1980). Differentiation of enteropathogenic campylobacter. *J. Clin. Pathol.*, **33**, 1122

96
Campylobacter jejuni and the broiler chicken process

J. G. CRUICKSHANK, S. I. EGGLESTONE,
A. H. L. GAWLER and D. G. LANNING

Public Health Laboratory, Exeter, U.K.

INTRODUCTION

In this study we have looked for *Campylobacter jejuni* at several stages in the broiler production process in an attempt to define sources. The chicken is regularly cited as the likely source of *C. jejuni* infections in man. The presence of campylobacters have been demonstrated in the intestines of chickens and their products[1,2,3,4], and surveys of commercially reared chickens indicate the isolation of campylobacters from 14%–91% of those examined[6,7,8].

Epidemiological evidence also suggests poultry as a source. Skirrow[5] reported six cases in which the organisms found had the same biotype as those isolated from the chickens they had been handling.

Hayek and Cruickshank[9] have reported a common source outbreak implicating chicken. In another outbreak 89 out of 123 Belgian military cadets developed enteritis 3 days after killing, skinning and cooking a chicken for their own consumption. *C. jejuni* was isolated from 34 of the men[10].

However, not all chickens appear to carry campylobacters as part of their normal gut flora[11] so it may be possible to maintain campylobacter free flocks similarly to salmonella free flocks (Lanning, personal communication).

The production of broiler chickens is organized to produce maximal growth rates. Provided the initial stock is free of campylobacters it should be possible to identify the stage at which colonization takes place.

MATERIALS AND METHODS

(1) Broiler process

There are four main stages in the broiler process – stock breeding, egg production, hatching and growing. Systems may vary in detail in different companies.

Breeding-stock companies provide stock of controlled genetic type. Day-old chicks are dispatched to the 'breeder houses' where fertile eggs for the hatcheries are produced. The chicks, which live on open deep litter, are vaccinated against a variety of infections and fed on a diet which is part commercial and partly re-cycled and pasteurized poultry slaughterhouse waste. Ventilation is common to all parts of the house. After mating, fertile-egg production starts at 26 weeks and continues until 60 weeks. Samples of blood and faeces are submitted at regular intervals for laboratory examination.

Eggs are taken to the hatcheries on chemically disinfected trays and the day-old chicks are sent in boxes with 'inserts' (paper or wood-wool) to the growing houses.

In the growing houses up to 20 000 birds are kept in a single room on deep litter. They are fed automatically from hoppers and given water *ad lib*. No other interference, apart from daily inspection and removal of dead birds, takes place until the 49th day when they are removed for slaughter.

(2) Bacteriology

Breeding stock is outside the control of commercial producers and was not investigated. Specimens of birds, eggs, faeces and 'inserts' were taken at intervals and examined using Skirrow's medium. Samples of environmental materials were similarly examined.

Twelve birds from each of 14 growing houses were examined separately over a 12-month period. Isolates were biotyped according to Skirrow and Benjamin[12].

(3) Serology

Antigens were prepared by heating cultures for 10 minutes and antisera were prepared in rabbits.

RESULTS

Campylobacter isolations are presented in Table 1.

Birds from three of the 14 growing farms harboured *C. jejuni*. Within an infected farm a high proportion, possibly all, were affected. Following normal cleaning and disinfection of the houses after removal of an infected batch, subsequent flocks in the same house did not become infected. In affected flocks there was no excess mortality and the average weights at the time of slaughter were the same as those of unaffected chickens. *C. jejuni* was also isolated occasionally from giblets.

SEROLOGY

Six sera from each of the 14 houses were obtained at slaughter and tested against three antigens. Seven sera gave positive results to various single antigens.

Table 1 Campylobacter isolations from various stages in broiler chicken production

Stage	Material tested	Isolation + or −	Time from start of stage to first isolation
Breeding stock	Eggs		
	Day-old chicks	Not tested	
Breeder houses	Day-old chicks	−	
	Older chicks	−	7 days
	Feed	−	
	Water	−	
	Ventilation dust	−	
Hatcheries	Egg – surface	−	
	Egg – substance	−	
Growing houses	Day-old chicks	−	
	Older chicks	−	7 days
	Feed	−	
	Water	−	
	Ventilation	−	
	Deep litter	+	3–4 days
	Rats, mice	−	
	Insert	−	
Abattoir	Cross contamination pre- and post-chlorine bath	+	

Therefore some campylobacters apparently invade sufficiently to give rise to antibody production and there are at least three antigenic types.

BIOTYPING

Using Skirrow's hippurate and H_2S tests, eight out of nine strains typed as *C. jejuni* 2.

COMMENT

C. jejuni is not an essential constituent of the bowel flora in chickens and the incidence of excreting flocks varies from place to place. Dr Nelson (V.I. Centre Gloucester – personal communication) has demonstrated experimentally that transmission does not occur either through the egg or by contamination of the shell. Natural-egg transmission was not demonstrated in our studies. However, within the closed environment of broiler production systems, birds may acquire the organisms within the first few days of life. The most likely sources for the organisms are: (a) feed and water, (b) ventilation ports – food and dust particles are carried through the ports and settle on the surrounding roof and attract wild birds which are known to carry *C. jejuni* and (c) contamination during transport.

Evidence that chicken campylobacters cause disease in man is largely epidemiological and further advances await the development of more discriminatory techniques than are available at present. However, it is of interest that while workers in one broiler factory did not show an increased incidence of absence from work or of gastrointestinal disease even early on in their employment, serological studies in another broiler factory indicate that a high proportion of the workers have antibody against *C. jejuni* (Dr D. Robinson, Manchester – personal communication). Therefore sub-clinical infections may be common in exposed populations.

CONCLUSION

At present it seems unlikely that efforts to prevent colonization of broiler chickens with campylobacters are justified on economic, veterinary or medical grounds.

References

1. Fletcher, R. D. and Plastridge, W. N. (1964). Difference in physiology of *Vibrio* spp. from chicken and man. Avian Diseases, **8,** 72–75
2. Smibert, R. M. (1965). *Vibrio fetus* var. *intestinalis* isolated from the intestinal content of birds. Am. J. Vet. Res., **30,** 1437–1442
3. Smith, M. V. and Muldoon, P. J. (1974). *Campylobacter fetus* ssp. *jejuni* (*Vibrio fetus*) from commercially processed poultry. Appl. Microbiol., **27,** 995
4. Smith, M. V. (1973). *Campylobacter fetus* ssp. *jejuni* from some commercially processed poultry products. Thesis Virginia Polytechnic Institute.
5. Skirrow, M. B. (1977). Campylobacter enteritis: a 'new' disease. Br. Med. J., **ii,** 9
6. Simmons, N. A. and Gibbs, F. J. (1977). Campylobacter enteritis. Br. Med. J., **ii,** 264
7. Bruce, D., Sochowski, W. and Ferguson, I. R. (1977). Campylobacter enteritis. Br. Med. J., **ii,** 1219
8. Ribeiro, C. D. (1978). Campylobacter enteritis. Lancet, **ii,** 270
9. Mayek, L. J. and Cruickshank, J. G. (1977). Campylobacter enteritis. Br. Med. J., **ii,** 1219
10. Brouwer, R., Mertens, M. J. A., Siem, T. H. and Katchaki, O. O. (1979). An explosive outbreak of Campylobacter enteritis in soldiers. Antonie van Leeuwenhoek, **45,** 517–519
11. Barnes, E. M. (1979). The intestinal microflora of poultry and game birds during life and after storage. J. Appl. Microbiol., **46,** 407–419
12. Skirrow, M. B. and Benjamin, J. (1980). Differentiation of enteropathogenic campylobacter. J. Clin. Pathol., **33,** 1122

97
Contamination of chicken meat with *Campylobacter jejuni* during the process of industrial slaughter

J. MEHLE, M. GUBINA and B. GLIHA

Ljubljana, Yugoslavia

INTRODUCTION

Since the recognition of *Campylobacter jejuni* as a frequent cause of enteritis in man the possible transmission from animals to human has been suggested. Chickens, particularly broilers, are thought to be a frequent source[1,2,3,4,5]. Preliminary studies indicated that campylobacters are transferred from gut to animal skin during the process of broiler slaughter. This study investigates the contamination frequency of broiler flocks and the contamination of meat after slaughter.

METHODS

Twenty-seven flocks each containing 15000–20000 chickens were investigated. A sample of ten animals was taken from every flock. The process of slaughter and final meat packing was followed continuously in two industrial slaughter-houses. The study comprised of three phases.

(1) Rearing phase
A group of 27 animals 30–50-days old were taken 10 days before the flock was slaughtered and the intestinal contents examined for *C. jejuni*.

(2) Industrial slaughter phase
After evisceration, samples of faeces, swabs of skin, swabs of the abdominal wall, and samples of the straining liquid obtained after meat washing were taken from 270 carcases.

(3) Phase of storage before sale
Fifty-four broilers were tested (two from each farm). Half of the broilers were

kept at 4 °C for 7 days and half were frozen at −25 °C for 3 weeks. Subcutaneous tissue, meat and skin samples were taken daily from broilers kept at 4 °C and weekly from those at −25 °C.

Tryptose agar with 10% sheep blood (TBA) was used for all isolations; plates were incubated at 37 °C for 2–3 days in a reduced oxygen-tension atmosphere. Colonies were identified as *C. jejuni* before counting.

Swabs of skin and abdominal wall were taken from a 100 cm^2 area, washed with 3 ml of saline which was passed through a 0.65 µm Millipore filter and 0.1 ml of the filtrate was inoculated onto TBA. Samples of the faeces were dissolved in 9 ml of physiological saline, the supernatant filtered and then centrifuged at 3000 rpm for 10 minutes. Viable counts were made from the filtrates.

Straining liquid was diluted 1:3, passed though a 0.65 µm Millipore filter and 0.1 ml was inoculated on TBA. Skin tissue was tested for persistence of *C. jejuni* under conditions of storage. Pieces of 25 cm^2 were washed in physiological saline which was in turn passed through a 0.65 µm and a 0.22 µm Millipore filter. The filtrate was spread on TBA and counts made after 2 days.

One cubic centimetre of subcutaneous tissue and muscles were tested by spreading over TBA.

RESULTS

C. jejuni was found in 19 of the 27 flocks (70%) in the rearing phase. This positive group was termed group A and the eight farms from which *C. jejuni* was not isolated at this stage was termed group B.

Table 1 presents the isolations of *C. jejuni* during the stage of industrial slaughter. Clearly the mechanical extraction of the intestines results in the widespread contamination of the surface of the carcase. The washing procedure does not eliminate the organisms. Table 2 presents the average number of organisms recovered from faeces, skin and straining liquid in birds

Table 1 Isolation of *C. jejuni* during the procedure of poultry slaughter

Sample	Faeces	Swabs of skin and abdominal wall	Straining liquid	Total
Group A (19 farms)				
Examined/farm	10	40	20	70
Cj positive	190	751	350	1321
Cj negative	—	9	—	9
Group B (8 farms)				
Examined/farm	10	40	20	70
Cj positive	—	—	—	—
Cj negative	80	320	160	560
Total examined samples	270	1080	540	1890

Cj = Campylobacter jejuni

Table 2 The number of *C. jejuni* isolated from samples of infected flocks

Samples	Number of C. jejuni
Faeces	$5 \times 10^5/\text{g}$
Swab of abdominal wall and skin	$280/100\,\text{cm}^2$
Straining liquid	$160/\text{ml}$

from the infected flocks. Table 3 shows the results of sampling from chickens from group-A flocks which had been stored after processing for 7 days at 4 °C or 3 weeks at 25 °C.

In group-B flocks no campylobacters were isolated at any stage of industrial processing or storage.

Table 3 The isolation of *C. jejuni* from chickens during storage prior to sale

Sample	4 °C Meat	4 °C Skin	−25 °C Meat	−25 °C Skin
Group A (19 farms)				
Cj positive	—	133	—	57
Cj negative	266	—	114	—
Group B (8 farms)				
Cj positive	—	—	—	—
Cj negative	112	56	48	24

CONCLUSION

Where flocks of chickens become colonized, all the birds are likely to be involved and gross contamination of the abattoir occurs.

References

1. Grant, I. H., Richardson, N. J. and Bokkenheuser, V. D. (1980). Broiler chickens as potential source of campylobacter infections in humans. *J. Clin. Microbiol.*, **11**, 508–510
2. King E. O. (1962). The laboratory recognition of *Vibrio fetus* and a closely related vibrio isolated from cases of human vibriosis. *Ann. N. Y. Acad. Sci.*, **98**, 700–711
3. Simmons, N. A. and Gibbs, F. J. (1979). *Campylobacter* spp. in oven-ready poultry. *J. Infect.*, **1**, 159–162
4. Skirrow, M. B. (1977). Campylobacter enteritis: a 'new' disease. *Br. Med. J.*, **2**, 9–11
5. Smith, M. V. and Muldoon, P. J. (1974). *Campylobacter fetus* ssp. *jejuni* (*Vibrio fetus*) from commercially processed poultry. *Appl. Microbiol.*, **27**, 995–996

98
Campylobacter jejuni in poultry products from retail outlets and in poultry slaughterhouses

B. J. HARTOG and E. DE BOER

Food Inspection Service, The Netherlands

We studied the occurrence of *C. jejuni* in chicken legs, wings, breasts and livers, and in processed products such as chicken fillet, sausages, mince, burgers and rolled chicken meat obtained from retail outlets.

Twenty-gram samples were suspended (1:10) in buffered-peptone water by means of a stomacher and 0.1 ml amounts of serial 10-fold dilutions were spread on Skirrow's medium with a pyruvate-bisulphate-ferrous sulphate supplement. The plates were incubated for 48 hours at 42 °C in anaerobic jars without catalyst, but with BBL GasPak hydrogen–carbon dioxide envelopes and the number of *C. jejuni* colonies counted.

Sixty-seven per cent of chilled chicken-livers contained viable campylobacters and in 36% the counts were $>10^3$ cfu/g. Campylobacters were isolated from just 4% of frozen chicken-livers. *C. jejuni* was also isolated from the peritoneal cavities of 32% of chilled-chicken carcasses and from 36% of frozen-chicken carcasses at the retail point of sale.

Investigations in four poultry slaughter-houses showed extensive contamination of equipment with campylobacters and that in 73% of chicken carcasses the organisms could be recovered from the peritoneal cavity. In two houses cooling water contained up to 3×10^3 cfu/ml and air sampling near the scalding tanks and in the evisceration areas yielded 5–6 cfu/m^3.

Cross-contamination occurs widely during the slaughter process but freezing helps to contain the organisms.

99
Campylobacter jejuni in raw red meats: a Public Health Laboratory Service survey

P. C. B. TURNBULL and P. ROSE

Central Public Health Laboratory, London

A survey was initiated to determine the contamination of raw red meats by *C. jejuni*. 2046 samples of minced beef, 1496 sausages (including sausage-meat), 376 samples of minced pork and 2278 of other meat samples were examined (total, 6169). 1236 of these samples were from abattoirs and the remaining 4933 from retail outlets including a few samples from meat factories.

Overall just 98 samples (1.6%) were found to contain *C. jejuni*. A higher isolation rate of 49/1236 (4.0%) was found among abattoir samples than among retail and other samples (48/4933–1.0%). Retail minced beef (21/2015–1.0%) and abattoir pork samples (32 of the 49 positive abattoir samples) accounted for the bulk of the 98 isolates.

Fifty-five of the 98 (56.1%) isolates were picked up on direct plating with approximate colony counts ranging from 1–20/0.1 ml meat slurry. The single exception was a pig spleen/bacon factory sample which contained 1200 colonies/0.1 ml.

No relationship was apparent between the number of samples examined by a laboratory and the number of campylobacter isolations made. Nor did isolation rates from meat samples correlate with numbers of patient isolations made over the same period in the different laboratories.

Some of the laboratories also looked for salmonella in the samples; 94/4002 (2.3%) were positive, but in only a single sample (minced beef) were salmonella and campylobacter found together. Isolation rates for salmonella were 75/3576 (2.1%) from retail samples and 19/426 (4.5%) from abattoir samples. Sausage-meat (28/962–2.9%), minced beef (21/1492–1.4%) and abattoir pork samples (12 of the 19 positive abattoir samples) accounted for the majority of salmonella isolations.

The analysis has revealed that: (1) the contamination rate of raw red meat by *C. jejuni* is, in general, very low; (2) when contaminated, counts are generally also very low; (3) enrichment was of some value although 14 of the 98 (14.3%) were direct plate positive/enrichment negative; (4) practice gained from looking for the organism and increases in seasonal temperatures over the period of the survey did not result in a noticeable increase in isolation rate and (5) there was no apparent correlation between salmonella and campylobacter isolations.

100
The occurrence of campylobacter on commercial red-meat carcases from one abattoir

W. R. HUDSON and T. A. ROBERTS

Meat Research Institute, Bristol, U.K.

Organisms of the genus *Campylobacter* have been associated with abortion in sheep and cattle, and with dysentery in swine. In recent years 'related' campylobacters have frequently been associated with human illness. The origin of these 'related' campylobacters is poorly understood and their possible occurrence on red-meat carcases was investigated at one abattoir.

Three-hundred carcases (100 cattle, 100 lamb and 100 pig) were swabbed at the end of the slaughter line immediately prior to chilling and the swabs examined for campylobacter using the technique described by Skirrow[1]. No campylobacters were found on beef and lamb carcases but 59% of pig carcases were positive.

A further 100 pig carcases were examined after chilling for 24 hours at 0 °C in 95% relative humidity. Swabs were taken from measured areas of the carcases – some from parts which were dry and some from parts which were damp due to contact with other carcases; 2% of samples from the dry areas and 26% from the wet areas yielded campylobacter. The numbers isolated were generally less than $1/cm^2$.

Sixteen of the isolates conformed to Véron and Chatelain's *C. coli* but differed from the majority of those isolated from human enteritis cases in their ability to grow at 30 °C, to produce H_2S and to resist triphenyltetrazolium chloride. These findings suggest that red-meat carcases are unlikely to be a major source of the organisms causing human campylobacter enteritis.

References

1. Skirrow, H. B. (1977). Campylobacter enteritis: a 'new' disease. *Br. Med. J.*, **2**, 9–11

101
Campylobacter infection in milking herds

D. A. ROBINSON

Public Health Laboratory, Manchester, U.K.

The commonest vehicle of *C. jejuni* infection in investigated human outbreaks in Britain is unpasteurized milk. In order to answer some of the questions concerning the place of the milk cow in the epidemiology of *C. jejuni*, a study of two milking herds was carried out.

Rectal swabs were examined every 2 weeks from all cows in both herds, and every week from animals found to be excreting campylobacter. Milk filters were examined three times a week. The study continued for 6 months in one herd and 12 months in the other. Summarising, the findings were:

(1) *C. jejuni* could be isolated from about 10% of each herd in the summer months, declining to zero during the winter and re-emerging in the spring.
(2) No symptoms associated with the infection were noted in any cow.
(3) The level of excretion by individual cows was low and intermittent.
(4) Calving induced a brief rise in the level of excretion.
(5) Several different serotypes were demonstrable within a herd at the same time.
(6) Individual cows were shown to excrete the same serotype for several months at a time.
(7) Transmission was demonstrated into, and between, calves and young heifers but not adult members of the herd.
(8) Campylobacters were not isolated from the milk filters from either herd at any time, despite persistent infection within the herds.

Conclusions:

(1) *C. jejuni* is a normal commensal of cows.
(2) It is possible that infection only occurs in calves, but that having become established it may remain for many months, if not for life.
(3) The presence of *C. jejuni* in the herd need not lead to contamination of the milk produced by the herd.
(4) As *C. jejuni* is a normal commensal, the control of milk-borne infection in man probably lies outside the responsibility of farmers or their veterinary advisers. Control of this problem can be achieved by pasteurization.

102
Aspects of *Campylobacter jejuni* in relation to milk

S. WATERMAN and R. W. A. PARK

Microbiology Department, University of Reading, U.K.

Milk has been implicated in outbreaks of campylobacter enteritis and although *C. jejuni* has been isolated from milk stocks on several such occasions, further tracing has been generally unsuccessful. One possible reason for failure to detect *C. jejuni* in suspect milk samples may be the sensitivity of these organisms to lactic acid, the concentration of which increases in milk during spoilage. Campylobacters initially present may be killed before samples are cultured.

Outbreaks of campylobacter enteritis associated with the consumption of supposedly pasteurized milk have occasionally been reported. However, studies to determine the heat sensitivity of campylobacters have shown that the organism is unlikely to survive correctly performed pasteurization.

Lander and Gill[1] produced mastitis experimentally in lactating cows with campylobacter. On the premise that the disease could occur naturally, but might have been overlooked in the laboratory, over 600 foremilk samples collected, with the help of Veterinary Investigation Centres throughout England, from cows with mastitis, have been screened for the presence of *C. jejuni* using an enrichment broth.

Campylobacters have not been isolated from these samples. Screening throughout a whole year should help to establish whether the udder is a source of human campylobacter infection.

References

1. Lander, K. P. and Gill, P. (1980). Experimental infection of the bovine udder with *Campylobacter jejuni/coli*. *J. Hyg.*, **84**, 421

103
A large milk-borne outbreak of campylobacter enteritis in Luton

P. H. JONES and A. T. WILLIS

Public Health Laboratory, Luton, U.K.

An outbreak of campylobacter enteritis which occurred in Luton has been investigated. The outbreak had an abrupt onset, lasted for about 3 weeks and involved mainly school children in the 2–4- and 5–7-year-old age groups. Epidemiological and microbiological data suggested that some 2500 children were infected. The source of the epidemic was almost certainly contaminated milk, although bacteriological proof could not be obtained. Biotyping of isolates[1] showed the involvement of two distinctive strains, one of which was dominant. Epidemiological evidence of limited person-to-person transmission of the infection was obtained; febrile convulsions as a prodrome of the illness was recognized for the first time[2]. Strains of *Campylobacter jejuni* and samples of patients' serum collected during this outbreak have enabled subsequent studies to be initiated on the serotyping of the responsible organism[3], on the serological response of patients infected with the organism[4] and on experimental infection of the bovine udder which demonstrated its potential as a source of *C. jejuni* in raw milk[5].

A search of the literature suggests that this is the largest documented outbreak of campylobacter enteritis.

References

1. Skirrow, M. B. and Benjamin, J. (1980). '1001' campylobacters: cultural characteristics of intestinal campylobacters from man and animals. *J. Hyg.* (Cambridge), **85,** 427–432
2. Havalad, S., Chapple, M. J., Kahakachchi, M. and Hargraves, D. B. (1980). Convulsions associated with campylobacter enteritis. *Br. Med. J.*, **1,** 984–985
3. Abbott, J. D., Dale, B. A. S., Eldridge, J., Jones, D. M. and Sutcliffe, E. M. (1980). Serotyping of *Campylobacter jejuni/coli*. *J. Clin. Pathol.*, **33,** 762–766
4. Jones, D. M., Eldridge, J. and Dale, B. (1980). Serological response to *Campylobacter jejuni/coli* infection. *J. Clin. Pathol.*, **33,** 767–769
5. Lander, K. P. and Gill, K. P. (1980). Experimental infections of the bovine udder with *Campylobacter coli/jejuni*. *J. Hyg.* (Cambridge), **84,** 421–428

DISCUSSION

In answer to questions on the source and epidemiology of the outbreak, Dr Jones said that it had not been possible to trace the source of the milk beyond the dairy, that the milk bottles appeared to be clean and that the pattern of infection could be explained on a single-exposure event.

Other points made were that two distinct strains of *C. jejuni* were involved and that a failure of the pasteurization process was quite likely the cause of the widespread dissemination. Of the 108 households checked, there were symptomatic infections in 16 that occurred at least 48 hours after the onset of illness in the index case, suggesting that some of these may have been secondary cases.

The infection of more than 1000 children, each drinking a third of a pint of milk, was considered by Dr Jones to indicate either a very low infective dose or massive contamination of the milk.

104
A water-borne outbreak of campylobacter in central Sweden

L. O. MENTZING

County Medical Officer, Karlstad, Sweden

During the first 2 weeks of October 1980, an explosive outbreak of gastroenteritis occurred in an area near Karlstad in central Sweden. Over 380 patients consulted local general practitioners (Figure 1). Of faecal samples from 263 patients, 221 were positive for *Campylobacter jejuni*. A total of 45 samples were also tested for growth of salmonella and shigella and all were seen to be negative.

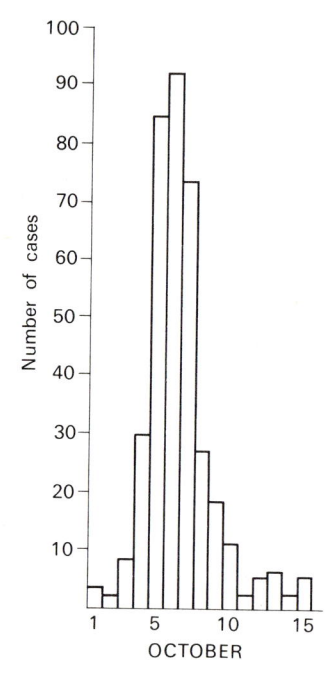

Figure 1 Campylobacter enteritis by date of onset, Grums, Sweden

Random samples of the population were interviewed by questionnaire. It could then be estimated that over 2000 people, of a total risk population of 14 600, were affected. Those who had fallen ill reported a history of diarrhoea (89%), abdominal pain (82%), nausea (57%), headache (56%), myalgia (55%) and fever (53%). Only 19% had vomited and 6% had noticed blood in their stools. The mean duration of the illness was 5.2 days, ranging from 1–16 days. Many of the patients suffered intense discomfort but few were seriously ill. Only seven were admitted to a hospital; one of these was a child. The attack rates by age and sex are presented in Table 1.

Table 1 **Attack rates during a waterborne outbreak of campylobacter enteritis by age and sex, Grums, Sweden, October 1980**

Age group (years)	Males No. cultured	%+	Females No. cultured	%+	Total %+
0–9	37	19	48	10	14
10–19	41	17	49	18	18
20–29	32	19	44	16	17
30–39	64	17	40	30	22
40–49	42	19	30	17	18
50–59	37	11	33	24	17
60–69	34	15	36	17	15
70–79	24	13	30	17	14
>80	8	13	11	9	10

Although the source of infection has not yet been identified, the geographical distribution of the outbreak and other epidemiological data indicate that the infection was spread by tap water. The water distributed in the area is unchlorinated ground water of good quality which is filtered through sand filters. The technical investigation is not yet complete, but it is strongly suspected that polluted water was accidentally introduced into the municipal water pipes in connection with reparation of water and sewage pipes or through unpermitted cross-connections with industrial process water.

DISCUSSION

Dr Wilson asked how many secondary cases there were in children presumably acquired from adults. Dr Mentzing replied that most such cases in adults were acquired from children, but 10 of the 26 were either in children or in adults acquired from adults. Dr Blaser commented that as secondary cases were defined as ones occurring 2–8 days after another case in the household, it is possible that some of these were actually primary cases with long incubation periods. Dr Blaser asked how the population was sampled and was told that every 15th name on a population census of the outbreak area, arranged by birth-date, was selected for interview. Commenting on Dr Dadswell's question concerning the lack of chlorination of the water supply, Dr Mentzing said that the water was of high quality and was sand filtered only.

Several points of cross-connection at which sewage from poultry or cattle farms could have entered the pipes after filtration were found subsequent to the outbreak. There was no information obtained on the amount of water drunk in relation to the infection rates but one child born during the outbreak became ill on day 5. Both parents of the child were ill.

105
Campylobacters from water

M. J. KNILL, W. G. SUCKLING and A. D. PEARSON

Public Health Laboratory, Level B, Laboratory and Pathology Block, Southampton General Hospital, Tremona Road, Southampton SO9 4XY

INTRODUCTION

In preliminary environmental studies *Campylobacter jejuni* was isolated from 56/114 (49%) samples of river water, from mud, droppings from a canary pen and the carcasses of a pigeon and fox[1]. This paper describes a longitudinal survey designed to examine natural waters from the area around Southampton for evidence of contamination with Campylobacter.

These investigations were initiated after reviewing the histories taken from patients who had campylobacter enteritis. This indicated that 30% had been involved in outside activities or had been in contact with sick animals or birds prior to their illness.

ENVIRONMENTAL SURVEY

Samples of water, mud and animal faeces were collected from sites on three of the rivers that drain West Hampshire (Figure 1). The survey took place over a 7-month period from June–December 1978. Fresh-water samples were taken from land-locked pools in the New Forest and from the higher reaches of the Rivers Test, Beaulieu and Lymington. Salt-water samples were taken from tidal sites on the Rivers Test and Beaulieu. The sampling sites were near to places where forest and farm animals graze and drink and where, in the summer, the children and visitors swim and play.

The River Test (sites A, B, C, P and D) flows through farmland. The sampling sites here were on the lower reaches of the river, extending from the tidal estuary (sites P and D) to some 3 miles upstream. Site C is a series of gravel ponds recently stocked as a fishing lake.

The Beaulieu River (sites E, F, G and H) rises in heathland in the New Forest and descends through deciduous and pine forests in an area where, in the summer, many visitors are allowed to camp and picnic. The river does not normally exceed 25–30 ft in width and 3–4 ft in depth, except below Beaulieu Village (site H) where it is tidal.

Southampton Area

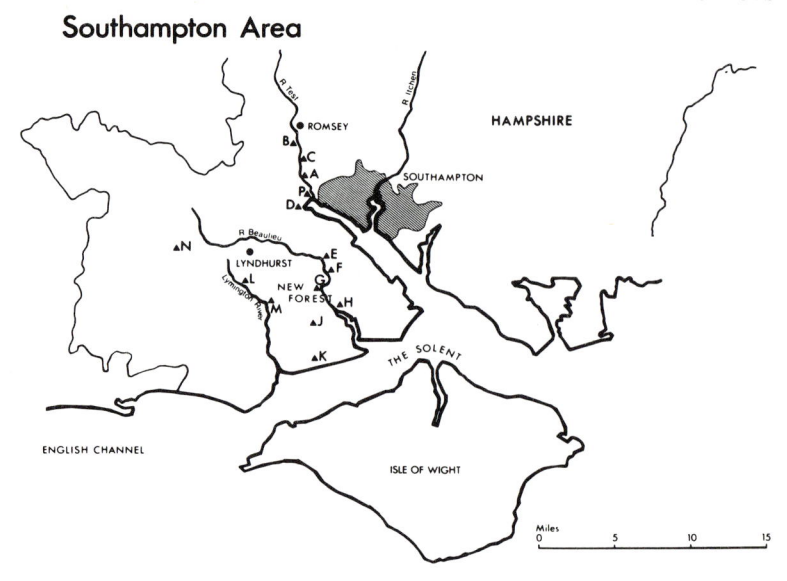

Figure 1 Map of sample sites

The Lymington River (sites L and M) flows through the New Forest where it was sampled at a popular bathing area. The sites were not tidal. New Forest pools (sites K, J, N and Q) are formed by drainage water from the forest and all are frequented by summer visitors. Site Q is an artificial lake situated in an area where fields are sprayed with human sewage.

MATERIALS AND METHODS

Samples of water were collected from these sites, initially at fortnightly and later at weekly intervals. Samples comprising 100 ml were collected in sterilized glass containers and held at room temperature until examination. The samples were examined as soon as possible after collection and at no time was the interval between collection and examination in excess of 6 hours. Mud and animal-faecal samples were collected in aluminium faecal pots and held at room temperature until examination.

Water samples were examined for the presence of campylobacter using a membrane-filtration technique in which a 0.45 μm pore-sized filter was placed onto an antibiotic selective medium (VPT)[2]. Plates were placed in anaerobic jars and incubated at 43 °C in micro-aerophilic conditions by evacuating the jar to 650 mm Hg and replacement with a mixture of 95% hydrogen–5% carbon dioxide. The membrane filter was removed at 24 hours and growth was examined at 48 and 72 hours by dark-ground microscopy for the presence of motile vibrios. Motile vibrios isolated as described above are referred to, for the purpose of this study, as heat tolerant campylobacters (HTC). The water samples were examined for the presence of *Escherichia coli* type I (faecal coli) using conventional membrane-filter techniques. Mud and animal-faecal samples were streaked directly on to VPT media and incubated under micro-aerophilic conditions for 3 days at 43 °C. The plates were examined daily and motile vibrios visualized by dark-ground microscopy. All strains isolated under these conditions and having the colonial and microscopical appearance of campylobacters were stored in liquid nitrogen after suspension of growth in a 50% mixture of glycerol and nutrient broth.

RESULTS

Heat-tolerant campylobacters were isolated from 251 of the 471 water samples (Table 1). Isolations were made throughout the study period excepting one day which coincided with marked flooding of the river. Repeated isolations were made from the sites on the Rivers Beaulieu and Test, and less often from the River Lymington and the Forest pools; site N yielded none at all.

Table 1 Isolation of campylobacter from natural waters

	No. examined	No. positive	% *Campylobacter isolated* (*total specimens*)
20 June	18	14	77.8
26 June	27	11	40.7
3 July	17	15	88.2
17 July	25	14	56.0
1 August	28	0	0.0
15 August	19	6	31.6
19 September	25	10	40.0
2 October	22	3	13.6
9 October	27	19	70.4
16 October	29	21	72.4
23 October	29	22	75.9
30 October	26	15	57.7
7 November	24	16	66.7
13 November	31	13	41.9
20 November	23	7	30.4
27 November	27	23	85.2
4 December	23	14	60.9
11 December	28	8	28.6
18 December	23	20	87.0
Totals	471	251	53.3

The relationship between the isolation of Campylobacter and the presence of faecal coli is analysed in Table 2. Campylobacters were detected only in water samples which had evidence of faecal contamination. Faeces from cattle and horses, and samples from cess pits and septic tanks were examined as possible sources for Campylobacter: none were found. One isolate was obtained from a mud sample taken in close proximity to the Beaulieu River at Site E.

Table 2 Relationship between isolation of HTC and faecal coliform levels in 471 water samples

No positive	0/20	148/246	37/76	40/79	16/29	10/21
Faecal coli levels/100 ml	Nil	1–100	101–200	201–500	501–1000	1000+

CONCLUSIONS

(1) Campylobacters were isolated from over 50% of the water samples collected from fresh and esturine sites on three river systems in West Hampshire.
(2) No isolations were obtained on a study day which followed a period of heavy rain.

References

1. Knill, M. J., Suckling, W. G. and Pearson, A. D. (1978). Environmental isolation of heat-tolerant campylobacter in the Southampton area. *Lancet*, **ii**, 1002–1003
2. Pearson, A. D., Suckling, W. G., Ricciardi, I. D., Knill, M. J. and Ware, E. (1977). Campylobacter associated diarrhoea in Southampton. *Br. Med. J.*, **2**, 955–56

DISCUSSION

Dr Blaser asked if the higher isolation rate for *C. jejuni* at low tide compared with high tide was due to dilution of contaminated fresh water with sea water or to increased salinity. Dr Pearson believed that it was mainly a dilution effect.

The fall in isolation rates in rivers after heavy rainfall seemed to suggest that the river was the primary reservoir and not the animal faeces washed into it.

The survival of campylobacter in water was questioned by Dr Davis. Dr Blaser replied that in his studies ten campylobacter/ml survived at 25 °C for only a few days whereas at 4 °C viable organisms could be recovered for up to 1 month.

106
Epidemiology of campylobacter infection

W. P. J. SEVERIN

Regional Public Health Laboratory, Enschede, The Netherlands

Campylobacter jejuni has been recognized to cause diarrhoeal disease in humans. In our area comprising 650 000 inhabitants the overall isolation rate from diarrhoeal stools in 1979–1980 was 7.7% as opposed to 12.7% in stools from patients aged 10–35 years. For salmonella these figures are 8.0% and 4.9%, respectively (Figure 1). This difference prompted us to obtain more epidemiological information.

In a retrospective survey in the period May–October 1979 questionnaires were sent to all patients (or their parents) and to one of their neighbours as control subjects. Respondents were asked about: close contact with farm animals; frequent contact with cats, dogs, cage-birds or other pets as well as recent diarrhoeal disease in these animals; consumption and method of preparing chicken, pork, beef, and mutton for the 4-day period before onset of the infection; visiting restaurants or snack-bars in the same period; home- or holiday-related onset of the disease and occurrence of diarrhoea in family contacts.

One hundred and two of the questionnaires were returned by both patients and their neighbours. Table 1 summarizes the findings.

Using the McNemar test for matched-pair analysis, the following significant differences were found:

(1) the presence of cage-birds (25 in patients *vs.* 12 in controls),
(2) the method of preparing chicken: longer – baking, roasting, boiling – versus shorter – fondue, barbecue, gourmet – cooking time (31 *vs.* 11 in patients, 27 *vs.* 0 in controls).
(3) Frequency of diarrhoeal disease in family (23 *vs.* 9).

Our study suggests that in order to prevent infection with campylobacter by chicken, careful preparation and thorough heating is needed, and that cage-birds should not be neglected as a source of infection.

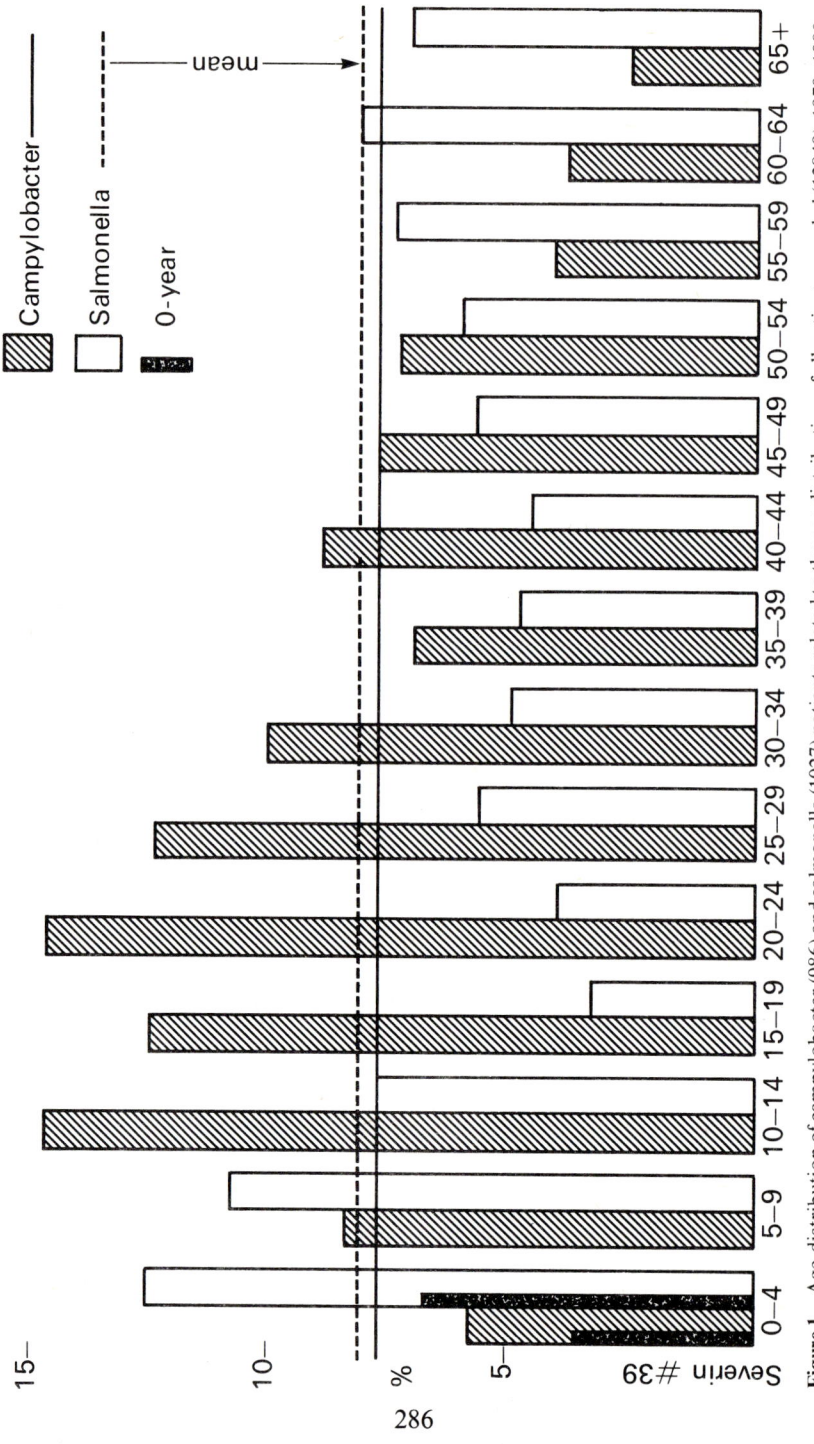

Figure 1 Age-distribution of campylobacter (986) and salmonella (1027) patients related to the age distribution of all patients sampled (12849), 1979–1980

Table 1 Epidemiological background of campylobacter patients and matched controls, Retrospective Mail Survey, Netherlands, May–October 1979

	Patients (n = 102)	Controls (n = 102)
Contact with farm animals		
cattle	10	5
sheep	6	3
pig	5	5
chicken	12	6
horse	7	5
Domestic animals		
dog	29	27
cat	14	9
cage-birds*	25	12
diarrhoea	7	9
Consumption and preparing (4 days preceding symptoms)		
chicken	51	37
ccoking time* long	31	27
short	11	0
pork	77	
beef	70	72
mutton	1	2
First symptoms		
at home	94	
elsewhere	2	
on holidays	6	
Family contacts (diarrhoea in the same period)*	23	9

* $p < 0.05$, McNemar analysis of matched pairs

DISCUSSION

Dr Ferguson asked if campylobacters had been isolated from the cage-birds and was told that as this study was purely epidemiological, isolation had not been attempted. Dr Severin stated in answer to Dr Feldman that the patients who showed markedly different age distributions for salmonella and campylobacter infections were derived from the same population.

107
Campylobacter outbreak in a military camp: investigations, results and further epidemiological studies

J. OOSTEROM and H. J. BECKERS

National Institute of Public Health, Bilthoven, The Netherlands

---

An outbreak of enteritis in a military camp prompted microbiological and/or serological examination of 54 subjects. Cultures of faeces of 51 persons revealed *Campylobacter jejuni* in 13 of them. An antibody titre of 1:160 or higher was observed, in the sera of 19 out of 41 persons, which in ten cases constituted the only evidence of infection.

An enquiry was conducted among 34 patients in order to establish the incubation time (average 4 days), the duration of the disease (average 4 days) and the nature of the symptoms. Attempts were also made to trace the source of infection and it was considered probable that raw hamburger had caused the outbreak.

Further epidemiological investigations concerning the possible sources of human infection have shown that poultry flocks were frequently infected (20/100), and that there was a high infection rate among pigs (182/300), sometimes with more than 10^4 cells per gram of faeces. No infection could be found in slaughtered cattle (0/200) or in raw milk (0/200). Experiments have shown that campylobacter is not killed by the intensive contact with air during the milking process and could survive in sterile milk, kept at 4 °C, for more than a month, whether this milk was vigorously shaken with air or not.

Ox bile in enrichment medium increased the isolation rate from all sources (Table 1).

Table 1. *The effect of ox-bile in an enrichment medium for campylobacter*

Examined materials	No. examined	No. positive (medium without bile)	No. positive (medium with 1.5% bile)
Chicken carcases	40	15	37
Chicken livers	22	6	19
Human faeces	176	11	12
Dog faeces	23	1	2
River and sewage water	29	0	4

108
Sero-epidemiological studies of *C. jejuni* infection

D. M. JONES, D. A. ROBINSON and J. ELDRIDGE

Public Health Laboratory, Manchester, U.K.

Using the complement fixation test, agglutination and the bactericidal test[1] the antibody response was defined in individual patients (Table 1) and in experimental infections of the cow and man[2] (Table 2). In the normal population between 2 and 5 per cent have been found to have complement fixing antibody to *C. jejuni*. The prevalence of antibody in workers processing ducks, chickens and cattle for food was found to be far in excess of the normal population[3] (Table 3).

The serological findings in point-source outbreaks due to milk-borne and chicken-borne infection (single serotype) established that at least 25% of those at risk in common-source outbreaks may be infected without the development of intestinal symptoms.

Table 1 Complement fixing antibody to *Campylobacter jejuni* in antenatal patients

	Serum titre		
	<2	4	>8
Urban*	196	3	1
Rural†	95	3	2

* Urban patients were from Manchester
† Rural patients were from Norwich

Table 2 Antibody response after experimental campylobacter infection in a volunteer

Day	CFT	Agglutination	Bactericidal
0	<2	<10	<2
5	<2	10	<2
10	16	160	<2
54	16	160	<2

Table 3 Complement fixing antibody to *C. jejuni* in poultry and meat-process workers

Establishment (animals processed)	Number workers examined	Antibody positive (%)
A (ducks and chickens)	28	68
B (chickens)	33	48
C (ducks)	15	60
D (ducks)	23	52
E (chickens)	34	27
F (cattle)	95	36
MAFF veterinary assistants	20	18

In the Luton outbreak two major serotypes of *C. jejuni* were involved and while many patients showed a serological response to only one of these serotypes, it was demonstrated that a number had a serological response to both, suggesting that infection with more than one serotype may occur concurrently. In another outbreak where students habitually consumed unpasteurized milk there was a high prevalence of symptoms (Table 4). The findings in this outbreak, taken together with the high frequency of antibody and low frequency of symptoms seen in the food-process workers, suggests that immunity to intestinal symptoms develops with repeated infection. This

Table 4 Antibody responses* of 11 agricultural college students to serotype 2/5 and serotype 6 using 3 serological tests

Student	Bactericidal 2/5	Bactericidal 6	Agglutination 2/5	CFT
1	<4	<4	<40	8
2	16	<4	160	4
3	32	<4	80	8
4	128	<4	640	32
5	128	<4	80	4
6	128	<4	80	16
7	128	<4	160	64
8	128	128	80	16
9	128	128	640	16
10	<4	<4	640	64
11	64	16	<40	8

* Reciprocal titre

situation may be analogous to that observed in developing countries where *C. jejuni* is often isolated in the absence of symptoms, although no antibody studies are yet available.

References

1. Jones, D. M., Eldridge, J. and Dale, B. A. S. (1980). Serological response to *Campylobacter jejuni/coli* infection. *J. Clin. Pathol.*, **33**, 767–769
2. Robinson, D. A. (1981). Infective dose of *Campylobacter jejuni* in milk. *Br. Med. J.*, **282**, 1384
3. Jones, D. M. and Robinson, D. A. (1981). Occupational exposure to *Campylobacter jejuni* infection. *Lancet*, **i**, 440–41

DISCUSSION

Dr Jones used as an antigen a sonicate of six different serotypes commonly found in the area, so as to provide the broad specificity necessary to determine the prevalence of infection in the community by means of a serological survey. Such means will also identify asymptomatic infections in an outbreak – emphasized by the Writtle outbreak in which 70% of the asymptomatic raw-milk drinkers had antibody. Dr Watson asked if auto-agglutination had been a problem. It had not.

109
Serological epidemiology of campylobacter infection

T. M. S. REID and I. A. PORTER

Regional Laboratory, City Hospital, Aberdeen

The complement fixation test provides a useful index of the prevalence of campylobacter infection[1]. Paired convalescent sera collected from asymptomatic and symptomatic culture-positive patients in the 'Aberdeen' milk-borne outbreak[2] were examined by complement fixation test. The antigen used was a sonicate of ten selected human isolates of *C. jejuni* including the strain isolated during the Aberdeen outbreak. Of the 88 sera tested all but three showed a CFT titre of 1/10 or greater. The three who lacked complement fixing antibody were nevertheless positive in the indirect immunofluorescent test using the outbreak strain as antigen. There was no difference in the mean titres of symptomatic and asymptomatic culture-positive patients. None of the sera from over 200 healthy blood donors in the affected area collected at the time of the outbreak gave a titre of 1/10 or greater. Follow up of these patients indicates that the CFT remains positive ($>1/10$) for not more than 3–4 months.

All sera referred to the Regional Laboratory from the Grampian Region over a period of 4 months have been screened retrospectively for evidence of campylobacter infection by the complement fixation test. Three per cent of these specimens showed a titre of 1/10 or greater; 68.5% of positive sera were referred on account of joint symptoms (pain, stiffness and swelling); 4.7% gastrointestinal symptoms (diarrhoea and abdominal pain); 4.7% pyrexias of unknown origin, and the remaining 22% from patients with diverse symptomatology.

References

1. Jones, D. M., Eldridge, J. and Dale, B. A. S. (1980). Serological response to *Campylobacter jejuni/coli* infection. *J. Clin. Pathol.*, **33**, 767–769
2. Porter, I. A. and Reid, T. M. S. (1980). A milk-borne outbreak of campylobacter infection. *J. Hyg. (Cambridge)*, **84**, 415–419

110
Duration of excretion period of *Campylobacter jejuni* in human subjects

E. P. WRIGHT

Public Health Laboratory, Luton, Beds.

There are few reports on the duration of excretion of *Campylobacter jejuni* in man. Wallace[1] describing a milk-borne outbreak found 58 (33%) of 178 culture-positive individuals were negative within 2 weeks of onset of symptoms, and 145 (99%) of 147 individuals were negative within 9 weeks. Svedhem and Kaijser[2] investigated 55 patients with campylobacter enterocolitis. After 2 weeks, 50% were negative and 90% of the patients had negative stool cultures after 5 weeks. To further study the duration of excretion a retrospective review of patients in Liverpool, England was undertaken.

PATIENTS AND METHODS

Laboratory records of the Liverpool Public Health Laboratory were reviewed from September 1977 to June 1980. During this period stool specimens from 260 patients had yielded *Campylobacter jejuni*.

Within this group 30 (12%) were known to have received chemotherapy either just before bacteriological diagnosis, or within 1 month of the onset of illness, and these patients were excluded from further analysis. The remaining 230 (male 117 and female 113), who were known not to have received chemotherapy, were divided into two groups for analysis.

Group A represents the entire series of unselected cases, some of whom were subsequently lost at follow up stage. Group B represents cases who were followed up until two or more consecutive stool specimens were negative (Table 1). Duration of excretion was estimated for each patient from the stated date of onset of symptoms to the last positive specimen. For the 15 (6%) patients who were symptomless, the duration of excretion was estimated from the dates of the first and last positive specimens. Faeces were examined using selective medium and incubated and identified under standard conditions[3]; no enrichment techniques were used. A patient was declared culture negative after two consecutive negative stools.

Table 1 Age distribution of culture-positive patients

Age group	0–11 months	1–9 years	10–19	20–29	30–39	40–49	50–59	60–69	Over 70 years	All ages
Number of patients (Group A)	6	24	34	71	24	25	24	6	12	230*
Number followed up until two negatives obtained (group B)	1	13	19	34	12	14	17	2	2	114

*Includes 4 patients whose ages were unknown

RESULTS

After the first negative stool culture, 83% of the patients continued to have negative cultures for campylobacters. The corresponding figure after two consecutive negative samples was 21%, and this criterion of two or more consecutive negatives was taken as an arbitrary and minimum indication of cessation of excretion for group B.

Most patients ceased excreting their campylobacter quickly so that in group A after 2 weeks, 72 of 230 (31%) remained positive, but after 4 weeks only 23 (10%) were still positive (Figure 1). In group B, 50 of 114 (44%) were positive after 2 weeks and 20 (17.5%) remained positive after 4 weeks. Only 5 (4%) were known to be positive after 6 weeks (Figure 2).

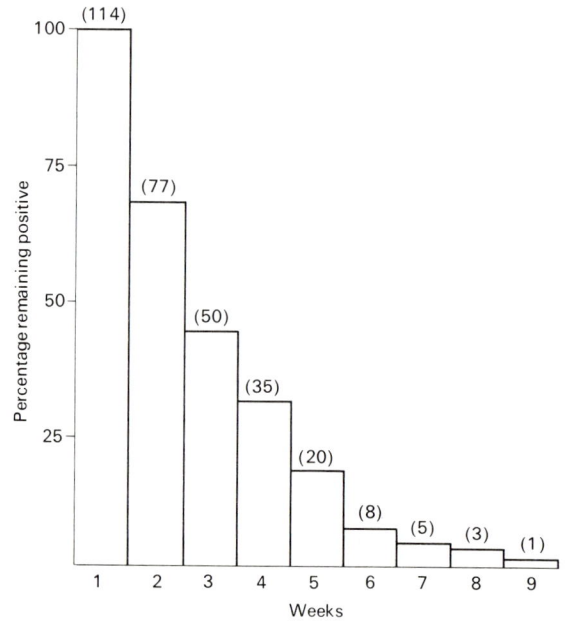

Figure 1 Rate of loss of campylobacters (Group A) (Total number of patients in parenthesis)

More detailed study of the five patients who were known to be still positive after 6 weeks failed to show any common factor to account for the prolonged excretion. There were no apparent differences in the duration of excretion for the different age-groups studied (Figure 3). The last known excreter was a female patient aged 59 years who ceased excreting after 9 weeks.

DISCUSSION

Nye and Roberts[4] described the association of prolonged salmonella excretion and infants below 12 months of age and adults over 60 years of age. This

EXCRETION PERIOD OF C. JEJUNI IN HUMAN SUBJECTS

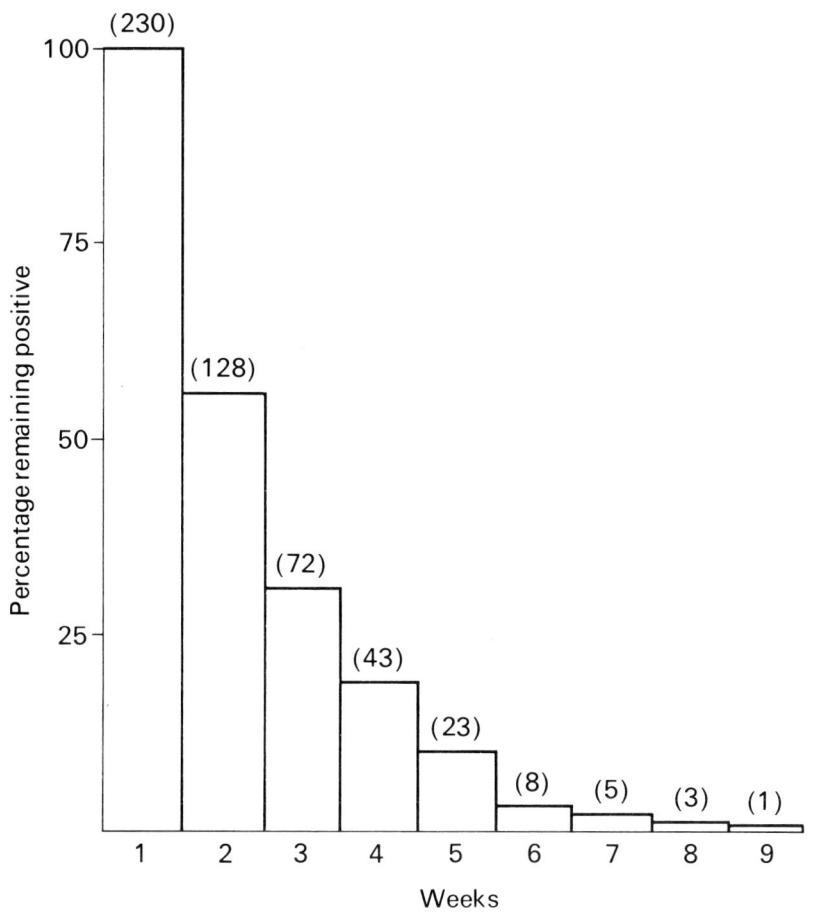

Figure 2 Rate of loss of campylobacters (Group B)

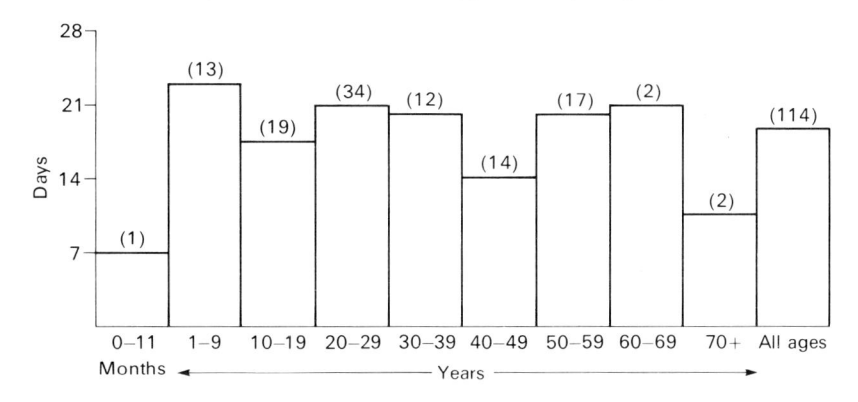

Figure 3 Mean duration of excretion (Group B)

association, however, was not apparent in the present study of campylobacter excretion, perhaps because of the small number of patients studied. Prolonged excretion of salmonella is associated with several factors including hypochlorhydria, a common feature in infancy, and of increasing prevalence after the fifth decade. Blaser et al.[5], reported that the survival of *C. jejuni* in hydrochloric acid was time- and pH-dependant with a 7-log kill within 5 minutes in solutions at pH 2.3.

Patients with salmonellosis treated with antibiotics are known to have a prolonged period of post-convalescent salmonella excretion[6]. Erythromycin rapidly produces culture-negative stools for campylobacters.

The recognition and mechanism of carriage in prolonged excretion of campylobacters still remain to be defined and possible associated factors such as hypochlorhydria, antimicrobial treatment, biliary carriage[7], use of enrichment techniques and serotype of the organism require investigation by prospective studies.

References

1. Wallace, J. M. (1980). Milk-associated campylobacter infection. *Health Bull.* (*Edinburgh*), **38**, 57
2. Svedhem, A. and Kaijser, B. (1980). *Campylobacter fetus* ssp. *jejuni*: A common cause of diarrhoea in Sweden. *J. Infect. Dis.*, **142**, 353
3. Skirrow, M. B. (1977). Campylobacter enteritis: a 'new' disease. *Br. Med. J.*, **ii**, 9
4. Nye, F. J. and Roberts, C. (1979). Prolonged excretion of salmonellae. *J. Infectn.*, **1**, 367
5. Blaser, M. J., Hardesty, H. L., Powers, B. and Wang, W.-L. L. (1980). Survival of *Campylobacter fetus* ssp. *jejuni* in biological milieus. *J. Clin. Microbiol.*, **11**, 309
6. Dixon, J. M. S. (1965). Effect of antibiotic treatment on duration of excretion of *Salmonella typhimurium* by children. *Br. Med. J.*, **ii**, 1343
7. Darling, W. M., Peel, R. N., Skirrow, M. B. and Mulira, A. E. (1979). Campylobacter cholecystitis. *Lancet*, **i**, 1302

111
Comparison of the epidemiological characteristics of human illness for salmonella and campylobacter

R. A. FELDMAN and M. J. BLASER

C.D.C., Atlanta

C. jejuni and *Salmonella* ssp. appear to share common reservoirs, such as poultry, and therefore these two organisms might be expected to have similar epidemiological characteristics. Both groups of organisms exhibit a warm-weather seasonal peak of cases, limited spread within families unless the index infection is an infant, an association with infected animals and the occurrence of common-source outbreaks associated with foods, unpasteurized milk and water.

However, several recent comparative studies indicate that there are also many differences between *C. jejuni* and salmonella infections.

(1) A laboratory-based study of patients with diarrhoea has shown that the highest percentage of stools positive for campylobacter was in the 10–29-year age-group (12%) while for salmonella there was little variation with age.

(2) In a study involving eight hospitals the median age of patients with campylobacter positive faeces was 24 years compared with 15 years for patients with salmonella infections. Only 6% of campylobacter isolates were from children under 1-year old whilst 23% of salmonella isolates were from children of that age group which is consistent with the infrequent occurrence of campylobacter outbreaks in newborn nurseries. The study also showed a higher percentage of campylobacter isolates from males (55%) compared to salmonella (37%). The seasonal peak for campylobacter occurred from April–November whilst it was from June–October for salmonella. Additionally there was a reduction in the duration of excretion following therapy in campylobacter infections in contrast to salmonella infections.

(3) In a study of Bangladeshi children campylobacter infections were considerably more frequent than salmonella infections.

(4) Unlike salmonella, campylobacter is rarely identified as an agent in nosocomial infections.

Some salmonella serotypes have distinctive epidemiological characteristics relating to vehicles, geographical distribution, age group involved and frequency of bacteraemia and meningitis. It is possible that with the introduction of adequate typing techniques for campylobacter, distinct epidemiological patterns for individual campylobacter types may be observed.

In conclusion the salmonella are a group of organisms with heterogeneous epidemiological characteristics and the same may be expected for *C. jejuni*. Careful investigation is necessary to uncover such important information as an infective dose and age specificity of secondary transmission.

112
Editorial discussion

The papers presented in this session demonstrate that different methods may be used to understand the epidemiology of campylobacter infection. Information was gathered by investigations of outbreaks, sero-surveys, case-control analysis and studies of actual or potential reservoirs of the infection.

From the diverse information presented several broad conclusions can be drawn.

(1) In the developed countries the majority of the population do not carry significant levels of serum antibodies to specific strains and appear to be non-immune (Jones *et al.*, Epidemiology, p. 290. Reid and Porter, Epidemiology, p. 293 and Svedhem *et al.*, Serology, p. 118).

Following infection antibody titres rise and therefore serological studies may be used to detect the prevalence of infection in a given population, and to determine the incidence and significance of asymptomatic infections (Jones *et al.*, Epidemiology, p. 290). Antigens with broad specificity are required to determine overall immune responses in general populations. The association of circulating antibody to campylobacter with clinical symptoms, such as arthritis (Reid and Porter, Epidemiology, p. 293), should provide a profitable area of research.

(2) In most outbreaks studied the incidence of illness in non-immune people exposed to an infectious inoculum is high (Mouton *et al.*, Clinical Aspects, p. 129, Mentzing, Epidemiology, p. 278; and Jones and Willis, Epidemiology, p. 276). In the majority of cases the illness was mild, with more severe symptoms such as bloody diarrhoea occurring in less than 10% of cases and only rarely requiring antibiotic therapy (Mentzing, Epidemiology, p. 278). The relationships between pathogenicity of the infective strain (Itoh *et al.*, Geographical Epidemiology, p. 5), dose (Mouton *et al.* Clinical Aspects. p. 129) and duration of excretion (Wright, Epidemiology, p. 294) with severity of disease, has yet to be established.

(3) Circumstantial evidence has implicated water (Mentzing, Epidemiology, p. 278) and milk (Jones and Willis, Epidemiology, p. 276) in large outbreaks of campylobacter enteritis. However isolates have not yet been recovered from these sources at the time of an outbreak. The techniques are available for isolating campylobacters from water (Knill *et al.*, Epidemiology, p. 281) where they are found as a ubiquitous contaminant especially in association with faecal coli. The isolation from milk is obviously more difficult (Waterman and Park,

Epidemiology, p. 275) although *C. jejuni* is apparently a normal commensal in cows and faecal contamination of milk may occur (Robinson, Epidemiology, p. 274). It is apparent that ingestion of campylobacter in milk does not reduce its pathogenicity (Jones *et al.*, Epidemiology, p. 290).

Epidemiological evidence also implicates several foods of animal origin as a potential source. Although isolation of *C. jejuni* from red meats was uncommon (Turnbull and Rose, Epidemiology, p. 271; Hudson and Roberts, Epidemiology, p. 273) it has been suggested that the use of enrichment media may increase the incidence of recovery (Oosterom, Epidemiology, p. 288). Poorly cooked chicken (Severin, Epidemiology, p. 285 and Mouton *et al.*, Clinical Aspects, p. 129) is a well documented source of infection. The incidence of campylobacter infection in chicken flocks produced under battery conditions is high and the killing and storage process produce contaminated meat (Cruickshank *et al.*, Epidemiology, p. 263; Mehle *et al.*, Epidemiology, p. 267; and Hartog and De Boer, Epidemiology, p. 270). As some flocks are free of infection the possibility of producing campylobacter-free stock should be investigated.

(4) The reservoirs for *C. jejuni* in the environment are extensive. The serotypes isolated from a wide variety of animals largely overlaps those common serotypes isolated from humans (Luechtefeld and Wang, Epidemiology, p. 249), and supports the hypothesis of transmission from animals to humans. The reservoir of infections in domestic animals such as dogs, cats and birds (Bruce, Epidemiology, p. 252 and Fenlon *et al.*, Epidemiology, p. 261) is being defined and epidemiological evidence now strongly implicates such animals in sporadic outbreaks (Severin, Epidemiology, p. 285 and Khan, Epidemiology, p. 256). The relevance of environmental isolates, such as those from water or animals, in terms of their pathogenicity for humans has, however, yet to be established.

SECTION IX
ROUND TABLE DISCUSSION ON PUBLIC HEALTH MEASURES

Participants: M. J. Blaser, J. G. Cruickshank, J. R. Davies,
P. C. Fleming, T. Itoh, B. Kaijser, A. D. Pearson
and M. B. Skirrow.

The major aspects of the discussion were concentrated on reviewing the available information on infective doses and potential sources of infection, determining the populations at risk and advising health authorities on treatment and the monitoring of water, food, etc.

The infecting dose

Some estimate of whether the infection is initiated by a large or small dose was considered essential before recommendations could be made. There is little direct evidence except several human challenge experiments which indicate that the infective dose can be as little as 500 organisms. No evidence was available from source material in outbreak situations. However, some circumstantial evidence has been obtained including the occurrence of waterborne outbreaks and the occasional person-to-person transmission which imply a small infective dose. The apparent absence of multiplication of campylobacters under normal conditions would also support this hypothesis.

In conclusion it is likely that a small dose can initiate infection however, as with other pathogens, the attack rate may be proportional to dose.

Infected source materials

There are well-documented outbreaks in which the source of infection was contaminated water or raw milk. Poultry has also been implicated and it is likely that other animal products will be found to be associated with infection. Ways in which methods of treatment would be appropriate if contamination was likely to have occurred were discussed.

Water

The prevention of water-borne outbreaks involves no specific measures related to the campylobacter hazard. Water for drinking and food preparation, which is derived from suitable catchment areas and is treated and distributed to conform with well-recognized standards, should carry no risk. Drinking polluted water and consuming raw shellfish from polluted waters carries a number of microbial hazards, including the risk of campylobacter infection.

Milk

Reported milk-borne outbreaks have been associated with raw milk and probable failure of pasteurization. The source of the organisms in milk is uncertain but adequate pasteurization would be expected to eliminate the risk. In areas where only raw milk is available the public should be made aware of the hazard of milk-borne pathogens and encouraged to heat the milk before consumption.

Poultry and other animal products

The prevention of food-borne infection relies on the application of good hygienic practice, both in the slaughterhouses and processing plants, to reduce cross-contamination, adequate cooking and the avoidance of re-contamination in the kitchen. The long-term aim should be to produce food, from animals and poultry, free of human intestinal pathogens but since campylobacter may be an intestinal commensal in many of the animal species used for food production, eradication of the reservoir may be the major difficulty. Further work is needed to assess the part played by contaminated animal feed and the role of the wild fauna, particularly birds, in the cycle of infection.

Foodhandlers and other excreters

There is no evidence to suggest that an asymptomatic excreter has been the source of campylobacter infection. There is no reason to exclude a convalescent excreter from foodhandling, provided that proper hygienic precautions are observed. It follows that there is no indication that routine examination of asymptomatic foodhandlers for campylobacter excretion is necessary. Other covalescent excreters, including children, need not be restricted in their activies once they are symptom-free. Those who have incomplete bowel control and are returning to sensitive environments, for example residential or day-care centres, pose a problem and it would be wise to exclude them from such environments until they cease to excrete campylobacters. In these circumstances the use of erythromycin in an attempt to terminate excretion might be considered.

Domestic pets

On occasion it has been shown that household pets have been the source of human infection. The greatest risk to humans may come from young animals, such as puppies and kittens, with diarrhoea. Sensible hygienic precautions should be taken in dealing with such animals.

Monitoring of foods

Until techniques for the detection of small numbers of campylobacter have been developed there is no merit in attempting to introduce food standards.

CONCLUSIONS

Most of the public health measures appropriate to the control of campylobacter infection apply equally to the control of other microbial infections which are derived from environmental and food sources. These include: the provision of safe water and milk supplies, good hygienic practice in animal husbandry and in the handling of raw foods, adequate cooking, kitchen hygiene and public awareness of the hazard.

The source of most campylobacter infections is not known and there is an urgent need for more work in this area. The development of a serological typing scheme to determine the distribution of different types in human infections, animals and the environment is essential. The significance of these serotypes could then be assessed and common-source outbreaks more readily recognized. Markers for pathogenicity should be investigated and the pathogenicity of environmental isolates should be determined. Improved techniques should be established for rapid diagnosis and for the detection of small numbers of organisms. Finally the role of erythromycin in treatment should be assessed.

SECTION X

CAMPYLOBACTERS — WHERE DO WE GO FROM HERE?

J. P. Butzler, J. H. Bryner, J. R. Davies,
R. A. Feldman, P. C. Fleming, M. B. Skirrow

Where do they come from?

Although there are well-documented common-source outbreaks associated with the consumption of contaminated water, milk and poultry, and some evidence for case-to-case spread and for human infections from domestic pets, most cases of campylobacter infection are 'sporadic'.

A better understanding of the routes of infection depends on the development of serological typing and of enrichment techniques. This should enable a more adequate investigation of cases, their contacts and suspected source materials.

How do they cause disease?

It is clear that not everyone who is infected with *Campylobacter jejuni* develops symptoms and not all cases present with diarrhoea.

Further work is needed to establish the dose-related attack rates, the extent of immunity resulting from previous infection and the role of the organism in other pathological conditions.

Markers for pathogenicity should be investigated since not all strains of *C. jejuni* may be pathogenic for man.

What should we be saying to clinicians?

C. jejuni entero-colitis is usually an unpleasant but self-limiting disease. In the majority of cases no specific treatment will be indicated since, by the time a bacteriological diagnosis is available, the diarrhoea will have responded to symptomatic treatment or remitted spontaneously.

The proper role of erythromycin in the treatment of *C. jejuni* infection is a matter for debate. It may be useful in selected cases where symptoms are severe or prolonged, or to limit the duration of excretion. Some erythromycin-resistant strains have been isolated and, although at present such strains are uncommon, irresponsible use of erythromycin may prejudice the value of this antibiotic in the future.

What should we be saying to health authorities?

In many countries *C. jejuni* is a major cause of infective enteritis in man, probably accounting for as many cases as other intestinal bacterial pathogens, in particular salmonellas and shigellas. Some of the areas where research would be most profitable are identified in Table 1.

There is a need to support research to develop an internationally recognized serotyping scheme so that full epidemiological investigations can be carried out. The importance of the large number of strains which can be isolated from farm animals and poultry and from environmental sources should be assessed.

Table 1 Areas of research needed

1. Identification of the antigens
2. Development of typing schemes
3. Diagnostic serology
4. Easier and cheaper isolation techniques
5. Field studies in developing countries
6. Epidemiology especially in modes of transmission
7. Natural history of disease in various areas
8. Controlled trials (efficacy of antibiotics?)
9. Monitoring of antibiotic resistance
10. Pathogenesis and pathogenic mechanisms

Research is also needed into better laboratory techniques for the isolation of the organism and for the detection of antibodies as a measure of past or current infection.

Campylobacter infection in man should be preventable by well recognized hygienic precautions in the treatment of water, milk and food.

CONCLUSION

The papers, demonstrations and discussions at this Workshop have demonstrated a world-wide interest in campylobacter infection. The extent and the limitations of present knowledge are clear.

It may be cynical to suggest that, if *C. jejuni* caused an economically crippling disease of livestock, there would be greater pressure to solve the remaining problems than there is to control an unpleasant but seldom life-threatening disease of man.

It is to be hoped that the next few years will see advances both in knowledge and particularly in its application to this aspect of preventive medicine.